D0151510

LISA ET LIBRARY RENEWALS 458-2440

DATE DUE

GAYLORD			PRINTED IN U.S.A.

WITHDRAWN
UTSA LIBRARIES

Health, Luck, and Justice

Health, Luck, and Justice

Shlomi Segall

PRINCETON UNIVERSITY PRESS
Princeton and Oxford

Library
University of Texas
at San Antonio

Copyright © 2010 by Princeton University Press

Published by Princeton University Press, 41 William Street, Princeton, New Jersey 08540

In the United Kingdom: Princeton University Press, 6 Oxford Street, Woodstock, Oxfordshire OX20 1TW

Library of Congress Cataloging-in-Publication Data

Segall, Shlomi, 1970–
Health, luck, and justice / Shlomi Segall.
    p. cm.
Includes bibliographical references and index.
ISBN 978-0-691-14053-7 (hardcover : alk. paper)   1. Social medicine.
2. Health services accessibility.   3. Equality—Health aspects.   4. Medical policy—
Social aspects.   5. Social justice.   I. Title.
RA418.S412 2009
362.1—dc22   2009012481

British Library Cataloging-in-Publication Data is available

This book has been composed in Minion with Myriad display

Printed on acid-free paper. ∞

press.princeton.edu

Printed in the United States of America

10 9 8 7 6 5 4 3 2 1

Library
University of Texas
at San Antonio

For my parents

Contents

Preface

I can probably trace the origin of this book to a specific point in time. It was when my friend and colleague, Nir Eyal, put to me the following question: If we both find luck egalitarianism so intuitively appealing (or is it simply that we were bowled over by Jerry Cohen's personality?), then why is it that the theory appears so counterintuitive when applied to health care? I could not imagine then that Nir's question would occupy me for quite a few years.

Over the course of those years I had many challenges, and even more assistance, offered to me by many friends and colleagues. First and foremost I am indebted to Nir as well as to Daniel Schwartz and Ori Lev, who read all the chapters of the manuscript and provided invaluable and systematic feedback. I count myself lucky to have these three as colleagues and companions.

Many of the ideas in this book were formed while I was a fellow at the Harvard Program in Ethics and Health (PEH). I cannot begin to express my gratitude to Dan Brock, who established and headed PEH and who brought me over from England to spend a couple of extremely fruitful years in Boston. More generally, Dan should be credited with shaking traditional bioethics from its slumber and urging people in the field to start thinking systematically about the ethics of population health. It was Dan's idea to invite ethicists, political philosophers, and economists to think together critically of the ethics of population health. That is precisely what I found at the PEH: Dan, Norm Daniels, Dan Wikler, Frances Kamm, Allan Brandt, Francesca Holinko, Graham Ball, Eric Cavallero, Neema Sofaer, Ole Norheim, Iwao Hirose, Greg Bognar, Sam Kerstein, Sigurd Lauridsen, Alexander Cappelen, and Bertil Tungodden have all provided a perfect setting for thinking about health, luck, and justice.

It was mainly the encounter with Norm that helped put flesh on the bare bones of this project. The depth and extent of Norm's work on justice and health is obviously unrivaled. Being in frequent conversation with him meant constantly challenging my own fledgling thoughts on the issues at hand. It is from the top of Norm's giant philosophical shoulders that I offer whatever modest contribution this book might make. Equally, it was my apprenticeship and friendship with Dan Wikler that got me thinking seriously on the issue of responsibility in health and health care. In health ethics, as Norm is with regard to justice, so is Dan with regard to responsibility, an expert without parallel. It is therefore obvious that in writing a book about justice, luck, and responsibility in health and health care I greatly benefited from the close contact with Norm and Dan.

Many other friends, colleagues, and mentors have commented on various chapters of the manuscript. Among those I would like to mention and thank Dick Arneson, Gustaf Arrhenius, Dani Attas, Bashir Bashir, Jodi Beder, Richard Child, Jerry Cohen, Avner de-Shalit, David Enoch, Marc Fleurbaey, Karen Grumberg, David Heyd, Katharina Ivanyi, Adi Koplovitz, Sarah Marchand, David Miller, Ike Okonta, Sheppley Orr, Avia Pasternak, Adina Preda, Miriam Ronzoni, Christian Schemmel, Harald Schmidt, Re'em Segev, Hillel Steiner, Zofia Stemplowska, Guilel Treiber, Peter Vallentyne, Kristin Voigt, David Weinstein, and Steve Winter. The manuscript, in whole or in parts, has also benefited from the work of an army of referees, to whose anonymous work I am grateful. Special thanks are due to Rob Tempio, my editor at PUP, who believed in this project from the first moment it was pitched to him. Rob has offered encouragement throughout and urged me to bring this project to fruition.

I am also grateful for permission to use here revised material from previously published articles:

"In Solidarity with the Imprudent: A Defense of Luck Egalitarianism," *Social Theory and Practice* 33, no. 2 (2007): 177–98.

"Is Health Care (Still) Special?" *Journal of Political Philosophy* 15, no. 3 (2007): 342–63.

"Why Devolution Upsets Distributive Justice," *Journal of Moral Philosophy* 4, no. 2 (2007): 259–74.

Financial support for this project was provided by the Harvard Program in Ethics and Health, by the Hebrew University of Jerusalem, and by the Israel Science Fund (Grant no. 436/08). The Widener Library at Harvard, Darwin's Café in Cambridge (Mount Auburn branch), and the Van Leer Institute in Jerusalem provided very congenial environments for reading, reflecting, and writing, and were thus invaluable for an otherwise easily distracted individual.

Finally, this project could not have been carried out without the unconditional support of my family.

Health, Luck, and Justice

Introduction

◾

What is the just distribution of health and health care? The answer this book seeks to offer is deceptively simple perhaps: Differences in health and health care are unjust if they reflect differences in brute luck.

The invocation of luck in accounts of egalitarian justice has become increasingly salient in recent years. In fact, "luck egalitarianism" can be said to be the main rival to John Rawls's dominant theory of justice. According to luck egalitarians, distributive justice requires correcting disadvantages for which individuals cannot be held responsible. In other words, the theory seeks to compensate individuals for the effects of bad luck on their lives. (I shall say more about the difference between Rawlsian and luck egalitarian justice in the first chapter). It may be surprising, perhaps, but despite the prominence of this egalitarian theory, to date there has not been any systematic attempt to apply luck egalitarianism to the study of justice in the distribution of health and health care.[1] In fact, some critics have commented in passing that the application of luck egalitarianism to health and health care leads to counterintuitive results.[2] That is precisely the challenge that this book seeks to meet: to offer and defend a luck egalitarian account of justice in health care and health.

The intersection of the luck egalitarian conception of distributive justice with health and health care raises two main ethical issues. First, how ought we to treat patients who have not taken good care of their health? According to luck egalitarians, distributive justice requires mitigating only eventualities for which individuals are not responsible. It follows, then, that luck egalitarianism arguably requires that patients that *are* responsible for their own illness (say, lung cancer patients who have smoked, or injured motorists who have driven recklessly) are not entitled to medical treatment. Could this be right? Most of us recognize that some people are "worse" patients than others. Some people have a less healthy lifestyle than others, they ignore their doctors' orders, they smoke, drink, and eat too much, and exercise too little. Such imprudent behavior not only worsens one's own health,[3] but also places unnecessary burdens on the health care system.[4] Why should the rest of us pay for their avoidable reckless behavior? If, in turn, health care *is* to be universal and unconditional, as egalitarians typically believe it should be, then what, exactly, justifies (on the luck egalitarian reading) medical treatment for citizens who are to blame for their medical needs? (By "unconditional health care" I simply mean a health care service that does not condition the provision of care on the prior prudent conduct of the patient. I elaborate on this in chapter 5.) That is the first of the two main issues with which this book is concerned.

The second issue is this. We often witness considerable disparities in health and life expectancy across society (let alone *between* societies, which is the subject of the final chapter). Not all of these inequalities can be explained in terms of access to health care (I shall say more on this in chapter 6). Some of the inequalities in health itself are due to social factors other than health care, and yet some other part of them is explained by genetic differences. Much of the inequality in individuals' health status, then, is owed either to social circumstances over much of which they have no control (social circumstances they were born into), or to natural genetic factors (which philosophers appropriately refer to as the product of a "natural lottery"). How, then, would a theory of justice that seeks to abolish the effects of differential brute luck from people's lives treat such inequalities in health and life expectancy? In other words, if health is, at least to some extent, a matter of luck, then what is it to distribute health justly, that is, independently of luck?

The first part of the book, then, deals primarily with health care, whereas the second part concerns health proper. A subsidiary concern for the book is to examine the interplay between political borders and the discussion in the first two parts. How does luck egalitarian justice in health and health care apply within and beyond the political boundaries of the state? The application of the theory of luck egalitarian justice in health care and health to the issue of political borders may serve two purposes. One is to point out some important policy implications of the theory, while a second is to reveal some further potential facets of the intersection of luck egalitarianism and health not yet explored in the first two parts of the book. The book is therefore divided into three parts (after the introductory chapter, discussing luck egalitarianism itself), dealing with health care, health, and the importance of political borders to these first two issues. I turn now to outline how the argument unfolds.

Chapter 1 begins by sketching the main components of the luck egalitarian conception of distributive justice. It then contrasts luck egalitarianism with the Rawlsian conception of justice. Later still it pursues and develops two important features of the luck egalitarian theory that seem to be in dispute among luck egalitarians. First, I attempt to establish that luck egalitarian justice considers only inequality, not equality, as potentially unjust. Second, I argue for a certain understanding of what are eventualities for which the individual is not responsible. The chapter is meant to provide a working definition of the theory of distributive justice to be employed throughout the book.

The main concern of the *first part* of the book, as I have said, is: How ought society to treat patients who can be said to be responsible for their own poor medical condition? The luck egalitarian conception of justice says that distributive justice does *not* require society to compensate members for disadvantages that result from their own voluntary actions. It is easy to see, then, why some political philosophers have suggested that the luck egalitarian conception of justice appears untenable when applied to health care. A luck egalitarian health care system will arguably not provide medical treatment to patients who can be said to be responsible for their ailment. That seems wrong: we are allegedly not required to treat an injured reckless driver or a smoker who contracts lung cancer, since their bad luck is what luck egalitarians call bad "option luck." That is, it is the result of these patients' "gambling," so to speak, with their own health. But to not treat these patients would clearly be harsh and wrong. This objection to luck egalitarianism is known as the "abandonment of the imprudent." It purportedly shows the luck egalitarian account of justice, and of justice in health care in particular, to be too narrow: it cannot justify treating the imprudent. (In a different way, the account may be said to be *too broad*: it arguably justifies treatments that go beyond what we traditionally associate with health policy. I address that worry in chapter 9.) The first challenge for the book, then, is to explain how a luck egalitarian account of justice in health care can defend itself against that "abandonment" objection.

Chapter 2 begins the defense of a luck egalitarian account of justice in health care by seeking to establish the need for a fresh examination of justice in that area. More specifically, it seeks to show that standard, responsibility-*in*sensitive accounts of justice in health care are inadequate. The chapter critically examines two prominent models for justice in health care: Norman Daniels's fair opportunity account, and Elizabeth Anderson's democratic capabilities account. I argue that these accounts have some decisive shortcomings in providing a theory of justice in health care. Among other problems, Daniels's emphasis on safeguarding opportunities for the pursuit of life plans ends up not justifying medical treatment for those who can be said to have completed their life plans, namely the elderly. The democratic capabilities account, in turn, has its own distinct faults: the fact that it makes the just claims of individuals for medical care contingent on the prevalence of a democratic regime, to name one. For these and other reasons I conclude that these two responsibility-insensitive accounts of justice in health care are inadequate.

After arguing against these two dominant accounts of justice in health care, I then turn in the rest of part I to developing and defending a luck egalitarian account of justice in health care, focusing on whether or not it can escape the abandonment objection and justify universal and unconditional health care.

In the past five years or so, philosophers sympathetic to the project of developing a luck-sensitive conception of justice have sought to address the abandonment of the imprudent objection by giving the luck egalitarian ideal a radical interpretation. These radical luck egalitarians, whom I term "all-luck egalitarians," propose an innovative interpretation, according to which imprudent patients need not be abandoned. The kernel of these philosophers' proposal is that justice requires taxing imprudent activities (smoking, say), and using the revenue to care for imprudent individuals who turned out to be unlucky (i.e., who have fallen sick). The idea, then, is one of pursuing justice between lucky and unlucky imprudent agents. In *chapter 3* I examine this proposal and demonstrate that it cannot offer a viable account of distributive justice in general, and one in health care in particular.

After rejecting the "all-luck egalitarian" attempt to address the abandonment objection, *chapter 4* turns to examine how standard luck egalitarians may respond to that objection. I argue that such recent responses by standard luck egalitarians are inadequate for one reason or another, and I then provide a different solution to the abandonment problem. That solution involves trading off the requirements of justice with those of other values. One moral requirement that is particularly relevant here is that of meeting a person's basic needs, including her basic medical needs. I show how the trade-off of luck egalitarian distributive justice with the more general requirement of meeting basic needs yields a plausible and attractive account of justice in health care.

Chapter 5 seeks to complete the defense of the luck egalitarian account of justice in health care. While chapter 4 effectively seeks to demonstrate that luck egalitarian justice does not require abandoning reckless patients, chapter 5 seeks to show how the concern for basic needs yields an attractive account of justice in health care. I develop an account of health care as a normatively nonexcludable public good. This understanding of health care spells a responsibility-sensitive, yet still unconditional, health care. The chapter concludes part I by demonstrating how luck egalitarians may justify a universal, *in-kind* provision of health care, whereas Daniels's account does not.

The *second part* of the book shifts the focus from health care to health proper. It seeks to offer an account of justice in the distribution of health, and moreover one that is sensitive to luck. Many people find it difficult to imagine how we would even begin to distribute health itself, let alone do it in a luck-sensitive fashion. We normally think of health *care* as something society can distribute more or less equally. But can we really redistribute health itself? We generally think of health as what economists call a nondivisible and nontransferable good.[5] Moreover, even if we could redistribute health, ought we to do so?

Two facts make that task not only possible but also urgent (I elaborate on this in *chapter 6*). First, even societies that feature universal and free access to health care may display considerable disparities in health. For example, people living in some neighborhoods of the Scottish city of Glasgow have a life expectancy that is twelve years shorter than those living in the more affluent parts of that city.[6] Unequal access to universal care, much as it obtains, cannot account for such striking disparities.[7] It follows that if we care about equality and about health, providing free health care to all cannot possibly be enough.[8] The second point is that epidemiologists have been telling us over the past twenty years or so that it *is* possible to mitigate the disparities in health by redistributing some other goods, such as income, housing, employment, and workplace autonomy. In fact, some philosophers have suggested that if we really cared about justice and health we would do well to scrap health care altogether and invest those resources in the social determinants of health.[9] So although health itself is a nondivisible and nontransferable good, the distribution of other goods (that *are* divisible and transferable) can affect the way in which health is distributed across society. This lesson, that inequalities in health itself ought to be of moral concern independently of inequalities in access to health care, and that they ought to be curbed by redistributing the social determinants of health, has now also been recognized by policy makers.[10] Giving attention to health in addition to health care therefore seems warranted, as I shall argue in chapter 6.

The rest of part II of the book, then, seeks to offer a luck-sensitive account of justice in the distribution of health proper. *Chapter 7* begins tackling that central task by inquiring what it may mean to redistribute health justly, and what it may mean to do so in a way that neutralizes brute luck inequalities. My discussion there contrasts a Rawlsian approach with a luck egalitarian approach to justice in health, and attempts to show that a fair distribution of health is one that safeguards individuals' opportunity to be as healthy as they choose to be.

A problem that is common to both Rawlsian and luck egalitarian approaches to health equity (or justice in health—I use the terms interchangeably) is the "leveling down objection." The problem, namely, is how to offer a fair account of justice in health that does not end up lowering some individuals' health prospects in the name of equality. In *chapter 8* I attempt to demonstrate that a modified luck egalitarian account, namely one that seeks to prioritize the health of the worse off rather than to equalize everyone's health, successfully averts that problem. To justify this prioritarian approach I inquire into the value of equality in health. I argue that it has only negligible instrumental value, and therefore that justice in health allows for priority (to the worse off), and does not necessitate a strictly equal distribution.

Chapters 7 and 8 combine to provide a "luck prioritarian" account of justice in health. More accurately perhaps, these two chapters discuss justice in the distribution of health *deficits* (e.g., illness broadly conceived). *Chapter 9* moves from discussing the distribution of health deficits to discussing the distribution of enhancements to full normal health. I argue in that chapter that a luck-sensitive account of egalitarian justice compels us to broaden our traditional concern in health from deficits to full health into enhancement of human functioning (e.g., through genetic intervention). I suggest that luck egalitarianism explains our intuitions about the role of medical intervention better than Daniels's "fair opportunity" approach.

The luck egalitarian theory of justice in health and health care having been outlined, the *third part* of the book applies the theory to the particular issue of political borders. There are two pertinent issues here: justice in the distribution of health and health care below state level, and beyond it. The first question asked is whether it is appropriate to delegate the responsibility to deliver health care to subnational regional authorities (say, from London to Edinburgh), while the second task is to examine our global obligations with regard to health.

Chapter 10, then, asks how we should allocate health care in plurinational societies. Does distributive justice require a unified health care system or a devolved one? Some have suggested that in culturally divided societies health care systems (and perhaps other welfare services as well) should be divided along regional lines. The argument grounding such proposals seems to run as follows: since members of homogeneous regional communities have relatively similar needs and tastes, it is easier for them to agree on a rather comprehensive distributive scheme. Against this suggestion, I argue that the policy of devolution in fact upsets distributive justice. A just health policy, I claim, need not cater to expensive communal tastes in medical consumption that were voluntarily developed.

Chapter 11 examines the implications of the luck egalitarian account of justice in health and health care for our obligation to meet the health needs of people outside our own political community. When, then, are inequalities in health and life expectancy that exist between nations justified? Luck egalitarian justice has a distinctive input here, I want to argue. It stresses that the nation one happens to be born into is a fact of pure brute luck, and thus should not affect one's health prospects. But there are further peculiarities to the global perspective on health that make that judgment somewhat more complicated. We now know, for example, that GDP is not such a good indicator of population health. As pointed out by Daniels in his most recent work, although the GDP per capita difference between Costa Rica and the United States is huge ($21,000), life expectancy is almost the same between the two countries. Correspondingly, in 1995 although Cuba and Iraq were equally poor (GDP per capita $3,100), life expectancy in Cuba exceeded that of Iraq (notice, prewar) by 17.2 years![11] These figures may suggest that the health of nations is not a matter of global justice, since it seems to be primarily determined by domestic policies. If so, a consistent luck egalitarian account, one that is committed to holding agents (in this case nations) responsible for their choices, does not identify an obligation on the part of the healthy and wealthy nations to boost the health of nations that are less healthy and wealthy. I attempt to show in this final chapter why that conclusion is largely unwarranted. There are four complicating conditions that may prevent us from holding residents of developing unhealthy nations responsible for their nations' poor health. These are: the question of whether or not the nation is a democratic one; the question of whether or not the global economic order allows developing nations to pursue policies that are good for their health; the question of holding dissenters accountable for health-related policies to which they actually objected; and the question of holding children responsible for policies they could not have affected. For all these reasons, I propose, it is seldom just to deny members of poor and unhealthy nations (what we may call) a "global health dividend."

The last two chapters mirror the division that is made earlier in the book between health care and health, with chapter 10 dealing with health care, and chapter 11 returning to health proper. More importantly, these two chapters provide insight into two potentially interesting aspects of luck egalitarianism touched upon but not quite explored earlier in the book. The crux of the matter in chapter 10 is the issue of communal (that is, of a subnational community) responsibility for collective tastes and preferences in medical care. A theory of justice that is sensitive to luck (the opposite of responsibility) may have an interesting input in that respect. Luck egalitarianism also has a unique input in dealing with global health. One difference between Rawlsian justice and luck egalitarian justice is that between what we may call a "political," on the one hand, and a "natural" or "cosmic" conception of justice, on the other. (I shall explain this distinction in the next chapter). Discussing global justice in health might help us bring out this difference between the two theories.

The defining feature of luck egalitarianism is no doubt the distinction it draws between eventualities for which we are responsible and ones for which we are not. In the course of the next eleven chapters I shall attempt to show that the centrality of that distinction to distributive justice is confirmed by many of our intuitions about justice in health care and health. If that proves to be the case, then this book may well say something not only about the nature of justice in health and health care, but also about the nature of justice itself.

1
∎

Justice, Luck, and Equality

Introduction

The purpose of this opening chapter is to provide the working understanding of luck egalitarianism as the theory of distributive justice that guides my account of justice in health care and health. I intend to do so by undertaking three tasks. The first, in section I, is to introduce luck egalitarianism as a conception of distributive justice to rival John Rawls's dominant account of egalitarian distributive justice. Juxtaposing the two conceptions of egalitarian distributive justice—the Rawlsian and the luck egalitarian one—is important not only for our understanding of luck egalitarianism as such, but particularly for discussing health, the reason being that the dominant account of justice in health and health care with which I shall largely contrast mine is Norman Daniels's Rawlsian account.

In the rest of the chapter I shall explore in detail two aspects of luck egalitarianism that are of importance for the discussion to follow. One concerns the question of whether or not luck egalitarianism counts only inequalities as unjust or equalities as well; the other concerns the correct interpretation of what precisely should count as a matter of bad brute luck, that is, instances where luck egalitarians would see a justice-based claim for compensation. These two aspects of luck egalitarianism are controversial points among luck egalitarians. Likewise, they both have consequences for the inquiry that I undertake in this book. Accordingly, I have chosen to expand on these two matters.

The first of these two points, as explored in section II, is this. Luck egalitarians typically agree that it is permissible to correct for differential brute luck. But they disagree whether it is a necessary condition that such differential brute luck lead to outcome inequality in order to make that correction mandatory rather than permissible. Here I shall attempt to defend the view that outcome equalities, even if they are the result of differential brute luck, are not as such unjust.

The second point of controversy, as discussed in the third and final section of the chapter, is this. Luck egalitarians hold that disadvantages for which the individual is responsible are not unjust. Yet they disagree on when exactly it is that individuals are responsible for certain disadvantages. A strict reading of luck egalitarianism would rule that disadvantages resulting from conduct that the agent could have avoided are not unjust. Another, more plausible, approach would say that the relevant criterion is that of innocent choice: any disadvantage that results from innocent choice is unjust. The version I favor and defend here speaks of disadvantages as being unjust (and thus meriting compensation) when they result from conduct or factors that it would be unreasonable to expect the agent to avoid. But first, let me introduce luck egalitarianism, and contrast it with the currently dominant conception of egalitarian justice, namely Rawls's.

I. Rawlsian vs. Luck Egalitarian Justice

Luck egalitarianism is essentially the idea that it is unfair for one person to be worse off than another due to reasons beyond her control.[1] Therefore, the point of egalitarian distributive justice, say luck egalitarians, is to level inequalities that are owed to differential luck. Luck egalitarians typically distinguish what they call brute luck from option luck. I shall elaborate this distinction shortly. For now suffice it to say that brute luck is the kind of luck over which we have no control, whereas option luck is luck the tempting of which we control, such as the luck that ensues from the decision to gamble.

Luck egalitarianism is generally traced back to Ronald Dworkin's two-part 1981 article "What Is Equality?"[2] However, it is possible to trace its origins even further back, to Rawls. Though he was not a luck egalitarian himself, it was Rawls who first noted that individuals are not entitled to their lots inasmuch as these are affected by factors beyond their control, such as their native talents.[3] Yet Rawls, nevertheless, denied a central role for responsibility and luck in his account of distributive justice. Famously, Rawls's main principle for allocating distributive shares, the "difference principle," does not differentiate between those who are responsible for the size of their shares and those who are not. Rawls's distributive principle would assign the same priority to a talented person who chooses not to work as he would to an equally poor (however that is measured) person who is hardworking but simply unsuccessful due to lack of marketable natural talent.[4] Luck egalitarians would want to say that this is unfair, and that we ought to assign priority to those who are worse off through no fault of their own. They in fact go much further than that and hold that the only point of distributive justice is to level disadvantages and inequalities that are due to brute luck. Thereby, they further distance themselves from Rawlsians, who argue that shares ought to be distributed according to how much worse off a person is, regardless of whether her position is owed to brute luck or rather to her own actions.

There are other points of departure at which Rawlsian justice diverges from luck egalitarian justice. One major difference is that Rawlsian justice is contractarian whereas luck egalitarianism is typically not. Principles of justice for Rawls are arrived at through the process of a social contract. Luck egalitarians (at least those who follow the luck egalitarianism of G. A. Cohen and Richard Arneson, as I do here, as distinct from that of Ronald Dworkin's), in contrast, see principles of justice as independent of what rational agents would choose under some circumstances that simulate impartiality. Rawlsian justice, thus, focuses on the relationship between individuals as members of a political community, members among whom the social contract obtains. This is why Rawlsian justice is sometimes characterized as "political," the implication being that the principles of justice it recommends are shaped by an image of the just relation between citizens, and what citizens can and cannot justify to one another. Luck egalitarian justice, in contrast, has no presumption of being contingent on what hypothetical individuals would or would not agree on. Rather than being "political," it is characterized as "natural" or even "cosmic," since luck could be seen as a product of nature or even of some cosmic intervention (whatever that may mean). This is not to say that luck egalitarianism has no political bite—far from it. The focus on luck, luck egalitarians would want to say, has a deep social and political basis, and not merely a natural one. Many of the disadvantages that most people would readily describe as unjust are ones that are the product of social circumstances over which a person has no or little control. Growing up in a deprived neighborhood or in a developing country is a social reality, not a cosmic one, and one that greatly determines a person's life chances. The emphasis on neutralizing bad brute luck is therefore not something that is detached from unjust social reality. Rather, luck egalitarians would typically say that the reversal of bad luck is the most radical way in which social injustice can be addressed, and therefore any theory that does not fully neutralize bad luck falls short of meeting the requirements of social justice. So while luck egalitarians do typically hold what we may call a natural, or nonpolitical, conception of justice, it is at the same time one that has profound political implications.

This difference between Rawlsian justice and luck egalitarian justice, as we shall see at various points in the book (especially chapters 2, 9, and 11), has significant implications for a theory of justice in health and health care. To give just a taste of it now, I want to draw attention to two implications of the Rawlsian theory of justice being "political." First, a "political" theory of justice allocates resources to its members based on what individuals owe each other *as members of a political community.* That is, it would allocate resources to individuals insofar as the allocation serves the purpose of preserving just and equal relations between members of that political community. Second, a "political" theory of justice, one centered on the political community, would draw a sharp distinction between what we owe members of our own political community and what we might owe people who are outsiders to it.

In order to outline some further points of departure between Rawlsian and luck egalitarian justice, allow me to say the following by way of introduction. It is possible to divide egalitarians of all colors according to the answer they provide to two central questions: What is it that justice requires redistributing? And how, precisely, ought this currency to be distributed? These are often referred to respectively as the "currency" and the "pattern" (or, simply, the "what" and the "how") of egalitarian distributive justice. The two main contenders for the correct currency of egalitarian distributive justice are resources and welfare. I shall say more on this shortly. As for the pattern of egalitarian distributive justice, the main options are equality, priority, and sufficiency. Equality simply signifies the allocation of equal shares. Priority requires not simple equality but rather assigning priority to those who are the worse off. Some argue that this, in fact, is the essence of the egalitarian ideal.[5] On this reading, the egalitarian ideal takes the pattern of assigning the next available benefit for redistribution to the person who is the worse off (in terms of whatever the relevant currency is). Those who believe that the *only* value in egalitarianism resides with benefiting the worse off, and not in equal distribution as such, are known as prioritarians. (Of course, one need not be a card-carrying prioritarian in order to recommend the use, on occasion, of the prioritarian pattern.) The third major pattern of egalitarianism is that of safeguarding some minimal level of resources (or welfare). In Harry Frankfurt's famous words, "what is important from the point of view of morality is not that everyone should have the same but that each should have enough."[6] This has come to be known as "sufficientarianism." As will become apparent, I shall appeal to and make use of all three patterns of egalitarian distribution in different parts of my argument. In other words, it is part of my argument that different patterns of egalitarian distribution are appropriate for different aspects of health and health care. For our immediate purposes, though, we need to examine how the differences regarding the pattern and the currency of egalitarian justice bear on the differences between Rawlsian and luck egalitarian justice.

Rawlsian justice is not necessarily committed to equality as such, but may rather espouse the prioritarian principle of maximin, that is, maximize the position of the worse off. Similarly, luck egalitarians may not necessarily advocate equality as such, but may rather couch their "luckism" in a prioritarian pattern. (I discuss this in detail in chapter 8.) Luck egalitarian distributive justice may thus adopt either the pattern of equality or that of priority. (As for sufficiency, luck egalitarians may adopt this pattern for nonegalitarian reasons; I explain this in chapters 4 and 5.) The luck egalitarian flexibility with regard to pattern of distribution is mirrored in a certain flexibility that it displays with regard to currency. Whereas Rawlsians see resources as the sole appropriate currency of distribution, luck egalitarians are famously divided between "resource" and "welfare" egalitarians. Dworkin, perhaps the original luck egalitarian (although he distances himself from the title), holds that resources are the appropriate currency of distributive justice. Other prominent luck egalitarians, namely Cohen and Arneson, speak of "access to advantage" and "opportunity for welfare" respectively, and are generally considered "welfarists." Despite Dworkin, luck egalitarianism today is mostly identified with the welfarist strand (perhaps Dworkin's denial of the title has something to do with this). For that and others reasons, the welfarist strand of luck egalitarianism is the one deployed here.

There is, by now, a substantial volume of literature on luck egalitarianism, and we shall refer to much of it later in the book. Yet, curiously perhaps, despite the magnitude of this literature, or perhaps because of it, there is still some ambiguity regarding what, precisely, the luck egalitarian ideal stipulates. I want to offer, and in the rest of this chapter defend, the following formulation as capturing the proper luck egalitarian sentiment:

> *It is unjust for individuals to be worse off than others due to outcomes that it would have been unreasonable to expect them to avoid.*

As mentioned, there are two elements, in particular, entailed in this formulation that it is necessary to defend here. (Some further points of contention between luck egalitarians will be addressed in chapters 3 and 4.) One concerns the requirement of there being inequality (the stipulation that some be "worse off than others"), and the other concerns the interpretation of brute luck as the idea of "reasonable avoidability." First, then, on my proposed formulation, luck egalitarian justice is properly concerned only with *in*equalities. It says only that it is unjust for individuals to be worse off than others; it does not specify whether it may be unjust for them to be equally well (or worse) off. In the next section, I shall defend that feature of my formulation of luck egalitarianism. In the final section, I defend the substitution of "responsibility" with the idea of reasonable avoidability in the luck egalitarian formula. I argue that instances of bad brute luck should be understood as an "outcome that it would be unreasonable to expect the agent to avoid." By defending the idea that egalitarian distributive justice should be concerned only with inequalities that are owed to differential brute luck, and that we ought to count as brute luck only instances where it would have been unreasonable to expect the agent to act otherwise, I thereby hope to defend a fine-tuned, indeed stronger, formulation of the egalitarian ideal (one that I then intend to apply to the study of justice in health and health care). My aim in the rest of this chapter is not, notice, to engage with critics of luck egalitarianism. That endeavor will be undertaken in many other parts of the book. Rather, whatever disagreements I engage with here should be understood as family quarrels among those who subscribe to the luck egalitarian credo.

II. Inequality vs. Equality

Luck egalitarianism (henceforth in this chapter LE) properly understood, I want to suggest, sees outcome inequalities as the sole concern of distributive justice. In contrast, outcome equality (in welfare or resources, or whatever the relevant currency of the outcome is) will not normally be of concern for a luck egalitarian. This might seem rather obvious. After all, LE concerns *egalitarian* distributive justice and so it is only natural that it should be concerned with inequalities. But in truth there is some vagueness about the matter: LE is sometimes formulated in a way that implies that it is concerned with inequalities *in luck* or in *brute luck advantage*. These, in turn, may or may not yield outcome inequalities. In this section, I will try to resolve that dispute and suggest that my formulation, namely that only outcome inequalities can be unjust, is the correct one. Notice that I leave the question of whether we ought to be egalitarians or prioritarians in our handling of those inequalities for later in the book. Here, I simply try to identify what it is that ought to be the object of concern for luck egalitarians, without specifying what it is that they recommend doing about it.

As indicated, the question I raise here is curiously neglected and overlooked. Arneson, for example, does not seem to address the question explicitly, but his ideal of equality of opportunity for welfare does seem to suggest that the focus is on opportunities rather than on outcomes. "Equal opportunity for welfare obtains among persons when all of them face equivalent decision trees."[7] Since two individuals may end up equally situated as a result of two unequal opportunity sets, it follows that outcome equality can be unjust according to Arneson. Cohen similarly writes that for him "the primary egalitarian impulse is to extinguish the influence *on distribution* of both exploitation and brute luck."[8] Thus, he allows that LE may be concerned with extinguishing the effect of brute luck from both inequalities *and* equalities. In contrast, Susan Hurley, in her discussion of Cohen's position, presents it as saying that only inequalities matter. "Egalitarianism should aim to neutralize *differences* due to luck, for which people are not responsible, whether these are differences in welfare or resource levels. But it should not aim to neutralize *differences* due to choice."[9] So, here it is inequalities that seem to be the sole concern of LE. Larry Temkin similarly seems to suggest that only inequalities matter when he expresses the luck egalitarian sentiment: "It is bad—unjust and unfair—for some to be *worse off than others* through no fault or choice of their own."[10] This sentiment, notably, says nothing about whether it is fair or not for some people to be equally well off as others.

In his recent response to Hurley, however, Cohen is even more explicit. "So, in deference to fairness, the relevant egalitarian says that she's against inequalities in the absence of appropriately differential responsibility (just as, she now realizes, she is also against *equalities* in the presence of appropriately differential responsibility)."[11] Moreover, Cohen now seems to be aware of the curious neglect of the matter in the luck egalitarian literature. The passage is worth quoting at length:

> Since there is a-symmetry in the luck egalitarian's attitude to plain, ordinary equality and plain, ordinary inequality—both are bad if and only if they are in disaccord with choice—it might seem that it is not luck but *equality* that plays no role in specifying luck egalitarianism. Why, indeed, is unjust inequality, rather than unjust equality, salient in statements of luck egalitarianism and in luck egalitarian sentiment? For several reasons. First, there is an historical reason: huge inequalities cried out for rectification at the bar of justice, given what was known about their origin. Nothing similar was true of any equalities. Second, there remains in contemporary society typically much more offensive inequality than offensive equality: there are reasons for objecting more strongly to the corporate welfare bum than to the able-bodied plain welfare bum who gets as much as the working stiff does.[12]

Cohen seems to say here that although as a matter of practical moral concern, inequalities (that are owed to luck) are in need of more urgent rectification than equalities (that are owed to luck), as a matter of principle, equalities can be as unjust as inequalities (when both are the product of unequal luck or responsibility).

It therefore seems that there is some ambiguity about the matter, but that at least some of the leading luck egalitarians consider equalities to be unjust as well. Subsequently, allow me to defend the opposite view, according to which equalities, even if owed to differential luck, are of no concern for justice. In order to make that case, I suggest contrasting LE with the ideal of desert, with which it is sometimes associated (or rather, confused). I claim that desert may hold that inequalities are actually required by justice, whereas LE does not. I further speculate that it is the confusion of LE with desert, both by proponents and by critics, that sometimes generates the thought that LE may condemn equalities as unjust.

Equality and Desert

Very crudely, then, the ideal of desert stipulates that distributive shares match individuals' respective levels of desert as they are revealed by their relevant conduct or performance.[13] According to the ideal of desert, it is therefore not unjust for a more deserving individual to be better off than a less deserving individual. Desert, on that understanding, could be assessed from two different normative perspectives, moral (e.g., how virtuous one is in helping others), or prudential (how prudent one is in looking after oneself).[14] Since LE is concerned, if anything, with prudence rather than virtue, I shall take the egalitarian version of desert that I have in mind to be accordingly concerned with prudence and not virtue (unless I state explicitly otherwise). Another distinction that it would be useful to bear in mind is the one between permissive desert and mandatory desert.[15] Permissive desert holds that the inequality between the abovementioned Deserving and Less Deserving is not unjust. Mandatory desert, in contrast, says that justice requires making sure that the individuals' unequal level of deservingness be matched by unequal levels of welfare (or whatever the currency of the distribution is). Finally, philosophers often distinguish between desert claims of the noncomparative and comparative kind. Noncomparative desert is the idea that for any level of meritorious conduct there should be a corresponding level of well-being. Comparative desert, in contrast, is the idea that how meritoriously a person conducts herself in comparison to others should determine how well off she should be compared to them. In distinguishing it from LE we ought to consider both kinds of desert.

Let us first contrast LE with noncomparative desert. I do so, I should say, only for the sake of argument, and therefore one should not deduce that my own view of LE is committed to noncomparative justice. In any case, a noncomparative view of LE would be saying that it is morally bad if a person is worse off than she could otherwise have been, and through no fault of her own. Noncomparative desert, in turn, says that it is bad for a person to receive less than she deserves. In that sense the two ideals are quite similar. But (mandatory) noncomparative desert also entails the view that it is equally bad if that person gets *more* than she deserves.[16] The equivalent sentiment for LE would be that it is morally bad for a person to be made better off (than she could otherwise have been) due to reasons that are beyond her control.[17] But, crucially, LE on my formulation denies that view.[18] LE may entail the view that benefits that are the consequence of good brute luck may be undeserved. As such they *may* be confiscated or taxed. Making some people worse off may therefore be a by-product, but never a direct requirement, of justice. In that respect LE differs from mandatory noncomparative desert, for according to the latter, justice requires stripping recipients of good brute luck of the corresponding benefits. That is an important difference between the two principles, it seems to me. (And whether or not noncomparative desert is an attractive idea to begin with is yet a different matter which I refrain from pressing here.)[19]

Let us turn to the comparative view of desert and see how it, in turn, differs from LE. On my formulation, it is unjust for individuals to be made worse off than others through no fault of their own. Accordingly, it is bad for someone to suffer worse brute luck than others, and to consequently be worse off than them. Proponents of desert hold a similar view. But proponents of (mandatory) desert also believe that it is equally bad when some are *equally well off* as others but through no merit of their own.[20] Luck egalitarianism on my formulation denies that there is anything unjust in that state of affairs. Where two individuals are equally well off, but where one is not as deserving (understood in terms of either prudence *or* virtue) as the other, desert would recommend making the less deserving person less well off (and restoring *in*equality), whereas LE would not.[21]

To flesh out the implications of these differences, consider the following example, fashioned after Peter Vallentyne.[22] Prudent and Lazy are two survivors on a desert (no pun intended) island. While Lazy lies on the beach, Prudent goes fishing and returns with a fish that she then proceeds to grill and enjoy on her own. Their respective levels of welfare are now, let us say, 10 for Lazy (hungry but rested), and 20 for Prudent. LE and desert agree that there is nothing unjust in this unequal state of affairs (call it A). Imagine now that a nice big fish washes up alongside Lazy, who, recall, is simply lying there.[23] This turn of events generates a new distribution (B), where now both Lazy and Prudent have 20 units of welfare. (On the one hand, assume, Lazy is more rested than Prudent, but on the other, the fish that washed ashore is not as tasty or big as the one that Prudent caught, hence the eventual equality in welfare.) Is there anything unjust about the new distribution (B)? Desert tells us that there is. The two individuals' equal level of welfare does not reflect their unequal levels of deservingness (understood, recall, in terms of prudence). Justice, then, requires that Lazy should transfer some of the fish (or some equivalent of it) to Prudent so that *in*equality is restored. It is indeterminate (at least according to the more plausible comparative desert view) how many units of welfare exactly Lazy ought to transfer. The only requirement is that some inequality ought to be restored between them, to match the unequal levels of deservingness. LE, on my formulation, does not entail that view, and properly so, I maintain. It denies that there is anything unjust about equality, including the equality that now obtains between Prudent and Lazy. More generally, LE is agnostic about the justice or injustice of any *equality*.

Potential Objections

It may be difficult at first to accept my suggestion that egalitarian distributive justice concerns only inequalities. Isn't it unjust, for example, for a rich person who lost much of his assets through reckless gambling to be as equally well off as a very prudent (though unlucky) poor person? Surely this is wrong, the critic might say. Recall, in response, that my formulation would stipulate leaving the prudent poor as she is only as long as there is no one else *in the entire society* (or whatever the relevant group is) who is better off than she is (and through no merit of their own). It seems to me that once attention is called to that fact, the sense of counterintuition raised by the comparison of the prudent poor with the imprudent (formerly) rich disappears. In a two-person society it is plausible to think of the equality that obtains between the reckless but lucky person and the diligent but unlucky one as a state of affairs that is not unjust.

As another objection, consider a hypothetical society composed of two individuals (or classes, for that matter), one diligent but untalented, and the other talented but lazy, existing in perfect equality. Equality is reached because, say, the diligent person works eight hours a day and ends up with as many resources (or whatever the currency is) as the talented person acquires in a four-hour working day. This state of affairs seems unjust and yet my formulation does not condemn it. Notice, however, that the eight-hour working day of the untalented is purely a matter of choice. As soon as she decides to reduce the length of her working day to seven hours, something she is perfectly entitled to do on my formulation, her bundle would accordingly drop to below that of the talented. When that happens, the demands of distributive justice would kick in and require a transfer from the talented to the untalented (since the latter is now worse off and through no fault of her own).

Consider another objection to the suggestion that egalitarian distributive justice concerns only inequalities. Suppose Jack and Jill occupy identical positions in a firm, but where Jill puts in twice as many hours (and, accordingly, let us also assume, produces twice as much output). Yet, at the end of the month Jack and Jill receive an identical pay check. Many would protest that an injustice has taken place here, and one that my formulation does not condemn. Notice, however, that it could have been the case that the firm actually stated in advance that no matter how much work one put in, everyone would be rewarded equally. (Think of the firm in question as a kibbutz, or indeed, as a department in a university.) If that were the case, then perhaps there would be no reason to think that Jill has been wronged after all. More accurately, there would not then be any reason to think that Jill has been wronged by *the firm* (or university, or kibbutz, or society). It might, in contrast, be that *Jack* has acted unjustly toward Jill, by not pulling his own weight equally. And indeed it is plausible that if Jack were a kibbutz member or a colleague in our academic department he would be an object of resentment for not pulling his weight. But crucially, we would not necessarily think that the university or the kibbutz has acted unjustly by providing him with equal pay. One would perhaps expect someone like Cohen to be sympathetic to the practice of un-differentiated pay in kibbutzim or among university faculty, which is why it might come as a surprise that he sees equality that reflects unequal deserving-ness as unjust.

Finally, even under circumstances where the policy of equal pay was not made public in advance, the equality between Jack and Jill, I claim, is not un-just. It is plausible to say that if the state of affairs (her getting as much as Jack despite working harder) is unjust, it is so because she has been discriminated against, or because her legitimate expectations have been frustrated. On that account, Jill has less than she could have had because of a discriminating inter-ference by the managers of the firm. The comparison with Jack only serves to *indicate* that. The equality between Jill and Jack is therefore not *constitutive* of the injustice that has been done to her; it is only potentially indicative of it. Thus, from the perspective of egalitarian *distributive* justice, there seems to be nothing wrong in the equality that prevails between Jack and Jill.

To sum up the point of this section, LE properly understood is *not* con-cerned with matching individuals' level of well-being to their respective levels of deservingness, and properly so. In contrast to desert, LE seeks to eliminate differential luck *only* when it generates inequalities. The next step of my in-quiry will examine that notion of differential luck, and will defend my inter-pretation of brute luck as the idea of reasonable avoidability. I turn to this issue now.

III. Reasonable Avoidability vs. Responsibility

One of the defining features of the luck egalitarian reading of justice is that society has no obligations of egalitarian distributive justice toward those who suffer bad option luck. Addressing the "harshness objection" to which such a position gives rise will occupy us in chapters 3 and 4. My concern here is rather to sharpen the distinction between option luck and brute luck. In other words, I want to specify when it is permissible, according to luck egalitarians, to deny people compensation for a disadvantage from which they suffer.

My suggestion is that we need to replace "responsibility" with a more plausible understanding of what constitutes a case of brute luck. (It is largely for that reason that the title of this book contains "luck" but not "responsibility".) My view is that we ought to understand "brute luck" as the *outcome of actions (including omissions) that it would have been unreasonable to expect the agent to avoid (or not to avoid, in the case of omissions).*[24] "Expectation" here is obviously to be understood as a normative expectation rather than an epistemic one.[25] We are not inquiring here into what people are *likely* to do, but rather what it is that society can reasonably expect of them.[26] Notice also that this unreasonableness criterion shifts the focus of attention from the individual to the society. It asks *not* whether the individual has acted in a reasonable way, but rather whether it is *un*reasonable for *society* to expect the individual to avoid a certain course of action. Thus, the burden of proof, as it were, is shifted away from the individual.

To see why this formulation is attractive, contrast it with a certain strict reading of LE. That reading says that individuals should only be compensated for eventualities that they could not possibly have avoided. This quite crude reading of the luck egalitarian ideal, which to my knowledge is endorsed only by Eric Rakowski,[27] has rightly been criticized for its not only harsh but also implausible conclusions. These include the view that we owe no disaster relief to people living in regions that suffer from some risk of floods or hurricanes (assuming they could have moved someplace else).[28] Contrast this with my proposed formulation according to which society ought to compensate for any undesirable outcome that it would have been *unreasonable to expect people to avoid*. People residing in certain parts of California are (often) responsible for choosing to live on a geological fault line. However, it would be unreasonable to expect them not to settle in these areas owing to the slight chance of being hit by an earthquake. In contrast, those who choose to camp on the slope of a volcano despite repeated warnings that it is due to erupt any day now *are* liable for any ensuing disadvantage. It would not have been unreasonable to expect them not to go camping there on that particular occasion. In responding to such examples, luck egalitarians may have so far acquiesced in allowing their critics to portray such actions as the decision to live near the Californian fault line as if they were some risky business venture. According to the latter line of thinking, if one chooses to take that risk (in return, say, for cheaper rent in those areas), then, one ought to bear the consequences of the risk alone if it were to materialize. But of course, as critics of LE have rightly recognized, choosing to reside in an earthquake-prone area is not at all like making a risky business choice.[29] If it is indeed unreasonably risky to live in some area due to risk of volcano eruption, then the state should typically not allow anyone to reside there (at least temporarily). In that sense, a geographical choice of residence is different from the decision to smoke, for example (as the latter does involve what most people would consider a legitimate trade-off between prudence and pleasure).

Likewise, the following example may also support my formulation. It is sometimes said that a strict reading of LE would result in the unacceptable judgment that we should deny women medical treatment for pregnancy and delivery, since they are (often) responsible for their condition (i.e., for getting pregnant). My suggested formulation escapes this absurd verdict. Although women who require medical care during pregnancy and delivery *are* (usually) responsible for their condition, it would be unreasonable to ask women (or couples for that matter), as a rule, to not get pregnant. The unreasonableness criterion also successfully explains the somewhat opposite case of providing treatment to women who may have aggravated the risk of breast cancer by their decision *not* to bear children.[30] Here again it would be unreasonable, traditional societies notwithstanding, to expect all women as a rule to *have* children (or to have more than one child).[31] The unreasonableness criterion thus seems to avoid some of the crudest "abandonment" cases that have typically embarrassed luck egalitarians.[32]

An obvious objection that might be raised at this point is one of circularity. The question I seem to ask, the critic might say, is: "What is it for which society owes individuals compensation?" And the corresponding answer I seem to provide is: "Outcomes that it would be unreasonable to expect individuals to bear on their own." In that case, the answer simply repeats the question without giving us any independent criteria with which to answer it. Yet, in response, I deny that that is the question that luck egalitarians seek to answer. Rather, the question they pose is: "What distributions are unjust from the standpoint of egalitarian distributive justice?" And the answer I attempt to give here is: "Inequalities that are due to actions that it would have been unreasonable to expect the disadvantaged individual to avoid." If so, the luck egalitarian need not provide any further independent criteria by which to judge what sort of conduct individuals ought to bear on their own. She simply states that her aim is to level inequalities that result from such conduct, *whatever conduct precisely that might be.* There is therefore no circularity here. The formulation of LE provided here gives a distinctive interpretation of the requirement of egalitarian distributive justice, namely that society ought to compensate individuals for whatever disadvantages result from conduct that it would have been unreasonable to expect them to avoid. If this were a circular position it would not be such a controversial one.

Now admittedly "unreasonableness" is an ambiguous notion, and that obviously has the weakness of leading to indeterminacy. However, I want to suggest that the formulation's ambiguity could also be a source of strength. The strength of the "reasonable avoidability" criterion is that it can give due consideration to the changing circumstances of each case. In conditions of extreme scarcity, for example, it may be reasonable to expect women (and their partners) not to get pregnant (if they can help it, of course), at least temporarily. We could envisage some extreme circumstances under which something like China's "one child" policy *is* a reasonable one to pursue. Under such circumstances, it would seem right to maintain that narrow considerations of distributive justice do not require providing for couples who bear more than one child the same benefits that we would provide under normal circumstances (provided, of course, that the denial of benefits to the parents does not harm the child, something which admittedly may be difficult). Or, suppose that a woman is warned by her physician of a high risk to her health should she choose to get pregnant. If she does opt for the pregnancy, then it would not be unreasonable, in my view, to see her as forfeiting a claim to treatment on grounds of egalitarian distributive justice. (She might, of course, nevertheless receive treatment on other grounds such as compassion, the concern for meeting basic needs, and of course the well-being of the child. See more on this in chapters 4 and 5.)

Consider some further familiar cases purportedly showing the counterintuitiveness generated by LE. Firefighters are responsible for incurring burns because they have chosen, by their own free will, to enter a burning building. But it would obviously be wrong to withhold treatment from them.[33] There might, of course, be some non–justice-based reasons to care for injured firefighters.[34] Yet, I would like to further suggest that there might also be a justice-based reason for doing so. It would clearly be unreasonable to expect a firefighter on duty to refrain from entering a burning building. (Of course, we might say that it would not have been unreasonable to expect that person to refrain from becoming a firefighter in the first place because she could have easily chosen a different career. However, it would be unreasonable to expect *everyone* in society not to become a firefighter, as there is clearly still a need for that line of work.) On the revised formulation, then, luck egalitarian justice would require treating firefighters who were injured in the line of duty. In contrast, it would deny justice-based treatment to a juggler who got burned jumping through a burning hoop (assuming it would not have been unreasonable to expect him to avoid doing so).

Take another counterexample leveled against the implications of luck egalitarianism, that of people who find themselves caregivers to a family member.[35] Sometimes people have effectively no choice but to stay at home and become such caregivers, at the expense of all sorts of opportunity sets that they might otherwise have had. We can think of cases where it would be unreasonable to expect the person in question to avoid becoming such a care-giver. Suppose that due to the special relationship she has with her mentally disabled and elderly mother, say, it is only she herself who is in a position to offer effective care under the circumstances. In that case, it would be wrong to deny her compensation for the loss of other opportunities (e.g., employ-ment, socializing) that she suffered. In other cases, by contrast, we might ad-mire the person for making the sacrifice of giving up a career or other op-portunities in order to stay at home with a family member. And yet, despite that, and because we feel it was not unreasonable to expect that person to act otherwise, we would deny her compensation. Moreover, we would feel that although her sacrifice is admirable, it would still be inappropriate for her to approach society for some compensation, precisely because she could have reasonably avoided that course of action.

Notice how the unreasonableness criterion functions better than another suggested criterion, the one concerning "innocent choice." It is sometimes said that the point of (luck) egalitarian justice is to compensate for innocent choices, and conversely, that justice does not require compensating individu-als for culpable choices.[36] "Innocent" and "culpable" are taken, on that ac-count, as referring to the type of motives that guided the agent on the course of action that has led to her disadvantage. Actions pursued for innocent and praiseworthy reasons ought to be compensated when leading to a disadvan-tage, whereas those done for reasons that are not innocent need not be com-pensated. It seems to me, however, that that criterion captures too much, and that, correspondingly, the "reasonable avoidability" criterion is better. Con-sider the example of incurring some loss (perhaps having your clothes ru-ined) during an attempt to rescue the neighbor's child from a fire. Suppose you are the closest person to the burning building, or that you are the most qualified individual among several who are equally proximate to the scene. Whether or not you are under some moral or legal obligation to rescue the child, it would clearly be unreasonable to expect you *not* to attempt to res-cue her. Thus, on my suggested reading, society owes you compensation for the loss you suffered in the course of that attempt (your slightly burnt clothes, say). Consider now a different example. Suppose you give half of your monthly salary to Oxfam in order to help the poor and starving in Africa. (We must suppose, for the sake of argument, that this is a supererogatory act, and not one required by justice.) It would be safe to assume that your choice in doing so is not only innocent but actually praiseworthy. Yet we feel that one would be wrong to ask to be compensated for the loss one suffered (e.g., the very losing of half of one's salary, some lost opportunities for investment, etc.) in the process of exercising that innocent, indeed praiseworthy, choice. Part of what constitutes the praiseworthiness of that action is the fact that it involved a certain cost to oneself. The praiseworthy action would therefore not be so praiseworthy if one asked for compensation for it afterwards. It is clear, then, that LE cannot be about compensating innocent choices. Consider, in contrast, how the reasonableness criterion handles examples of this kind. Even though your decision to give half of your salary to Oxfam is an innocent and even praiseworthy one, it would still *not be unreasonable* to expect you to refrain from doing so. Thus, no compensation is owed to you as a matter of distributive justice.

The Oxfam example shows, among other things, why placing the unreasonableness criterion on society rather than on the individual provides a better account. It is irrelevant to determine, from the point of view of justice, whether or not it is reasonable for the individual to give half her salary to Oxfam. It may, for example, give her much more satisfaction to do so than it would to spend that money on herself, and thus it would be perfectly reasonable. It is irrelevant, from the point of view of justice, for other people to determine whether the action has been reasonable or not. We are far more concerned with making such (normative) judgments with regard to what society can reasonably expect. Whether or not it is reasonable for the individual to give half her salary to Oxfam, it is *not un*reasonable *for society* to ask her to refrain from doing so (given the projected detrimental effect upon her).[37]

Here, finally, is a counter objection to my Oxfam example. Suppose Mother Theresa neglected her own health while dedicating her life to the poor and starving of Calcutta.[38] Surely it would have been wrong to deny her compensation (or medical treatment). On the "innocent choice" account she deserves compensation, whereas on my account she does not. In chapter 4, I will argue that luck egalitarians ought to bite the bullet and hold that society ought to treat her, but for reasons external to egalitarian distributive justice. (In this incidence, it might be out of gratitude, or out of the concern to provide an incentive to other people to follow her example, but more generally it would be out of the concern for meeting basic needs.) It would not, however, according to the "reasonable avoidability" account, have been unreasonable to expect Mother Theresa to take good care of her health while attending to the poor of Calcutta.

Conclusion

Luck egalitarianism has emerged in recent years as a leading interpretation of the demands of egalitarian distributive justice, and is now the main rival to the dominant Rawlsian account. My aim in this chapter was not to address the weighty criticisms leveled against the theory by its (mainly Rawlsian) opponents. Rather, I wanted to introduce the main differences between the luck egalitarian and the Rawlsian conceptions of justice. In addition, I sought to address two residual family quarrels among luck egalitarians. Namely, I have argued, first, against some key luck egalitarians, that egalitarian justice properly concerns only inequalities, and never equalities, and second, that luck egalitarians ought to understand bad brute luck as eventualities which it would have been unreasonable to expect individuals to avoid. By doing so, I hope to have provided a working understanding of luck egalitarian distributive justice, one that I seek to employ throughout the rest of the book.

Part I

Health Care

2
■

Responsibility-*Insensitive* Health Care

Introduction

Luck egalitarians hold that inequalities are unjust when they are the outcome of individuals' unchosen natural and social circumstances. Accordingly, they hold that justice only requires compensating individuals for disadvantages for which they cannot be held responsible. Arguably, it follows that luck egalitarians must deny our obligation to provide assistance to those who come to need it through some fault of their own, e.g., an emergency service to a reckless driver or a liver transplant to a persistent alcoholic. Many believe that these counterintuitive cases demonstrate that luck egalitarianism cannot provide a theory of justice in health care. This is known as the "abandonment of negligent victims" objection.[1] The account of justice in health care that luck egalitarianism provides is, in this sense, too narrow. (An objection claiming that luck egalitarian health policy can be, in a different sense, too wide, will be discussed in chapter 9.) The first part of the book seeks to meet this challenge, and show not only why luck egalitarian justice can escape the abandonment objection and justify universal and unconditional health care, but also that it does so in a way that is superior to other contending egalitarian theories.

I begin addressing this task by first looking at those contending theories. Namely, I examine the plausibility of accounts of justice that give no role for considerations of personal responsibility. I assess how plausible the accounts of justice in health care are that these approaches generate. In this chapter I shall examine two responsibility-insensitive accounts of just health care: Norman Daniels's fair opportunity for life plans account, and Elizabeth Anderson's democratic equality account. Both avoid the abandonment dilemma, but both have difficulties, for different reasons, in justifying universal health care. A third account of just health care that purports to sidestep the abandonment objection is examined in chapter 3. While the two accounts examined in this chapter overlook considerations of personal responsibility, the one examined in the next chapter goes in the exact opposite way, in that it pays full attention to matters of personal responsibility and luck, more than a standard luck egalitarian account would. I attempt to show that, ultimately, all three accounts are unsatisfactory, and then move in chapters 4 and 5 to defend a (standard) luck egalitarian justification of universal health care.

I turn in this chapter, then, to examine standard accounts of justice in health care. As mentioned, I examine two such accounts, one more worked-out than the other: Daniels's fair opportunity account, and Anderson's (and others') democratic equality account.[2] I would like to suggest that these two accounts face certain difficulties, quite a few of them decisive, in providing an account of just health care. The first section offers an objection to Daniels's fair opportunity account, and the second section deals with an important counter-objection. Section III presents the democratic equality account and examines its ability to provide an account of justice in health care.

I. The Fair Opportunity Account

Norman Daniels's is unquestionably the most worked-out account of justice in health care. Daniels has developed his fair opportunity account over many books and articles, spanning over more than twenty years. Any attempt to provide a complete assessment of that opus within the limited scope of this chapter is doomed to failure. Instead, I shall focus on the main essentials of his theory here, touching on other aspects of his theory in the chapters to come (particularly in chapter 9, but also in chapters 5, 7, and 11).

Daniels's theory of justice in health care is premised on the claim that health has "strategic importance" in our lives.[3] Health is strategically important, according to Daniels, because it contributes significantly to our ability to pursue and realize our life plans. Put differently, health greatly affects one's share of the "normal opportunity range," the range of opportunities one can normally expect to have in one's particular society, given one's particular talents.[4] Due to this strategic importance of health, society ought to provide health care in an egalitarian way, and one that also would restore health to the greatest extent possible.

Daniels's account is essentially an attempt to provide a Rawlsian account of justice in health care, something that Rawls himself never attempted. As Daniels pointed out, in Rawls's "original position" no one is ever sick! Not surprisingly, then, Rawls himself never bothered with a theory of the just distribution of health care. That is the lacuna that Daniels sought to fill. The main dilemma in confronting this task was to decide under which of Rawls's principles of justice health care should be regulated. Famously, Rawls's theory of justice consists of three lexically ordered principles: the principle of equal liberties, the principle of fair equality of opportunity (FEOP), and a principle regulating the distribution of all other social primary goods (the difference principle, or DP). Social primary goods are nonnatural goods in which all individuals have an interest, whatever else they want for themselves. Thus, the obvious principle for distributing health care would have appeared to be the lexically inferior DP. The kernel of Daniels's innovative approach was to resist that intuitive move, and place the distribution of health care under the lexically prior FEOP.

The reason behind Daniels's decision to place the distribution of health care under the auspice of the FEOP is the observation that health is crucial for the pursuit of jobs and careers. Being ill or handicapped drastically affects one's range of opportunities, career-wise. Thus, bringing all members as close to being healthy as possible contributes to the pursuit of equal opportunities for jobs and careers. Now, Daniels slightly revises the FEOP when applying it to the distribution of health care. Namely, he expands the principle's domain from jobs and careers to life plans more generally. The term "life plan" is commonly used in political philosophy to describe both careers and other projects (broadly conceived) that we might wish to pursue during our lifetime. (I shall return to analyze "life plan" in more detail in the next section.) Notice that the main implication of placing the distribution of health care under the FEOP rather than under the lexically inferior DP is that the former mandates a strictly equal distribution whereas the latter permits an unequal distribution of health care, provided that doing so would benefit those who are the worst off. Importantly, Daniels's Rawlsian account gives no room for considerations of personal responsibility, and therefore does not distinguish prudent patients from imprudent ones. This aspect of the theory has the happy result of avoiding denying medical treatment to imprudent patients, thus maintaining an unconditional provision of health care.

Over the current and next section, I shall argue that, *contra* Daniels, an account of justice in health care cannot be based on the concern for fair equality of opportunity to pursue life plans. If my argument is sound, then Daniels's attempt to provide a responsibility-insensitive account of health care proves inadequate.

I can think of two main objections to Daniels's theory, one of which has already been put forward forcefully and convincingly in the literature, so I shall merely mention it.[5] That objection begins by pointing out that the poor have worse opportunities to pursue their life plans compared to the rich. If *equality* of opportunity for pursuing life plans is what we are after, then that justifies providing superior health care to the poor and disadvantaged. Indeed, perhaps it justifies providing health care only to the poor, and this way inequality of opportunity would be curtailed. Far from justifying universal care, then, the fair opportunity account may actually justify *selective* care.[6] Many people, however, believe that health care ought to discriminate against neither the poor *nor the rich*. For one thing, such discrimination might be harmful to individuals' sense of self-respect.[7] There is therefore something wrong about an account of justice in health that yields such a recommendation. Daniels may thus try and incorporate the concern not to harm people's sense of self-respect (which is, after all, "perhaps the most important primary good" according to Rawls)[8] into his account of health care. He may contend that given our obligation to boost the opportunities of the worse off, and given our concern not to harm the self-respect of all members of society, including the better off, we ought to provide the best possible care to everyone in society, and then help the worse off boost their opportunities in some other areas of life (education, income). Health care thus makes a limited but still important contribution to equality of opportunity.[9] One might wonder, though, how harmful selective health care actually is for the self-respect of the rich. A selective service such as Medicaid, for example, is seldom seen as disrespectful of the rich. If anything, it is the exact opposite that is sometimes suggested (namely that it potentially stigmatizes the poor).

This criticism of Daniels's fair opportunity account therefore does not seem all that false. It tells us that his account leads to selective rather than universal health care. But suppose we decided, whether for reasons of self-respect or for other reasons, not to allow discrimination between the poor and the rich in health care. Even then, I want to suggest, there may be other problems with the ability of Daniels's fair opportunity argument to provide an adequate account of justice in health care.

The second objection, then, the one that I would like to put forward, is based on the following familiar premise (a premise that Daniels, we shall see below, also accepts).[10] Most patients treated by health care systems are individuals in the twilight of their lives. Furthermore, it is also the case that the bulk of health care resources are spent on these elderly patients. An oftencited figure is that, in the United States, 30 percent of health care expenditure is currently spent on patients in the last six months of their life.[11] Let us suppose, for now, that that current practice is consistent with a just system of health care (I will investigate shortly the implications in case it is not). For those elderly patients, health care cannot be said to provide opportunity, equal or otherwise, to pursue *life plans*. The effect of successful treatment of patients who are in the last weeks of their lives is not so much that of giving them opportunity to pursue their life plans, but rather that of alleviating their pain and suffering and extending their lives as long as humanely possible.[12] To be sure, "the last six months of a person's life" is a figure known to us only after the fact. In other words, in the case of some of these (typically younger) patients, medical care was truly intended as a means of restoring healthy functioning, so as to allow them to continue pursuing their life plans, but was simply unsuccessful. Still, it is safe to say that the elderly constitute most of those patients on whom so many resources are spent in the twilight of life.[13]

Now, I certainly do not want to suggest that people have no important pursuits that they wish to carry out in the last years (or even months) of their lives.[14] Rather, my claim is only that these pursuits cannot fall under what political philosophers normally call a "life plan." It seems safe to say, then, that the lion's share of health care resources are *not* currently geared toward providing patients with an opportunity to pursue their life plans. Therefore, it is either the case that the opportunity account does not provide a correct account of justice in health care, or, that our practice of spending this amount of resources on the elderly should be revised in accordance with a theory that emphasizes opportunities to pursue life plans.[15]

Daniels does, indeed, opt for the latter. He argues that we have reasons to limit the amount of resources spent on life-saving treatment when the patient is over 75.[16] He also provides a persuasive case for rationing health care resources in that way, one based on the idea of rationing health care throughout one's life, and on the plausible assumption that most people will have lived out their life plans when they reach the age of 75. The latter assumption is a plausible one precisely because 75 is more or less the lifespan that most people in developed countries expect to reach, and so the rational thing would be to structure one's life plan to fit with that range of life expectancy.[17] It is therefore justified, according to a theory that takes individuals' ability to realize their life plans as its currency, to cut off expensive life-sustaining medical treatment at that age. But even assuming that rationing life-saving treatment in that way is justified,[18] Daniels's account still remains exposed. My objection, recall, was not that Daniels's account demands providing *less* provision to the elderly (or that he limits the cost of expensive life-sustaining treatment they are entitled to). It is rather that a theory premised on pursuing life plans fails to justify *any* health care (to patients over 75[19]) whatsoever.[20] Even the provision of aspirin to individuals who can be said to have completed their life plans must, if we hold Daniels to his theory, be justified on grounds other than opportunity to pursue life plans, and therefore other than justice. That seems problematic.

It may be useful to compare, in this respect, health care with education. Daniels himself points out that aside from health care we should note also "the strategic importance of education for protecting equal opportunity."[21] And yet my objection does not seem to be as effective in the case of education, and properly so. There may be various reasons for providing subsidized programs of adult education, but it does seem that as far as egalitarian justice is concerned, we are required to provide education mostly at some earlier stages of life. That judgment seems acceptable enough with regard to education but, crucially, not so with regard to health care. For, in difference to education, we commonly think that society *does* owe it, as a matter of justice, to provide health care to the elderly, even when they can be said to have completed their life plans.

II. Opportunities and Life Plans

One way in which Daniels can avoid the objection just made is to say that it is part of everyone's plan of life to "lead a long and pain-free life" or to "take it easy once one retires and read lots of novels." If these kinds of pursuits were to be included in what it means to pursue a life plan, then medical care for the elderly could still be justified as a means of pursuing one's life plans.[22] Projects of this kind (e.g., "leading a long and pain-free life") fall under what we may call a *broad* interpretation of a "life plan." That broad interpretation of a life plan, I will argue in this section, is unavailable to Daniels. If so, my objection to his account of justice in health care stands.

As mentioned, Daniels develops his justification of health care by extending John Rawls's FEOP "for jobs and careers."[23] Jobs and careers are strategically important for Rawls, Daniels notes, because "major rewards in our society derive from jobs and offices."[24] That is why Rawls subjects "access to jobs and offices" to the FEOP rather than to the (less demanding) DP. Daniels correctly notes that major rewards also follow from pursuing the type of life plan we choose to lead. It is that fact (and only that fact, I submit) that makes Daniels's extension of the FEOP to cover life plans (rather than just jobs and offices) a plausible one. But Daniels attempts to extend the FEOP further, and in a way that Rawls's does not allow him, or so I want to suggest.

Consider what Rawls says of the rationale behind his FEOP:

> if some places were not open on a basis fair to all, those kept out would be right in feeling unjustly treated even though they benefited from the greater efforts of those who were allowed to hold them. They would be justified in their complaint not only because they were excluded from certain external rewards of office but because they were debarred from the realization of self which comes from a skilful and devoted exercise of social duties. They would be deprived of one of the main forms of human good.[25]

It follows, according to Rawls, that society ought to distribute some goods more equally than even the difference principle (DP) would allow. That is, some goods are of such importance that the opportunity to attain them should be distributed equally (among individuals of equal talent) even if that entails some measure of leveling down in economic terms.[26] Rawls provides various reasons for thinking that access to these positions is of greater importance than access to other social primary goods (to which the less demanding DP applies). These reasons include keeping a check on the economic inequalities allowed by the DP, increasing efficiency through meritocratic competition, and ensuring equal access to the financial rewards that jobs bring. In addition, and perhaps most plausibly,[27] the priority of the FEOP over the DP is premised on ensuring equal access to the potential intrinsic rewards of having a (rewarding) job—rewards such as self-realization and increased self-esteem.[28]

Note, again, that for Rawls, the FEOP guarantees equal opportunity for jobs and offices not across the board, but between people of equal talent.[29] Famously, unlike the DP, the FEOP is not designed to correct for the natural lottery of talents, but is aimed, rather, at eliminating social barriers to individuals exercising their talents. It is a principle that demands fair *competition* for jobs and careers.[30] As mentioned, Daniels broadens Rawls's FEOP from jobs to the pursuit of life plans more generally.[31] However, he retains everything else in Rawls's principle. So whereas Rawls is concerned with equality of opportunity for jobs between individuals of equal talent, Daniels is concerned with equality of opportunity to pursue *life plans* between individuals of equal talent.[32] This is a plausible move for Daniels to make, and he is right to broaden the FEOP from jobs to the more general "life plans," since some of our life plans may not be, strictly speaking, jobs or careers. Such life plans would include publishing a book of one's poems (not for financial gain), getting to be selected to represent one's country in some international event, and so forth. We may refer to these pursuits as life plans in the *narrow* sense of the term. But Daniels's formula cannot be taken to imply "life plan" in the broad sense of the term mentioned earlier. Daniels is barred from using the broad interpretation of life plan, which is, as we said earlier, the only kind of interpretation of life plan that can be applied to most people over 75. The reason is this. Why should we take people's talents into consideration when contemplating life plans of the kind of "leading a long and pain-free life" or "taking it easy once one retires and reading lots of novels"? *Talents—equal or not—do not come into play here.* There are obvious reasons that make talents irrelevant here. To begin with, these pursuits are not tasks and therefore talents do not determine the quality of their execution. But more importantly, these pursuits do not constitute competitive positions, contrary to the rationale behind Rawls's FEOP.[33]

Now one way in which talents *could* affect the distribution of those broadly defined life plans, thus countering my argument, is in the following.

The ability to spend one's golden age playing with one's grandchildren (or reading lots of novels) could potentially depend on one's talents, for the very ability to retire may depend on the financial assets one has accumulated throughout one's life. The extent of one's financial assets, in turn, often depends on the type of job(s) one has held throughout one's life. And *that* is affected, even in a just Rawlsian society, by one's talents. This is one way in which talents could affect the range of broadly defined life plans available to any given person, so the objection goes. To put the point in Daniels's terminology, spending one's retirement reading lots of novels could be part of people's fair (i.e., talent-relative) share of the normal opportunity range.

To be sure, in our nonideal societies the ability to retire and spend time playing with one's grandchildren does depend on one's financial ability (and, by derivation, on one's talents). But it is far from obvious that Daniels can justifiably allude to such reasoning in defense of adopting the broad interpretation of "life plan." Recall that under the FEOP, the distribution of opportunities (to pursue life plans) should be independent and lexically prior to inequalities in the distribution of income (and other social primary goods). Now admittedly, FEOP does allow for access to life plans to be relative to talent (in fact, it *requires* it to be so). For example, a person does not have a valid complaint when she is not allowed to play for the Boston Symphony if she does not have the relevant musical talent. But FEOP does *not* justify disqualifying a person from playing for the Boston Symphony on the grounds that she could not afford the $100 registration fee required for the Symphony's trials. (If anything, FEOP mandates eradicating precisely such social barriers to the exercise of one's talents.) And, it is no defense at all to claim that the person did not have the required registration fee because her (other) limited talents did not allow her to earn that sum of money prior to the trials. Such a claim goes directly against the rationale for the FEOP as a lexically prior principle to the DP. The only way to make "life plans" in the broad sense of the term sensitive to talents, then, would entail subverting the rationale of governing health care through the lexically prior FEOP. "Life plan," in Daniels's scheme, therefore cannot be broadened to cover the type of broad life plans that apply to the elderly without thereby undermining the rationale for subjecting health care to the lexically prior FEOP.

Justifying the provision of health care through the FEOP rather than through the DP means, then, that Daniels's account of justice in health care is in conflict with the rather uncontroversial practice of treating patients who can reasonably be said to have completed their life plans.[34] Thus, this attempt to provide a responsibility-*in*sensitive justification of universal health care proves unsuccessful. Let me move now to examine the other responsibility-insensitive account of just health care mentioned, the one offered by Elizabeth Anderson.

III. The Democratic Equality Account

In contrast to Daniels's opportunity account of just health care, it should be noted, the democratic equality (or capabilities) account is offered primarily as a general theory of egalitarian justice, and not as one particularly tailored for health care. It is also important to stress, by way of preface, that some recent invocations of that theory of justice have been formulated specifically as a reaction to the luck egalitarian emphasis on personal responsibility and luck. As such, the fact that "democratic egalitarians" do not abandon imprudent patients is not merely a fortunate by-product of their theory but rather one of its very reasons of being. In a nutshell, those advocating the ideal of justice as based on equal democratic capabilities hold that the point of distributive justice is to allow citizens to participate as equals in democratic politics and civil society. Resources are therefore to be distributed in such a way as to guarantee equality in the distribution of basic democratic capabilities. The purpose of health care, it follows, is to restore individuals back to full health so as to facilitate their capability to participate in politics and civil society on an equal footing. Let me then first say something about "democratic equality" as a general theory of justice, and then examine its ability to provide an account of just health care.

As mentioned, democratic equality (DE) is a theory of egalitarian justice that has resurfaced in recent years mainly as a reaction to luck egalitarianism. As such, it is of particular interest to anyone who wants to defend a luck egalitarian account of health care. DE maintains that instead of comparing individuals' respective bundles of goods (or the absence thereof [what Elizabeth Anderson, perhaps its chief proponent, calls searching for "relative deficiency"]),[35] the point of egalitarian justice is to provide everyone with a sufficient level of functioning. More specifically, justice requires an equal distribution of only those goods and capabilities that are needed for the sake of equal citizenship and equal access to civil society,[36] as well as "whatever capabilities are necessary to enable them [individuals] to avoid or escape entanglement in oppressive social relationships."[37] DE is therefore not concerned with equality as such but rather with equal capabilities to participate in democracy and civil society.

Having been originally formulated in opposition to luck egalitarianism, it is, as mentioned, no coincidence that DE easily averts the abandonment objection. By guaranteeing to citizens a basic set of capabilities that would enable them to participate in society, democratic equality eschews considerations of personal responsibility in determining what a just distribution is. It explicitly rejects drawing a distinction between democratic capabilities that are undermined due to chance and those that are undermined due to the person's own fault. Democratic egalitarians seek to guarantee a certain level of capabilities universally and across the citizenry, thus consciously ignoring considerations of personal responsibility. Accordingly, DE arguably mandates restoring citizens to full healthy functioning, so as to allow citizens full and equal capability to participate in politics and society. DE thus seems to justify universal and unconditional health care. My claim, however, is that though it avoids the abandonment problem, DE nevertheless displays a number of other, perhaps even more decisive, weaknesses in providing a theory of justice in health care. Let me, then, offer five critical comments about the ability of DE to justify health care entitlement.

Richard Arneson points to the following, perhaps obvious, initial problem with DE as a general theory of justice. Concerned as it is with equality in relationships, it gives little consideration for noncomparative, that is, absolute levels of goods. "Whatever exactly participation as equals requires, it evidently does not require much by way of desirable quality of life. We could function as democratic equals while life is bleak, even squalid, for all of us."[38] More to the point of health care, people can be of equal democratic capabilities when they are all equally physically incapacitated. DE is therefore compatible with no provision of health care whatsoever (provided its absence renders everyone equally ill). At the same time, we should notice that the charge that its exclusive focus on relative distribution allows for such leveling down is not something that is unique to DE. For that weakness is shared by all egalitarian theories, including luck egalitarianism (more on which in chapter 8). Still, the point to bear in mind here is that contrary to what they may believe, democratic egalitarians do not guarantee a minimal level of health to all citizens, and their theory is in fact compatible with very low health (and thus with no health care).

Here is a second reservation about DE. Democratic egalitarians' aversion to comparing the relative bundles that individuals possess, something egalitarians usually deem indispensable for distributive justice, leads them to advocate guaranteeing a certain sufficient bundle of goods with which to achieve equality of democratic capabilities. Their method, presumably, is to look at each society and evaluate what it is that members of that particular society require for achieving equality of status and of democratic capabilities with each other. It seems to me, however, that democratic egalitarians are wrong to think that one could articulate what that bundle of goods consists of without paying attention to relations of inequality within the society in question. It is impossible to know what resources are needed for the purpose of political equality if we do not know the relative distribution of important resources in a given society. The attempt to satisfy a decent baseline through some checklist of sufficient provision, while disregarding inequalities of income and other socioeconomic goods will therefore inevitably fail. Now, someone like Anderson may reply that sufficiency is not, strictly speaking, an absolute term, but rather one that potentially has a strong relative element. What is sufficient or adequate for members of a society to have would in many cases depend on the relative position of other members in that society. As long ago pointed out by Adam Smith, the fact that all other members of one's society wear a linen shirt makes owning one part of the bundle of goods required for a minimally decent life in that society.[39] Sufficiency therefore does have a relative element. But while it is true that the level of sufficiency may be determined with an eye to relative distribution, sufficientarianism, by definition, still allows for inequalities that exist above that level of sufficiency, however high it may be set. Thus, paying attention only to some level of sufficiency might still result in substantial inequalities. As such, sufficiency may not be enough (as Paula Casal succinctly put it)[40] in guaranteeing political equality (let alone equality in all other aspects of social life).

Nowhere is this more apparent than in the case of health. As the epidemiological literature on "the social determinants of health" reveals, one's health is affected, not only by the absolute level of the resources available to one, but also by its relative value.[41] Whichever variable explains the link between inequality and low health—whether it be stress,[42] low status,[43] or lack of cohesion[44]—the implications are that a concern with health compels us to flatten inequalities in the goods that determine it, and to not be content with some level of sufficiency. Thus, a concern for equal health-related democratic capabilities compels us to aim at an *equal* distribution of those goods that affect our health, and is therefore not satisfied with allowing inequalities above some level of sufficiency. Moreover, the implications of pursuing a sufficientarian distribution, as recommended by DE, would be, when it comes to health, not only unjust, but also bad, and bad for everyone. That is, satisfying only some level of sufficiency is liable to make everyone worse off, healthwise, than they otherwise could be. Consider the following. We know that in societies that display unequal distribution of socioeconomic status, even those who are better off are worse off health-wise than they themselves could have been had society been more egalitarian. In other words, we now know that inequality itself is bad for our health. And crucially, inequality is bad for *everyone's* health. The well-off members of society in the nonegalitarian yet affluent United States are worse off (health-wise) than their comparable class in equally affluent yet far more egalitarian Scandinavia.[45] Allowing inequalities beyond some level of sufficiency may therefore be detrimental to everyone's health. Thus, any attempt to guarantee a just distribution of health would have to be based on attending to socio-economic inequality itself, not to guaranteeing some level of sufficiency.

There is another problem entailed in trying to stipulate some level of sufficient well-being that would allow individuals to participate in politics and civil society on equal terms. Presumably, the thought is that below some level of subsistence, say if one is homeless, illiterate, or ill, one cannot be an effective participant in politics and civil society. But consider the following dilemma. Suppose that due to scarce resources we can assist only one of two patients who are below the minimal level required for effective participation. The treatment will be equally effective and will bring about exactly the same amount (in absolute terms) of improvement for both patients. Furthermore, both patients would enjoy an improved quality of life and, moreover, of life that is worth living. However, since one of them is worse off health-wise, the treatment will fall short of tipping him over the sufficiency threshold, which it would for the other, better-off patient. DE, which seeks to be effective in guaranteeing to as many people as possible the chance to be fully participating members of society, is thus compelled to recommend assisting the better-off patient first. However, this is counterintuitive from both egalitarian and commonsense perspectives. (This is known as the "threshold fetishism" of sufficientarianism.)[46] It appears then that the sufficientarian element of DE leads it here to anti-egalitarian and counterintuitive consequences.

Here is a third drawback of DE. Like any other capability-based theory, DE is concerned only with the level of the said capabilities. It is indifferent to the potential unequal *costs* for different people of operating these capabilities. The classic example here is that of pain.[47] Jack and Jill may have a certain equal capability, but Jill may incur greater pain in exercising the capability in question (going up a hill, say). Consider DE's stipulation that people should have equal access to the polling booth (or to the concert hall, say, when access to civil society is concerned). DE is satisfied, then, if both Jack and Jill have the capability to walk to the polling booth. DE is, however, blind to the fact that Jill's journey is more arduous and painful than Jack's. If there were an expensive medicine that could alleviate the pain Jill incurs while walking, a democratic egalitarian state would not subsidize it (except when that pain is debilitating). Surely, this does not seem just. Notice, in contrast, how a luck egalitarian account avoids that counterintuitive result. The luck egalitarian view is not premised on providing this or that capability or opportunity. Rather, it holds that any disadvantaging medical condition that is owed to bad brute luck ought to be treated. Jill's pain is clearly a medical condition,[48] it is clearly a disadvantage, and thus in cases where it is a matter of bad brute luck, luck egalitarian justice would require treating it.

A fourth objection to democratic egalitarian health care is that it would not cover medical conditions that neither enable political and civil participation nor eliminate oppressive relationships. A case in point would be the ability to procreate. To be sure, infertility *can be* the cause of oppressive personal relationships, but in cases where it is not, democratic equality is under no obligation to provide fertility treatments. According to democratic egalitarians, the bad luck of being born infertile (or the bad luck of having an infertile partner) is no cause for justice-based treatment or compensation. That, again, seems counterintuitive.[49] Contrast this, again, with the way in which a luck egalitarian view of health care would approach the issue. Admittedly, it is debatable whether or not infertility is a departure from full *health*, but it *is* nevertheless a clear departure from the normal functioning of the human species (and so, Daniels's account, notice, is not vulnerable to this particular objection[50]). It is also a condition that often makes a person's life worse than it otherwise could have been. Thus, when infertility is the result of bad brute luck, luck egalitarian justice would recommend covering its treatment.

My fifth and final critical point of democratic egalitarian health care is that it is contingent on there being a democratic regime in place.[51] If, in a given society, democracy were to be suspended, citizens would lose their entitlement to health care (among other things).[52] This does not seem right. Equally wrong is the case of citizens who declare no interest in participating in the democratic process. Democratic egalitarians are compelled to deny such people the entitlement to health care, which again seems counterintuitive.[53]

Democratic egalitarians may in response say that part of what democratic egalitarian justice *stipulates* is democracy itself. Part of what constitutes a just society is having a democratic regime and democratic institutions. Furthermore, according to democratic egalitarians such as Anderson and Scheffler, democracy is not only intrinsically the most just political regime, but it is also the best guarantee against oppression, and the regime under which individuals are most likely to stand to each other as equals. Democracy, therefore, is not a contingent element of the democratic egalitarian theory. But notice that the fact that democracy itself is not contingent to DE does not deny that *egalitarian distributive justice*, as recommended by DE, *is* contingent on democracy. DE recommends distributive measures only insofar as these measures facilitate equal capability to participate in a democratic society. If democracy itself is absent, unjustly no doubt, distributive measures would then still become redundant.

To see why what I have just said is a weakness for a theory of distributive justice, imagine a society where democracy has been suspended. Imagine (although I concede that it might require some stretch of the imagination) a society that is just, except for the fact that, for some reason, free discussion, along with elections and all such manner of democratic participation, has been suspended. Suppose also that the society in question is ruled by an enlightened dictator for a fixed period of four years, say, until the restoration of civil peace and stability. (Think of something like the Union under Abraham Lincoln during the American Civil War, although this is in many ways not quite the case [if only for the fact that Lincoln insisted on the unprecedented move of running an election in the midst of a civil war].) Under those circumstances, the suspension of democracy is undeniably a violation of DE. Yet my concern is with the status of all other requirements of distributive justice, requirements that under this nonideal situation become redundant. Surely, that cannot be right. Or think of another nonideal situation, requiring less by way of imagination perhaps, where convicted criminals are barred for life from participation in politics.[54] In all these examples, standing "equal before others in discussion" is, willy-nilly, no longer feasible. The same is true for the "obligation to listen respectfully and respond to one's arguments,"[55] which no longer seems to matter. It seems odd, in these undoubtedly unjust cases, that the remainder requirements of distributive justice should also cease to obtain.[56]

The point is equally true if we consider equality of status rather than equality in democratic capabilities as the source of justice-based claims. This would require more, by way of imagination, but imagine a society based on a caste system that seeks to be just in all matters but those of social status. If social equality is no longer a goal, as in such a society, then out goes with it an egalitarian distribution of health care. But surely that is wrong. Grounding distributive justice in equal social status therefore also appears to be misguided.[57] Of course, distributive measures would still be required here if it were the case that providing egalitarian health care (or some health care) goes some way toward reducing the inequality in status or in compensating for the absence of democratic rights. That, as a matter of fact, may actually turn out to be the case. But at the same time it is not obvious that this is true also as a matter of principle. Provision of some health care *may* make one feel a more equal member of society, but it may as well not. For example, medical treatment, and even *entitlement* to medical treatment, does not make foreign students, guest workers, and tourists into full members of society (more on this point in chapter 5).[58]

Here is another possible response democratic egalitarians may have to my fifth objection. They may say that distributive measures are still justified even when democracy is suspended, since justice tells us to maintain individuals' democratic capabilities in anticipation of the restoration of democracy. The same can be said about the entitlement of those who declare no wish to participate in politics. Democratic equality may still require that such individuals be cared for medically as part of the package of resources that ought to be provided in order to maintain their capability for participation, should they change their mind. A first thing to note in reply is that that defense would have to rely on there being a real chance of democracy ever coming back or of a chance to participate in the future, which is a problematic assumption, at least in the said case of convicted criminals. Secondly, the counter-objection confuses the following. Suppose that capability X is required for citizens to be equally capable to practice democracy. It still does not follow that in the absence of democracy capability X needs to be *maintained*, and moreover maintained equally. For example, gagging one segment of the population and restricting its freedom of expression for five years, say, is certainly bad for democracy. But crucially, doing so is not necessarily detrimental to these individuals' capacity for democratic participation. It may actually be the case that during those five years of oppression the democratic urge and energies of these individuals are boosted by the sense of injustice perpetrated against them.

A concern for maintaining democratic capabilities during the absence of democracy does not readily lend itself to an entitlement to health care during that time. Thirdly, even allowing the need to maintain certain functionings in anticipation of the return of democracy, or for a potential change of mind regarding one's willingness to participate, the suggestion is still problematic. Think again of the example of physical mobility. Suppose that right now Jack needs a wheelchair in order to move about. And suppose that because of a current shortage, it will be cheaper to supply it to him in five years' time, coinciding with the time democracy is scheduled to be reinstated. In short, it would be cheaper to supply it then, rather than go into the trouble of providing it to him right now. The anticipation of the return of democracy does not give us a reason to supply Jack with the wheelchair today. DE is consistent with his being immobile for the entire period during which democracy is suspended.

I therefore conclude that DE cannot provide a plausible account of justice in health care. Note that I have only rejected democratic egalitarians' view that citizenship in a democratic society is the basis of just health care (and distributive justice more generally). I did not deny the significance of democratic capabilities and of equality of status altogether. These may have both intrinsic and instrumental values. As such, democratic capabilities and equality of status may serve as sources of many distributive claims and obligations. In that respect I find David Miller's position on this matter to be more plausible than Anderson's (and Scheffler's). Like the latter, Miller takes equality of status to be a source of distributive claims. But unlike them, he takes these claims to be independent of distributive justice, and in any case not the basis of distributive justice.[59] It seems to me that the flaw in democratic egalitarians' (such as Anderson and Scheffler) theory is that they conceive of egalitarian distributive justice simply as "the distributive implications of taking equal citizenship seriously."[60] Instead, we ought to think of that relationship in precisely the other way around. Providing the material resources needed for equal democratic citizenship is required by distributive justice, but it is only part of what it means to take individuals' equal moral worth seriously.[61]

This concludes my examination of the ability of a theory of justice founded on providing equal democratic capabilities to provide an account of justice in health care. Although we should certainly be concerned with equal status and equal access to politics and civil society, such concerns cannot ground egalitarian justice in general and justice in health care in particular.

Conclusion

Standard accounts of justice in health care eschew considerations of personal responsibility. As such they overcome a major obstacle to justifying universal health care, namely that of denying treatment to imprudent patients, to which luck egalitarianism is (as of yet) susceptible. Yet, these standard accounts of just health care, Daniels's fair opportunity account and Anderson's democratic equality account, face their own serious shortcomings and inadequacies. The fair opportunity account, I have argued, cannot justify medical treatment to individuals who have completed their life plans, namely the elderly. The democratic equality account, in turn, proved critically flawed on various scores. Among other things, its contingent reliance on democratic capabilities does not seem to sit well with our intuition that health care is a matter of distributive justice no matter how it affects our ability to participate in politics and in civil society.

3

■

Ultra-Responsibility-Sensitive Health Care

"All-Luck Egalitarianism"

Introduction

In the preceding chapter we reviewed two accounts of justice in health care. The first was premised on ensuring equal opportunity for individuals to pursue their life plans, whereas the second was based on guaranteeing to citizens the capabilities to participate as equals in a democratic society. Both theories, we saw, cope well with the dilemma of providing treatment to irresponsible patients. The former seeks an equal starting point in the pursuit of life plans, regardless of considerations of personal responsibility. The latter seeks to guarantee equal capability to participate as citizens, again, in disregard to the patient's prior conduct. Despite their ability to escape the abandonment dilemma, we saw, these theories fail on other, more fundamental grounds.

If luck egalitarians are to do better than these Rawlsian theories in providing an account of justice in health care they would first have to overcome the abandonment objection. There is a relatively recent, radical variant of luck egalitarianism that is purportedly successful in doing so. I shall try and demonstrate in this chapter why, despite my overall sympathy with luck egalitarianism, I find this particular version of it untenable. Then, in the next chapter, I shall begin reviewing more standard luck egalitarian responses to the abandonment objection and locate my own favored account somewhere among those. To put this differently, if the previous chapter dealt with responsibility-insensitive accounts of justice, the account under examination here is ultra-responsibility-sensitive, as we shall see. My favored account, to be developed in the next chapter, is again located somewhere in between.

The said version of luck egalitarianism that allegedly does not abandon irresponsible patients is what I term here "all-luck egalitarianism" (I will shortly explain that term). Several philosophers (whom I group under that term) have recently suggested a way through which responsibility-sensitive egalitarianism can provide universal health care, without succumbing to the abandonment objection. According to this radical variant of luck egalitarianism, egalitarian justice requires pooling the costs of medical treatment among those who make similar gambles with their health. An example we could use to illustrate this is smoking and smoking-related diseases (but we could equally think of reckless driving, say). According to this proposal we should pool the costs of smoking-related diseases between lucky smokers (ones who did not contract those illnesses) and unlucky ones (ones who did). The revenue collected from such a tax would be used for treating the unlucky smokers. If all-luck egalitarians are correct, their proposal would succeed in providing a responsibility-sensitive account that at the same time avoids abandoning imprudent patients to their dire fates. As such, this account would be superior to the standard luck egalitarian account, which is arguably vulnerable to that objection.

In this chapter I would like to examine this all-luck egalitarian proposal, point out its merits, but ultimately argue that it is faulty in ways that make the standard luck egalitarian view superior. In the first section I present the all-luck egalitarian ideal of justice, and outline the virtues of the account of universal health care that it supports. Section II then offers some preliminary difficulties inherent in the all-luck egalitarian view. Section III then explains more specifically what is problematic in the ideal of neutralizing luck as such, and why that ideal does not necessarily justify treatment to unlucky smokers (and imprudent patients more generally). Finally, section IV speculates on how all-luck egalitarians got things wrong, and where they part ways with standard luck egalitarianism. Having rejected all-luck egalitarianism and its ability to meet the abandonment objection, I conclude that luck egalitarians still lack an adequate response to the abandonment objection.

I. A Test Case: Justifying Medical Treatment for Smoking-Related Diseases

In order, first, to understand the attraction of the view under consideration here it is useful to see how it overcomes the abandonment dilemma. We said that luck egalitarians struggle to justify funding treatment for reckless patients. According to luck egalitarianism, we said, justice requires neutralizing the effects of bad luck on individuals' lives, but doing so only when the individual in question has not tempted luck, as it were. This bad brute luck is distinguished from bad option luck, which is, as we said, the bad luck that may ensue as a consequence of conscious and voluntary risk-taking or gamble. The abandonment objection says that luck egalitarianism may lead to harsh and arguably counterintuitive consequences, namely with regard to those suffering bad option luck. Crucially, luck egalitarianism does not require society to provide medical treatment to individuals who are responsible for their own medical condition (say through an unhealthy lifestyle). These patients, say smokers, have suffered bad option luck, and thus do not deserve compensation or treatment. Furthermore, luck egalitarians must say that if society *does* extend medical treatment to smokers, it can *only* do so at the price of unfairness toward nonsmokers. Nonsmokers who are asked to subsidize the effects of smoking are being exploited by smokers, who could have avoided smoking but didn't. Alternatively, if luck egalitarians seek to avoid this harshness objection by *forcing* smokers to take out special insurance (medical and otherwise) or to pay taxes on cigarettes, they then run the risk of paternalism (something many liberals find objectionable).[1]

The proposal under consideration here approaches the dilemma of treatment for reckless patients differently. At the core of it is a new and radical interpretation of the egalitarian ideal. According to this relatively new reading, since luck is morally arbitrary, differential option luck should be considered as unjust as differential brute luck. This relatively recent interpretation has been put forward by, among others, Michael Otsuka, Kasper Lippert-Rasmussen, Thomas Christiano, Marc Fleurbaey, Bertil Tungodden, Alexander Cappelen, Ole Norheim, and Nicholas Barry.[2] I should say that while all these philosophers see differential option luck as morally arbitrary, not all of them are committed to the view that inequalities that are owed to differential option luck ought to be neutralized. I think it would be correct to say that at least the last five mentioned are; according to the latter, justice requires neutralizing all differential luck, whether brute or option. That is why I suggested terming that position as "all-luck egalitarianism." Standard luck egalitarians (to whom all-luck egalitarians sometimes refer as "brute-luck egalitarians"), by contrast, are committed only to neutralizing inequalities that are owed to differential brute luck.

All-luck egalitarianism (henceforth ALE) has an obvious appeal for philosophers who prefer their egalitarianism to be on the responsibility-catering side. For, to eliminate the effects of luck, good or bad, brute or option, from people's lives is, effectively, to hold them responsible for the choices they make, not for the lucky or unlucky consequences of their choices. People who smoke the same number of cigarettes for the same period of time may have been born with a different genetic propensity to contract a smoking-related illness (say, lung cancer or a cardiovascular disease). Thus, what distinguishes their radically different fates is merely luck,[3] and luck, we all agree, is morally arbitrary. To neutralize luck is to hold all smokers equally responsible for their decision to smoke. One way of doing so is to impose taxes on cigarettes, the revenue of which can fund treatment of smoking-related diseases.[4] Taxes on cigarettes thus mitigate the effects of luck on determining which smokers get sick and which don't. (They do so, obviously, not by redistributing the illness but by redistributing well-being more generally.) The same argument can, of course, be applied to other cases, such as that of reckless drivers. Suppose two equally reckless drivers, one of whom ends up smashing into a tree, injuring herself and her passenger, while the other equally reckless driver somehow ends his joyride safely. What distinguishes their radically different fates is merely luck. On the all-luck egalitarian suggestion, speeding tickets are a way to make the lucky reckless driver foot part of the bill for treating both the unlucky reckless driver and her passenger.

This is an attractive argument. Notice how all-luck egalitarians appear to avoid the harshness objection, to which standard luck egalitarianism is susceptible. According to ALE, individuals suffering bad option luck need *not* be abandoned. Rather, they ought to be helped by those enjoying good option luck. In our test case of smoking, this means that unlucky smokers ought to be helped by unaffected (i.e., lucky) smokers. Notice, secondly, that the all-luck egalitarian proposal sidesteps the harshness objection *without* recourse to exploiting nonsmokers. The proposal is to fund medical treatment of, say, cancer patients who smoked through taxing *other smokers*, not through taxing the general population, which is made also (or even mostly) of nonsmokers. The third attractive feature of the all-luck egalitarian argument is that it also seems to avoid the charge of paternalism. Taxes on cigarettes are not intended here as deterrence against (or punishment for) smoking. In imposing taxes on cigarettes, the state is not presuming to tell smokers how to lead their lives. Rather, in so doing the state merely pursues the requirements of justice (between lucky and unlucky smokers). Thus, the policy is justified, arguably, on grounds of fairness, not paternalism.

This is, as I already conceded, an attractive proposal. I said in my introductory chapter that responsibility-catering egalitarians have long struggled to justify medical treatment to imprudent patients. Now all-luck egalitarians seem to have found an innovative solution. However, as I shall attempt to demonstrate, their proposal encounters several crucial difficulties and ultimately proves unsuccessful.

II. Some Preliminary Problems with All-Luck Egalitarianism

The first thing to note is that although ALE copes with the harshness objection better than standard ("brute") luck egalitarianism does, it still does not escape it fully. I said that the all-luck egalitarian view avoids the harshness objection by pooling risks between equally reckless patients, such as lucky smokers and unlucky smokers. But what if it so happens that in a given society, and over a given time span, all (or even most) smokers turn out to be unlucky (i.e., fall ill)? In that case there will be no (or not enough) lucky smokers whom we could call upon in order to help those unlucky ones. It is therefore the case that all-luck egalitarians' ability to solve the harshness problem is contingent on a more or less equal distribution of good and bad luck among all smokers in society. But that would surely not always be the case.

There are other, more fundamental problems with ALE in general, and with its ability to avoid the abandonment of imprudent patients in particular. The main problem stems from the all-luck egalitarian interpretation of the egalitarian ideal as requiring that "individuals who make the same choices should also have the same outcomes."[5] Here is an initial, relatively minor, problem with that formulation of the egalitarian ideal. The principle that says that "individuals who make the same choices should also have the same outcomes" is satisfied in the following scenario. Suppose A and B smoke ten cigarettes a day, and C and D smoke twenty cigarettes a day. The all-luck egalitarian principle as stated requires that A and B end up with the same outcome, and also, that C end up with the same outcome as D. The principle, however, is silent on whether A and B taken together should have an outcome that is *better* than (or, even as good as) that visited on C and D. In fact, the principle is satisfied with C and D (those who smoked more) ending up with better health than A and B! It follows that, in order to give it a sympathetic reading, we ought to reformulate the all-luck egalitarian ideal. The reformulated principle ought to say something like: "It is unfair for one individual to end up worse off than another if she has made at least as prudent decisions as that other person." (We shall revisit this formulation in chapter 7.) This reformulation would avoid the conclusion that it is just, on the all-luck egalitarian view, for those who smoke less to end up with worse health than those who smoke more.

Here, however, is a substantial problem with the all-luck egalitarian policy of aiding unlucky smokers (and other imprudent patients). A principle of justice that seeks to *match outcomes to choices* would justify much more than (the arguably attractive policy of) taxes on cigarettes. It would require, for example, ensuring that those who make identical casino gambles would end up reaping the same spoils. This could be done by pooling all identical bets between all gamblers. Of course, one problem with doing so is that it would seem to defeat the whole purpose of gambling. If you buy a $5 lottery ticket (or casino chip), say, and end up, as a consequence of risk pooling, with a 100 percent chance of winning a reward of, well, $5, then there is not much "gambling" going on here. Yet, this is precisely what ALE would require us to do. On that score, the all-luck egalitarian principle seems mistaken, because it does not normally strike us as *unfair* that some gamblers get higher prizes than other gamblers.[6]

It may be suggested, in response, that there is an important difference between what Lippert-Rasmussen calls "gambling proper" and gambling with

your health, which may fall under what he calls "quasi-gambling." The difference between the two is that the thrill of gambling is intrinsic to the former
but not to the latter.[7] Arguably, it is right to expect gamblers proper to bear
the cost of their bad luck alone, whereas it would be wrong to do so in the
case of quasi-gambling, such as gambling with one's health. One thing to note
here is that though there is something intuitively correct in the distinction
Lippert-Rasmussen makes, it is at the same time not one that is as clear-cut as
it may initially seem. It is certainly true that it would be wrong to characterize
all imprudent patients as gamblers proper. Most people probably "gamble"
with their health, so to speak, not for the thrill of gambling but for reasons of
oversight, laziness, and weakness of will. And yet, it is possible to think of
examples where people behave recklessly with regard to their own health for
the thrill of gambling. Think of those pursuing various types of "extreme"
sports, or of (typically) young people smoking precisely because it is bad for
them (even though they might not like the smell and taste of tobacco at all).
And, on the other hand, many of what Lippert-Rasmussen calls "proper gamblers" do so not, or not just, for the thrill of gambling but for the (perhaps
false) prospect of winning. Surely it is true for many casino gamblers that the
higher the (perceived) prospects of winning, the greater the incentive to gamble. Arguably, then, the incentive to gamble in such cases actually intensifies
the less risky the gamble is. That would seem to suggest that for many casino
gamblers the thrill of the risk is marginal if not actually antithetical to their
decision to gamble.[8] Lippert-Rasmussen's (otherwise) fine distinction cannot, then, prevent ALE from compensating (at least some) casino gamblers
for their losses. That seems to me counterintuitive.

Alternatively, perhaps what Lippert-Rasmussen's distinction drives at is a
point about legitimate expectations. It is reasonable to expect casino gamblers to shoulder their own losses. No blackjack loser can complain that her
legitimate expectations have been frustrated if she fails to be reimbursed by
state officials upon checking out of her Las Vegas hotel. But the same cannot
be true, one might say, for quasi-gamblers; say, people who gamble with their
health. But if that is so, I would argue, it is so for contingent reasons. It simply
happens to be the case in certain societies that individuals are not yet aware
that gambling with one's health is like gambling proper in the sense that it
denies one a legitimate expectation for a justice-based compensation. The
fact that not all members of society currently adhere to the luck egalitarian
credo is simply an (unfortunate?) accident of history. There does not therefore seem to be a justice-based reason to treat the two cases of gambling differently. A related idea that might be driving Lippert-Rasmussen's point is
that it would be absurd for someone who has chosen to gamble for the very
thrill of risking a loss to then approach society (or other, successful, gam-

blers) for compensation in the occasion that the risk materialized. It is very much a chutzpah to ask for compensation for a loss the thrill of which you courted. Now, admittedly it is somewhat less presumptuous to ask for compensation for losing a "quasi-gamble," i.e., a gamble to which the risk is not intrinsic. But even though somewhat less so, it still seems inappropriate for the gambler to do so. If that quasi-gamble was genuinely something the person could reasonably have avoided (which is how I suggested, in chapter 1, we understand "brute luck"), it seems wrong that society or other (lucky) quasi-gamblers would owe her compensation when the gamble goes sour.[9]

One final reason I could think of why someone like Lippert-Rasmussen might think that it is right to compensate for quasi-gambles is that it is in society's interest that people take such gambles. Some prudent business ventures or career choices involve a gamble. That gamble is typically a quasi-gamble, that is, one that is taken not for the sake of risk but in spite of it. It is socially desirable, for all sorts of reasons, that people take such gambles. Thus, it is right to compensate individuals for losses when such risks materialize. Consider the example offered in this context by Lippert-Rasmussen.[10] Suppose Ned and Oliver have two courses of action open to them: (A) 100% chance of receiving 100, or (B) 95% chance of receiving 100, and 5% chance of receiving 200. It would not only be unreasonable, but actually irrational, for anyone *not* to gamble in this case (i.e., opt for B). Suppose, then, that both individuals gamble and Ned ends up with 200 and Oliver with 100. It seems to me that in that case justice requires taxing Ned (lucky), and splitting his earnings with Oliver (unlucky). But notice that it is possible to say that on that occasion, Oliver actually suffered bad *brute* luck, not bad option luck. For Oliver could not have reasonably been expected to act otherwise. Thus, he acted prudently, and it is generally agreed that any resulting bad luck from action that is prudent ought to be considered as bad brute luck.[11] The case of Ned and Oliver does not, then, lend support to leveling *option* luck inequalities. Accordingly, we see, the relevant distinction is not one between gambles proper and quasi-gambles, but one between risks that it would be reasonable to expect one to avoid, and ones where it would be unreasonable to expect one to do so.

III. What's Wrong with Neutralizing Luck as Such?

Let me now move to my main worry about the ability of ALE to meet the abandonment objection. Here, again, is the position under examination. What justice effectively requires, according to ALE, is that there ought not to be a shortfall in well-being between individuals who exercise an identical level of prudence (or imprudence). So think again of our two smokers who have smoked an identical number of cigarettes for an identical number of years. Let us also assume that the two smokers are identical in all other relevant features, such as that it is equally easy (or difficult) for them to quit smoking. Suppose one of them contracts a smoking-related disease while the other one does not. The difference in outcome is merely a matter of luck, and luck, so all-luck egalitarians tell us, ought to be neutralized.

Notice first that imposing taxes on cigarettes is not the only way to pursue justice between these smokers. Instead of pooling the burden of smoking-related expenses ex-ante it is equally just, following all-luck egalitarians, to do so ex-post. Admittedly, doing so would be less practical than ex-ante taxation. But crucially, it is equally justified to tax lucky smokers at a certain point in the future, once it has been revealed who turned out to be the lucky smokers and who were not so lucky. Ex-post taxation would, then, equally rectify the alleged injustice involved in two smokers exercising an identical level of prudence yet ending up with such radically different fates.

The all-luck egalitarian ideal therefore does not necessarily require ex-ante pooling of risks. But, moreover, on a closer look it does not necessarily require *any* pooling of risks. To see this, consider again the case of the lucky and unlucky smokers. Why precisely is it unjust for two individuals who make the same gamble with their health to end up with unequal levels of well-being? Is the problem really that they have such unequal fates while exercising an identical amount of recklessness? If that were indeed the case, neutralizing luck, and thus equalizing their fate, could then be carried out *by making the healthy smoker sick*. In other words, to equalize the respective fates of the two smokers does not require pooling risks between them, but can also be carried out by (and thus justify) causing the healthy smoker to be affected by lung cancer, say through radiation (supposing that this was medically possible). This form of leveling down is one way of neutralizing the effects of luck, good or bad, from determining the smokers' *unequal* fates. If we take ALE to its logical conclusion, making the lucky smoker as unhealthy as the unlucky smoker would be an equally just course of action as that of providing medical treatment to the unlucky one. But that surely does not seem right.

Notice that the implications of ALE do not seem right even when something other than health is leveled down. Consider this. It is equally just, according to ALE, to leave the unlucky smoker to her dire fate while at the same time simply stripping the lucky smoker of her good fortune, say by requiring her to burn some of her money, or give it to charity. Doing so would be wasteful or inefficient perhaps, but crucially, it would comply with the requirement of equalizing the fates of the lucky and unlucky. ALE understood as leveling differential-option-luck-inequalities can thus be achieved not only through pooling luck, but also through leveling down. Notice, furthermore, that ALE can also be satisfied through leveling *up*. Making sure that equally reckless conduct would yield an equal level of well-being can be attained by raising the welfare of the unlucky smoker to that of the lucky smoker (if not by curing her sickness then at least by compensating her financially). This, again, is consistent with the ideal of ALE understood as leveling differential-luck-inequalities.

ALE can be met, then, not only by pooling luck between lucky and unlucky smokers, but also by leveling their respective welfare down or up. If that is the case, lucky smokers may have a valid complaint against the state if it opts for the pooling strategy. The reason is this. We said that ALE does not *require* pooling luck between lucky and unlucky smokers, but only *permits* doing so. The lucky smoker may thus point out that ALE also permits another course of action, and one that serves her better, namely the option of leveling up. Suppose then that out of the three courses of action made permissible (but none of which made mandatory) by ALE (pooling, leveling down, and leveling up), society opts for the one that is not optimal for the lucky smoker (not to mention the unlucky smoker). In that case, the lucky smoker may have legitimate grounds for complaint against the state. Since pooling luck is only permissible but not required, and since other options are available, it would be wrong to harm the lucky smoker. After all, she may say, it is not her fault that Unlucky Smoker got sick. It follows that ALE does not justify pooling luck, even in the cases where it initially looks attractive to do so.

To sum up the point, the all-luck egalitarian principle is satisfied by worsening the health (and more generally, the lot) of the lucky smoker, which is surely unacceptable. Notice that standard luck egalitarianism is not vulnerable to leveling down in this particular case. Since standard luck egalitarianism advocates leveling only brute luck inequalities, it is therefore not concerned with equalizing the fates of the lucky and unlucky smokers. Thus, it avoids (at least) this form of leveling down. (I shall have more to say on the general case of luck egalitarian leveling down in chapter 8.)

All-luck egalitarians could potentially avoid the problem just encountered by revising their principle in the following way. They may say that the object of egalitarian justice is not to neutralize luck as such,[12] but rather to neutralize only *bad* luck. (Notice that that revised position would still deviate from standard luck egalitarianism, which seeks to compensate only for bad *brute* luck rather than for all instances of bad luck as such.) That principle of justice requires improving the lot of the ill smoker, while *not* recommending inflicting the lucky smoker with lung cancer (or burning away some of her money).

However, adopting that interpretation would generate other problems that the original all-luck egalitarian principle initially sought to avoid. Namely reformulating the all-luck egalitarian ideal in the abovementioned way cannot justify taxes on cigarettes, and for obvious reasons. Neutralizing *bad* luck alone does not imply pooling the effects of luck between lucky smokers and unlucky smokers. It simply implies eradicating the effects of bad luck from the lives of unlucky smokers. It does not specify, nor justify, eradicating the effects that good luck has on the lives of lucky ones. As such, the revised principle does not justify pooling risks between lucky and unlucky smokers. So the revised principle at best justifies treating unlucky smokers, but without specifying that other smokers, as distinct from society as a whole, should help pay for their treatment.

IV. All-Luck Egalitarianism, Moral Luck, and Desert

ALE may have another attraction up its sleeve: it could be seen as a counterargument to the thesis of moral luck. The thesis of moral luck says that there is a genuine moral difference between being guilty of murder and being guilty of attempted murder. Such a moral difference, if it indeed exists, would help justify the difference in punishment in the two cases, something most people find intuitive, both in practice and in principle. But, interestingly, the claim about moral luck looks less convincing in tort cases. Recall our earlier example of the two equally reckless drivers, one ending up injuring herself and a passenger, the other managing to avoid crashing despite very reckless driving. What differentiates the radically different fates of the two reckless drivers is pure luck. All-luck egalitarians would have us make the lucky reckless driver contribute toward treating the unlucky driver, and also toward compensating the passenger. But why exactly would that be just? What grounds does the unlucky reckless driver have for a claim *against the lucky reckless driver*? I can see none. I also do not see grounds for a claim that the unlucky driver may have *against society*, asking it to mitigate her personal bad (option) luck by redistributing the burden of the accident with the lucky driver. The unlucky driver may plausibly say that it is unfair that while she acted exactly in the same way as the lucky driver she ended up so much worse off. But society may plausibly retort that the undesirable fate she endures was something she could have foreseen and something that it would have been reasonable for her to avoid. Thus, she has forfeited any claim against society or against other drivers (whether reckless or not). So while I disagree with the common approach to moral luck (by such philosophers as Bernard Williams and Thomas Nagel) according to which there is some moral difference between lucky and unlucky drivers,[13] I also disagree with its critics who say that the absence of such moral difference requires equalizing their fates.[14] When individuals drive in a reckless way that they could reasonably have avoided, they then forfeit any claim for compensation both from society and from fellow reckless drivers. We might have forward-looking reasons for taxing or penalizing *all* reckless drivers, but we do not have, I have argued, backward-looking considerations of fairness for doing so.

Now, some may be troubled by the conclusion that egalitarian distributive justice on my reading has nothing to say about the resulting very significant inequality between the lucky and unlucky reckless drivers. If nothing else, it ought to bother us that the unlucky reckless driver should face such a dim prospect as a consequence of a momentary lapse of judgment. To quote Arneson: "His 'punishment'—the quality of life he gets after the accident—does not fit his 'crime'—the brief lapses of judgment."[15] Indeed it does not. And were we concerned with matching levels of well-being to levels of personal desert, such an outcome would have been troubling. But whether or not desert is an attractive idea, LE, I said in chapter 1, is concerned with a narrower slice of morality. It seeks only to account for *egalitarian* distributive justice. Fitting "punishments" to "crimes" (or rewards to merit) does not fall under that purview. As such, the fate of the unlucky reckless driver may be troubling for all sorts of reasons, but not for ones of egalitarian distributive justice.[16]

If it is *not* right to target lucky smokers and require them to foot the bill for the medical costs of unlucky smokers, then who should? Should this burden fall to unlucky smokers alone? That, we said, might be harsh. Should the burden fall, instead, on society as a whole? That, we also said, seems unfair toward nonsmokers. We are back, therefore, at the dilemma with which we started, namely, how to justify not abandoning imprudent patients.

All-luck egalitarians, it turns out, cannot avoid the abandonment problem without generating other counterintuitive outcomes (such as leveling down, health or otherwise). In anticipation of the next chapter, let me briefly inquire into where all-luck egalitarians part ways with standard luck egalitarianism, and why consequently they get things wrong. Contrary to ALE, standard luck egalitarians are not committed to neutralizing the effects of luck as such (which, as we just saw, would in any case make little sense). Nor are luck egalitarians committed to neutralizing the effects of bad luck as such. They are committed, rather, to compensating individuals for disadvantages for which they are not responsible (that is, could not have reasonably avoided). Despite ALE, then, it is not the case that luck egalitarians advocate compensation for bad *option* luck. Option luck follows, by definition, from risks that are taken voluntarily. A person who suffers bad option luck is, we could say, "in the business" of risk-taking. It is the consequence of that type of business that she may reasonably be expected to bear. Luck is indeed arbitrary, as all-luck egalitarians rightly point out, but *tempting* luck, as it were, is not. And what we owe each other (as a matter of distributive justice), according to standard luck egalitarians, extends to neutralizing luck only in the cases where it has not been tempted.

Admittedly, my response to the all-luck egalitarians' argument illustrates, perhaps, that the term *luck egalitarianism* may be somewhat misleading. (It is worth recalling that although most luck egalitarians have come to endorse the label, the term "luck egalitarianism" was first coined by a critic, namely Elizabeth Anderson.)[17] Furthermore, some of what luck egalitarians (and Arneson in particular) say may lead others to interpret the luck egalitarian ideal in the all-luck egalitarian way. In particular, Arneson's formulation of the egalitarian ideal as requiring what he calls "equal opportunity for welfare" is especially prone to provoking such misunderstanding. Arneson writes, for example, that "Equal opportunity for welfare obtains among persons when all of them face equivalent decision trees—the expected value of each person's best (= most prudent) choice of options, second-best, ... nth-best is the same."[18] The ideal of "equal opportunity for welfare" characterized this way may be understood to require that individuals who exercise an identical amount of prudence (or imprudence) should end up having the same amount of welfare. That interpretation does, admittedly, imply equalizing the fates of the two smokers, for they have exercised an identical amount of (im)prudence. But other things Arneson says indicate that it is standard (brute) luck egalitarianism that in fact motivates him—for example, when he writes in the same place that "The argument for equal opportunity rather than straight equality is simply that it is morally fitting to hold individuals responsible for the foreseeable consequences of their voluntary choices."[19] And, in another place, Arneson explicitly notes that (in difference to ALE) his egalitarian ideal is vulnerable to (something like) the abandonment objection.[20]

Other luck egalitarians are typically clearer about their commitment to the luck egalitarian ideal in its standard interpretation (that of compensating cases of bad brute luck alone), and about rejecting ALE. Cohen in fact says that his ideal of "equal access to advantage" is preferable to Arneson's "equal opportunity for welfare" precisely because it is closer to "the right reading of egalitarianism, namely that it proposes to eliminate involuntary disadvantage, by which I (stipulatively) mean disadvantage for which the sufferer cannot be held responsible."[21] Dworkin also explicitly states that the point of equality is not to eradicate bad luck, but rather to compensate individuals for outcomes for which they cannot be held responsible. If a person starts a chain of events, whereby she takes deliberate risks (against which she chooses not to insure), then justice does not require compensating her for the bad consequences that may follow.[22] This shows that Dworkin does not subscribe to ALE.[23]

To conclude this final section: ALE differs substantially from standard luck egalitarianism. And while ALE attempts, but ultimately fails, to avoid the abandonment objection, standard luck egalitarianism remains explicitly vulnerable to it.

Conclusion

I hope to have shown that the all-luck egalitarian justification for treating imprudent patients (e.g., unlucky smokers) yields counterintuitive results. Mainly, the principle that states that "individuals who make the same choices should also have the same outcomes" would justify not only treating imprudent patients but also making healthy imprudent people (e.g., lucky smokers) sick. I have then demonstrated that a revised principle, one seeking to neutralize the effects of *bad* luck, would be problematic for a different reason. Such a principle could not justify taxation that targets imprudent individuals that are healthy (lucky smokers). My conclusion, therefore, is that all-luck egalitarianism does not succeed in justifying treatment to imprudent patients, and as such fails in providing a responsibility-sensitive account of universal health care.

4

■

Tough Luck?

Why Luck Egalitarians Need Not Abandon Reckless Patients

Introduction

Let us take stock of what has been discussed so far. I started this first part of the book by presenting the abandonment dilemma, namely, how to sustain a responsibility-sensitive account of egalitarian justice that is yet able to justify universal and unconditional (i.e., one that does not deny it from imprudent patients) medical care. We saw that the fair opportunity account and the democratic equality account, although able to justify universal care, cannot, for different reasons, provide a truly egalitarian account. All-luck egalitarianism, for its part, proved unsatisfactory for the somewhat opposite reasons (e.g., it justifies pooling casino gambles). Can (standard) luck egalitarianism escape the abandonment objection and justify universal health care? Over the next two chapters I will attempt to advance an argument to that effect. In this chapter I shall argue that luck egalitarianism is not committed to abandoning imprudent patients.[1] (In the next chapter I will say why, positively, we ought to provide treatment to such patients. In doing so I will have completed the luck egalitarian account of unconditional and universal health care.) I argue that luck egalitarianism can escape the abandonment objection if, when applied to health care policy (and social policy more generally), it is complemented with other moral considerations (including other considerations of justice), such as those of meeting basic needs.

The abovementioned abandonment objection is largely credited to Elizabeth Anderson.[2] Anderson claims that luck egalitarians are harsh on victims of option luck (such as those taking risks with their health), for they abandon such victims to their dire fates.[3] In response to Anderson, I claim that luck egalitarians can escape this objection unscathed. While I agree with her that the solution cannot be found from within luck egalitarianism, I will demonstrate that the luck egalitarian account of distributive justice does not forbid helping imprudent patients.[4] In order to do so I first look at recent luck egalitarian responses to the abandonment objection. I examine five such responses (section I). After concluding that these responses cannot, for different reasons, meet the abandonment objection fully, I go on to discuss what alternative account could meet that objection. For that purpose, I need to justify the use of what is essentially a nonegalitarian reason (to treat the imprudent) in defense of a theory that concerns egalitarian distributive justice (section II). In section III I examine and rebut three potential objections to my proposed strategy for responding to the abandonment objection (that of trading off egalitarian justice against other, nonegalitarian, considerations). In section IV I suggest that the concern for meeting basic needs is one such consideration that could complement luck egalitarianism and, as such, potentially lay to rest the abandonment objection. The concluding section returns to examine, but rebuts, the possibility that the standard I use to help luck egalitarianism provide a complete guide to health care could be applied also to its rivaling accounts (Daniels's and Anderson's).

I. Luck Egalitarian Attempts to Deflect the Abandonment Objection

How might luck egalitarians respond to the abandonment objection? Here are five such attempts.

The first luck egalitarian response I want to look at here has some affinity with the all-luck egalitarian position surveyed in the previous chapter. It is similar in the sense that it also questions the distinction between brute and option luck. This response therefore similarly questions the alleged luck egalitarian commitment to abandoning those who suffer bad option luck (e.g., unlucky smokers). However, it is somewhat less radical and so, consequently, is its conclusion. The response, as offered by Peter Vallentyne, says that in some cases, the rational thing to do, that is, the course of action that yields the highest expected utility, does involve taking some risk. To flatly deny compensation in all cases of bad option luck, regardless of the "quality" of the risk, is to discourage individuals from taking calculated risks, and is therefore inefficient and wasteful. Efficient, and thereby just (*pace* Vallentyne), institutions would therefore compensate for bad option luck (in cases where taking a gamble is the rational course of action).[5]

Vallentyne's argument cannot, however, meet the abandonment objection fully. As Vallentyne himself points out, his argument does not "eliminate" the abandonment objection, it only "softens" it, for it does not recommend compensating *all* cases of bad option luck. Specifically, he acknowledges that we should not compensate for bad option luck when taking the risk in question was irrational (that is, not the course of action yielding the highest expected utility).[6] Note also that Vallentyne's contribution is in demonstrating that it is efficient (and thereby, arguably, just) to provide incentives for risk-taking when doing so is the prudent course of action. Vallentyne does not argue, then, that luck egalitarians are committed to compensating risk-taking when to do so would be *im*prudent. It therefore seems that Vallentyne's proposal cannot be used for meeting the abandonment of the imprudent objection. It rather redefines (correctly, I think) what counts as imprudence (where some risk-taking *is* prudent, and therefore should be compensated).[7] In effect, then, Vallentyne's proposal is consistent with the criticism that depicts luck egalitarianism as abandoning the *imprudent* (rather than abandoning all victims of bad option luck), and thus cannot serve as a response to it.

Here is a second luck egalitarian response to the abandonment objection. As a response to that objection, Ronald Dworkin advocates adding a residual layer of mandatory social insurance to his famous (voluntary) hypothetical insurance, so as to cover incidents of bad option luck that lead to destitution and loss of basic capabilities. This mandatory scheme insures individuals against ending up lacking the most basic of capabilities needed to lead a decent life, regardless of the personal history that led them to require such assistance.[8] Critics such as Anderson, however, dismiss Dworkin's solution by arguing that it is paternalistic, and as such, disrespectful of those it aids.[9] Dworkin (in later writings) deflects that accusation by saying that his proposed health insurance, although compulsory, compensates incidents of bad option luck that individuals behind a veil of ignorance would most likely choose to insure against and is therefore not clearly paternalistic or badly so. Since everyone wants to avoid leading a "horribly grim" life, it follows that individuals are not averse to an insurance scheme that guarantees them basic resources such as adequate unemployment benefits and basic health care.[10] But in meeting the paternalism objection, I want to argue, Dworkin creates another, related, problem for himself.

As stated, Dworkin's mandatory insurance compels individuals to insure against becoming destitute. Deviating from ("brute") luck egalitarianism, Dworkin proposes to insure against destitution (illness, hunger, homelessness, unemployment) whether or not these eventualities are the agent's fault. So whereas luck egalitarianism consists of, in a sense, insurance against welfare deficits that are owed to reasons beyond individuals' control, Dworkin proposes supplementing that ideal with insurance against becoming destitute out of imprudence or negligence. That is to say, drivers are, according to his proposed scheme, insured not only against crashing into a tree but also, specifically, against crashing into a tree due to reckless driving. Having insured against such a scenario, citizens are thereby entitled to medical treatment (and compensation more generally) in the event of recklessness. The problem with Dworkin's response, however, is that it is in tension with the plausible idea that society may (and should) condemn imprudent behavior. If the reason we treat Jack is that he has insured against falling ill or injured, either intentionally or negligently, then what complaint can society have against Jack when payday, so to speak, arrives and medical treatment is due? Yet, we often think that, whatever treatment or compensation society does eventually extend, it still has some valid complaint (or a grudge) against Jack if his destitution was caused by his own avoidable recklessness. Society is often entitled to penalize, or at the very least frown upon, an individual such as Jack for abusing the insurance scheme through his imprudent conduct. If this is how we generally conceive of the imprudent, it cannot be the case that the justification for treating them is their antecedent contribution toward social insurance. Under Dworkin's scheme we would be denied our complaint against someone like George Best, the late footballer, who after receiving a publicly funded liver transplant was spotted having a drink. After all, he would have insured, under Dworkin's compulsory insurance scheme, precisely against the very scenario of harming his own health (indeed we compelled him to do precisely that!). Dworkin thus denies society its rightful complaint or grudge against the imprudent patient. I shall henceforth call this "the grudge objection" to Dworkin's mandatory insurance argument.[11]

The present objection need not rule against adopting Dworkin's mandatory insurance (indeed I shall recommend something akin to it in section IV). The grudge objection is not an objection to the means through which compensation for victims of option luck is to be (partly) financed, but only to the moral grounds given for our obligation to do so. In fact, it is possible for Dworkin to avoid the grudge objection (as well as the accusation of paternalism) without much difficulty. In section IV I will attempt to demonstrate exactly how he can do so. For now, we must acknowledge that if luck egalitarian health care is to avoid Anderson's abandonment objection, aiding the imprudent would have to be justified differently.

A third luck egalitarian suggestion for meeting the abandonment objection relies on pointing out that it is unfair to hold individuals responsible for the degree to which they are responsible agents to begin with. In a postscript to his canonical 1989 article, Richard Arneson suggested that people's capacity for prudence varies along with natural talent and upbringing, and therefore a modified version of luck egalitarianism should take account also of the degree to which people's imprudence is itself a matter of bad luck.[12] A somewhat similar solution is offered also by John Roemer in his famous "pragmatic theory of responsibility." Roemer proposes to identify "types" of individuals clustered around their ability to act prudently (schoolteachers are generally more prudent than steelworkers, say), identify a mean rate of prudent behavior within those types, and treat conduct that is less prudent than that mean as imprudent behavior for the purposes of distributive justice.[13] If imprudence is, to an extent, itself a matter of bad brute luck, it would follow that the imprudent should be compensated, thus avoiding the abandonment objection.

Meeting the abandonment objection, it is important to note, is perhaps not Arneson's and Roemer's main motivation in advancing the above argument. My evaluation of that particular argument's ability to meet the abandonment objection is therefore not intended as a criticism of the argument itself. What I do want to say about Arneson's and Roemer's proposal is that even though this type of modification brings luck egalitarianism closer to meeting the abandonment objection, it is unable to do so fully: Arneson and Roemer only relocate the boundary between prudence and imprudence (and hence between option luck and brute luck), rather than show that imprudence is impossible (and that all luck is brute). Had they shown that, perhaps they would have answered the problem of imprudent agents pointed out by Anderson. Arneson's and Roemer's reinterpretation still leaves a spectrum of cases of genuine option luck, and therefore does not entitle its victims to luck egalitarian compensation. Thus, the abandonment objection still stands.

A fourth potential response to the abandonment objection relies on the plausible premise that, in reality, option luck almost never occurs. Option luck understood as "a deliberate and calculated risk,"[14] taken with full information, hardly ever occurs in real life. Rather, almost all disadvantages suffered in contemporary market societies have an element of bad brute luck about them.[15] Being unemployed, for example, almost always entails a structural element that is beyond one's control. It would follow that in contemporary societies, the abandonment objection does not arise, simply because there are no pure cases of bad option luck that would be ignored by luck egalitarians. If anything, the abandonment objection is worth worrying about once we have reached an egalitarian utopia.

Let us suppose then that the abandonment objection arises only in fully egalitarian societies. Notice that even then, the objection still represents an embarrassment to luck egalitarians, whose theory is an attempt to say something of universal truth with regard to the requirements of egalitarian justice. But even setting that thought aside, it is still doubtful that this fourth response can go all the way in rescuing luck egalitarianism from the abandonment objection. Consider this. The response only concerns the moral arbitrariness of luck, and thus of the need to compensate risk takers. But the abandonment objection refers not only to cases of reckless risk-taking, but also to cases of deliberate waste and self-harm. That is to say, the broad category of option luck includes not only risk takers but also individuals who deliberately inflict disadvantages, including illnesses, upon themselves. They do so not as a result of a risk badly taken but out of a conscious decision to bear the costs of a certain course of action in order to enjoy some other advantage that that course of action may bring. Smokers, for example, are not all necessarily risk takers, as they may simply be willing to sacrifice the later years of their lives for the pleasure of smoking throughout their (shorter) lives. Here again luck appears to be irrelevant. Daniels's fair opportunity approach and Anderson's democratic equality approach would support treating patients with that kind of history, while luck egalitarians arguably are committed to abandoning them. It appears, therefore, that this luck egalitarian response does not cope well with such self-inflicted harm cases.[16] The claim that option luck hardly ever occurs cannot, then, help luck egalitarians to meet fully Anderson's abandonment objection.

The final luck egalitarian response to the abandonment objection that I shall look at invokes the requirements of *autonomy*. Since it holds that individuals should be compensated for losses for which they are not responsible, luck egalitarian justice must demand, to be consistent, that individuals be held responsible for their actions. To meet that purpose individuals must be autonomous, for surely people cannot be held responsible when lacking the autonomy to do otherwise. And, in order to safeguard such autonomy, certain threshold requirements must be satisfied (minimal healthy functioning, adequate nutrition, the social basis of minimal self-respect, etc.). Indeed, it is essential for a luck egalitarian regime to observe these threshold requirements, for, once victims of bad option luck are allowed to slip below the material prerequisites of autonomy, their subsequent choices and actions invariably fall under the brute luck category, as the agents cannot be held responsible for the resulting disadvantages. Thus, a luck egalitarian regime would have to compensate these individuals continuously, which is surely wasteful. For that reason, it is imperative that those who suffer bad option luck do not fall below the subsistence level required for autonomous conduct.

This purported luck egalitarian response to the abandonment objection is attractive. However, upon reflection this autonomy response turns out to be a *non*egalitarian consideration (and therefore it cannot constitute a luck egalitarian response). To explain: it is not a requirement of luck egalitarian justice that victims of option luck be raised to the level of autonomy. For it is not unfair to abandon them, according to this reading; it is only inefficient.[17] Since it offers a potential solution to the abandonment objection nevertheless (only not an egalitarian one), I will return to consider this response in section IV when considering nonegalitarian solutions to the abandonment objection.

It may be the case that the five responses examined here do not exhaust the array of potential luck egalitarian replies to the abandonment objection. However, if they do, and if, as I have argued, these luck egalitarian responses cannot meet the abandonment objection fully, then any attempt to rescue luck egalitarianism from that objection would have to be an external one (i.e., a non–justice-based reason). I turn to examine that suggestion now.

II. Value Pluralism

We saw that egalitarian considerations cannot help luck egalitarian justice escape the abandonment objection. In section IV I shall attempt to provide some reasons for thinking that luck egalitarians can meet the abandonment objection, and justify treatment for imprudent patients by employing reasons that are independent of distributive justice. But before I do so I need to say something about the permissibility of employing such nonegalitarian considerations[18] to meet an objection that targets luck egalitarianism's very understanding of what egalitarian justice requires.

In order to do so we need to delve into the nature of distributive justice, and more specifically remind ourselves what component of justice luck egalitarianism attempts to interpret. For egalitarians, equality, the idea that we all have the same fundamental moral worth, informs all aspects of morality.[19] Among those aspects of morality justice is a target of obvious special attention. And within justice, fairness (or distributive justice, I use the two interchangeably) is the focus of attention for luck egalitarians. Fairness is the component of justice that is (at least for egalitarians) comparative.[20] To illustrate, a society in which freedom of expression is denied is, arguably, an unjust society. But a society in which some have freedom of expression and others don't is (also) *unfair*. It is distributive justice (or fairness), then, that luck egalitarians focus their attention on.[21] Here, for luck egalitarians, equal moral worth entails that persons should not end up worse off than others due to reasons that are beyond their control.[22] Luck egalitarians, then, aspire to say something about distributive justice alone, rather than about the whole of justice, let alone morality.[23]

It is essential to observe that in designing institutions we are likely to entertain other considerations of justice besides those of fairness (as well as other moral considerations besides those of justice).[24] These considerations may include utility,[25] concern for self-respect,[26] privacy,[27] publicity,[28] autonomy,[29] compassion, promise keeping, cultural diversity, and so forth.[30] These considerations inform our thinking about political and social institutions, and may constrain the extent to which we implement our egalitarian conception of distributive justice. To illustrate, we may sometimes have reasons to allocate to an individual more than her fair share because not to do so would undermine her self-respect.[31] Further nonegalitarian reasons (for allocating to someone more than is required by fairness) include our reasons for rewarding someone for altruistic conduct (e.g., so as to create incentives to follow her example),[32] or allowing certain types of (equality-upsetting) gifts.[33] These may all constitute reasons to depart from the luck egalitarian conception of fairness, and are all considerations that political philosophers must entertain while debating the merits of any given policy (at least ones bearing on resource allocation), and health policy more so than others. Political philosophy, we may sum up, is a complex undertaking, in which we must trade off the requirements of distributive justice with other considerations of justice, and other moral considerations in general.[34]

I noted that fairness must be traded off against other moral considerations (and in particular, other considerations of justice), but there is more than one way in which that could be carried out. In some cases, other considerations may simply trump those of fairness. When that happens, we inevitably adopt policies that we know to be, to some extent, unfair. Allowing a certain measure of gift-giving, minimizing intrusion into people's privacy, and considerations of efficiency are all examples of considerations that may lead us to adopt policies that we acknowledge to be less than fair. But in some other cases, a trade-off (between fairness and other moral considerations) need not result in adopting unfair policies. That happens when considerations of fairness prove indeterminate (for one reason or another). Fairness, on that occasion, does not tell us to allocate a resource X to person Y. But considerations of fairness also do not forbid us from doing so. Allocating X to person Y in this case is *neither fair nor unfair*. And, taking into account other considerations, say those of self-respect or meeting basic needs, would tell us to pursue some specific policy where fairness itself was proven to be indeterminate. When luck egalitarians say that equality (or fairness) should be traded off against other considerations, they advocate, I believe, both of the above forms of trade-off. For the purposes of my argument, though, I need only commit to the latter, and less demanding, form of trade-off. The abandonment objection points to the sort of case, it seems to me, where luck egalitarian distributive justice is indeterminate. Here, luck egalitarianism does not recommend (that is, is silent on) policy X, but that policy, in turn, proves to be desirable for other reasons.[35] It is here that trading off luck egalitarian distributive justice with other considerations produces a determinate and desirable policy. In other words, the combination of luck egalitarianism with other considerations may tell us to provide medical treatment for the reckless driver rather than abandon her.[36]

Those who level the abandonment objection at luck egalitarians seem to ignore the complex nature of political philosophy as described here. Critics of luck egalitarianism (and especially Elizabeth Anderson) seem to burden distributive justice with instructing almost every conceivable aspect of our political morality. Anderson claims to demonstrate that "luck egalitarianism generates injustice,"[37] but in fact she shows (at best) that luck egalitarianism leads to just policies that are undesirable for other reasons. Despite Anderson, we see now, the view that luck egalitarian distributive justice does not compel us to provide treatment to reckless drivers and unlucky smokers is compatible with the view that we should nevertheless do so, due to some other moral consideration.

There is nothing peculiar in the realization that society's pursuit of distributive justice might involve certain costs in terms of other aspects of justice, and other moral values more generally. Consequently, one must accept that distributive justice sometimes needs to be traded off against these other values. Luck egalitarianism is compatible with the view that equality (or egalitarian distributive justice) does not trump all other considerations of justice, let alone all moral considerations.

III. Three Objections to Luck Egalitarian Value Pluralism

Let me mention now three potential objections to the argument just made. The first objection rejects the notion of value pluralism (at least in its luck egalitarian manifestation) altogether. The second objection accepts value pluralism (even in the way it is employed by luck egalitarians), but claims that luck egalitarians cannot be value pluralists. And the third objection accepts value pluralism, and accepts that value pluralism is compatible with luck egalitarianism, yet denies that luck egalitarian value pluralism answers the abandonment objection.

The first objection, then, rejects value pluralism altogether, or at least objects to its deployment with regard to distributive justice. The objection seems to target especially luck egalitarians, where the rather radical implications of their theory (such as abandoning the imprudent) may entice its proponents to dampen the theory's harsh effects. And one way of dampening those harsh effects is to trade off the demands of egalitarian distributive justice with other values such as utility. David Miller, for example, says that because luck egalitarians (and Cohen in particular) start off with an egalitarian principle that is quite strong and has extreme implications, they (luck egalitarians) are forced to argue that while equality is what (distributive) justice requires, justice itself should be traded off against other values. The problem with that strategy, Miller says, is that it leads to justice being routinely flouted. Doing so is objectionable, he says, and for the same reason that it is objectionable to suppress justice in the name of security (say through imprisonment without trial). Following value pluralism, Miller concludes, "the egalitarian comes to acquiesce in a social system that routinely flouts justice as he sees it, so that justice becomes little more than a utopian aspiration, something we might aspire to if citizens could transform their day-to-day motivations from self-interest into a wish to serve their fellows. But this surely won't do. Justice must be something we take seriously here and now."[38]

I disagree with Miller. Justice in the egalitarian guide to policy is no more a utopian aspiration than is the principle of maximizing autonomy under a Westphalian state system, or our concern for privacy in an inevitably bureaucratized information society.[39] As we saw earlier, luck egalitarian arguments interpret only a certain scope of what we call justice (let alone morality), and therefore do not deny the validity of all those other considerations. And it is precisely because we take *all* these different considerations seriously that we need to trade them off against one another.[40]

The second objection to luck egalitarian value pluralism accepts value pluralism, but argues that value pluralism is at odds with luck egalitarianism, or at least with the position of one of the prominent luck egalitarians, namely Dworkin. Dworkin's conception of equality as the "sovereign virtue," it is said, excludes trading off the requirements of equality with other values. If equality is indeed the sovereign virtue, then how can other values and considerations possibly trump it?[41] But this objection seems to me to confuse egalitarian *distributive justice* with equal *concern*. The sovereign virtue, according to Dworkin, is the latter.[42] And, it is probably safe to say that trading off different values is something that can be carried out in a way that still shows equal concern for all citizens. Thus, there is no reason why luck egalitarians in general and Dworkin in particular may not trade off distributive justice with other values.[43]

The third objection, as mentioned, targets the employment of the value pluralist strategy in responding to the abandonment dilemma. The claim is that the answer to the abandonment objection must come from *within* egalitarian justice, and for the following reason: "If all citizens have equal moral worth, then there is something troubling about allowing anybody to fall to an extreme level of material deprivation when others have sufficient resources to prevent this."[44] That is why, arguably, it is egalitarian principles themselves that should rectify this injustice. If so, nonegalitarian considerations cannot save luck egalitarianism from the abandonment objection, so the argument goes. Now, one can think that there is something troubling about allowing anybody to fall to an extreme level of deprivation, and one can also think that this would be troubling because of the equal moral worth of all persons. One may hold these truths and yet still disagree with the conclusion implied by this current objection. It is simply not true that every time someone hurtles toward deprivation, this happens due to a failure to treat that person fairly. It may be (and probably almost always is) bad that someone is destitute, but it is not necessarily unfair.

Let me pause and summarize what has been established so far in this chapter. In the first section I rejected several possible luck egalitarian responses to the abandonment objection. These responses attempted to provide a luck egalitarian reason for treating imprudent patients. I then argued, over the next two sections, that luck egalitarians could meet the abandonment objection by complementing fairness with a nonegalitarian value. I now turn, finally, to examine what nonegalitarian value can possibly count as such reason for assisting those suffering the effects of bad option luck. Such a reason could serve as the basis of the luck egalitarian commitment to provide medical care to imprudent patients.

IV. A Potential Solution?

One potential nonegalitarian response to the abandonment objection is the autonomy argument mentioned at the end of section II. (The argument said that it is mandatory to treat the imprudent, for it would be wasteful to allow individuals to fall below the level of subsistence needed for autonomous agency.) Another, perhaps even stronger reason to treat the imprudent is that we must not allow basic needs, including medical needs, to go unmet. The obligation to meet basic needs is a well-entrenched moral requirement in ethics and political philosophy.[45] It is based on the recognition that individuals have a deep interest in having their needs met. The more basic the need is, the deeper the interest of the individual is in having it met. We commonly think that there is some urgency about meeting needs, urgency that is not necessarily there when we consider meeting people's mere preferences.[46] We consequently think that individuals would be harmed if their basic needs are not met.[47] Since it is plausible to think that we owe each other equal protection from harm, this is often seen as capable of grounding a universal entitlement to health care.[48] Health care, on this account, is simply part of the social minimum that society ought to guarantee to its citizens.[49] In the next chapter I shall say more about how the reliance on meeting basic needs fits with my overall luck egalitarian account of justice in health care. For now I merely want to establish that coupling the moral requirement to meet basic needs, including basic medical needs, with luck egalitarian distributive justice allows for a comprehensive ethical guide to health care, and one that escapes the abandonment objection.

The requirement to meet basic needs whomever they belong to can be seen as following from individuals' equal moral worth, and the equal respect society ought to show toward them (which is Dworkin's luck egalitarian "sovereign virtue"). This is a moral requirement that is external, and prior (in the sense of being more fundamental), to the one of egalitarian distributive justice. The moral requirement to meet basic needs coupled with luck egalitarian distributive justice thus requires us to treat imprudent patients who are needy. In this way, luck egalitarian health care avoids the abandonment objection. It is relatively easy, notice, for the sort of luck egalitarianism I defend here to allow the concern for basic needs to complement the requirements of egalitarian distributive justice. For, as I said repeatedly, my version of luck egalitarianism is distinct from the ideal of desert. It does not insist on punishing individuals or on matching the level of their well-being to the level of their deservingness (prudence-wise). It is therefore not a requirement of justice, on my account, that the imprudent be left to suffer. The account thus lends itself to being coupled with the rather straightforward concern for meeting basic needs.

Notice that by supplementing the requirements of egalitarian distributive justice with those of meeting basic needs we are thereby adding a layer of sufficientarian distribution to the egalitarian one required by luck egalitarianism. We already encountered this combined pattern when discussing Dworkin's proposal for avoiding the abandonment objection. The compulsory insurance scheme he proposes is in fact a sufficientarian layer of distribution that supplements the egalitarian distribution represented by his hypothetical insurance. In difference to Dworkin, though, I suggest that that sufficientarian distribution is justified on grounds of the moral requirement to meet basic needs, and not on grounds of the prior insurance. (Doing so avoids the grudge objection mentioned in section I. I elaborate on this in the next chapter.)

How, then, does the requirement of meeting basic needs combine with the luck egalitarian conception of fairness to form a coherent ethical guide to policy? Recall that in section II we concluded that fairness could sometimes be indeterminate. More specifically, we said that treating the imprudent is, under the luck egalitarian conception of fairness, neither fair nor unfair. The requirement of meeting basic needs, in turn, tells us to meet all members' basic needs irrespective of how (im)prudent their antecedent conduct was. Thus, the combination of indeterminate luck egalitarian fairness with the concern for basic needs yields a coherent guide to policy that avoids the abandonment objection.

Now notice that even when luck egalitarian distributive justice is supplemented with a sufficientarian concern for meeting basic needs, it does not escape the following dilemma. Often, given the scarcity of resources, we must give priority to treating one patient rather than another. Suppose two patients are in equal need but one of them is so out of her own fault while the other is not. Suppose the situation is one of a car crash, where one of the injured individuals is the reckless driver and the other, equally needy, is her innocent passenger. Though both are equally needy, considerations of luck egalitarian justice would determine that the innocent passenger should be assigned priority and get treated first. Now, some may be troubled by that conclusion, for it implies, at least in the example as I construed it, that a small measure of recklessness may lead to what amounts to a death sentence (when resources are scarce). This may seem harsh toward the reckless driver. To quote Arneson again: "His 'punishment'—the quality of life he gets after the accident—does not fit his 'crime'—the brief lapses of judgment."[50] It seems then that even coupled with the concern for meeting basic needs, luck egalitarianism is unable to escape being harsh.

Let me make two points in response. The first point is that this objection is not peculiar to luck egalitarianism (although luck egalitarianism might, admittedly, exacerbate the problem here). Second, I would like to suggest a possible way out of this dilemma for luck egalitarians. Here is the first point. Suppose we supplemented luck egalitarianism with the considerations of autonomy (as suggested at the end of section I). In the example above, autonomy will be harmed if we leave either patient untreated. Considerations of autonomy therefore do not forbid assigning priority to the innocent driver. In fact, even responsibility-insensitive accounts of justice in health care (such as Daniels's and Anderson's) are not immune from the need to justify *not* giving priority to the innocent passenger. It would represent an equal loss of democratic capabilities, or an equal loss of opportunity to pursue one's life plan, to leave either injured motorist untreated. Assuming that we are forced to choose between the two, we would then need a justification for not using considerations of self-responsibility as tie-breakers here.

The dilemma of whether or not to assign lower priority in treatment to those who have brought the medical condition upon themselves is therefore not peculiar to luck egalitarians. Whatever justification one offers for providing health care, one would still have to decide whether or not to allow considerations of personal responsibility to affect the way in which medical resources, which are inevitably scarce, are distributed. For example, the dilemma of whether or not to assign priority in anti-retroviral therapies to AIDS patients who have been infected by contaminated blood (as the Chinese government has recently decided) is one that all theories of justice, and not just a luck egalitarian one, have to address.[51] It does not matter, for that purpose, whether one justifies health care on grounds of providing opportunities for life plans or safeguarding basic democratic capabilities. In the absence of reasons to the contrary, health care systems would be justified in assigning priority to a patient who has been harmed by the health care system itself.[52] It is plausible to think that we have reasons to prefer a patient who is needy out of other people's fault over one whose need is no one's fault (not to mention the one whose need is her own fault). In short, the need to justify neutrality (with regard to considerations of personal responsibility) in medical care is a challenge facing all theories of justice in health care, and not just luck egalitarianism.

Interestingly, Daniels himself is actually not committed to such neutrality, or so I want to suggest now. That is to say, he is in fact not at all averse to allowing considerations of personal responsibility to affect the way in which scarce medical resources are allocated. Consider this. Daniels holds that we ought to assign priority in medical treatment to "meeting a group's health needs if they are the result of unjust social practices" (say, in the case of racism toward blacks in the United States).[53] If we are presented with two equally needy individuals, it is right, according to Daniels, to assign priority to the one who belongs to a group that has been systematically disadvantaged. It is quite reasonable to assume, though, that our obligation to someone who has suffered a personal harm is stronger than the one we owe someone who suffered a collective harm. And it is also plausible to think that if anything, and other things being equal, our obligation to assign priority in medical treatment is stronger toward someone who has suffered harm at the hand of the health care system (the person infected while donating blood) than it is toward someone who suffered harm outside the health care system (see note 52). If both these assumptions are plausible, then it turns out that Daniels is actually committed to assigning priority in treatment to a patient, the less responsible she is for her condition. If we hold that the patient whose need is society's fault has priority over the one whose need is no one's fault, then we implicitly also hold that the patient whose need is no one's fault has priority over the patient whose need is her own fault. And if so, Daniels implicitly endorses the moral relevance of the patient's own responsibility in allocating scarce goods. Not only, therefore, is it the case that the challenge presented by the scarcity of medical resources is not peculiar to luck egalitarianism. It now turns out that the latter's solution to that dilemma, namely factoring in whether or not the patient was at fault, is something that a leading rivaling theory (Daniels's) is also committed to.

Still, assigning absolute priority to the innocent passenger over the reckless driver in the case of only one available rescue might seem harsh on the reckless driver. Although she is at fault for the accident, and certainly more so compared to her passenger, we still feel uneasy about allowing this difference to result in something that may well amount to an automatic death sentence. There is indeed a simple and obvious way around this problem (and that is the second point I promised to make) and that is to apply, at least in principle, a mechanism of weighted lottery. Suppose we agree that the reckless driver is more at fault compared to her innocent passenger. And suppose we also agree that she does not deserve an automatic death sentence for what could be a rather small amount of imprudence (not stopping at a stop sign, say). We could then accordingly toss an imaginary coin between the two patients, one that is slightly weighted in favor of the innocent passenger. Thus, we are able to have a responsibility-sensitive account that is not unduly harsh (in circumstances of scarce resources).

No doubt more should be said about how basic medical needs ground a universal entitlement to health care. That will be my task in the next chapter. My intention here has only been to point out that such a strategy could potentially answer the abandonment objection regarding the provision of health care to the imprudent. If persuaded by my argument in this chapter, the reader ought only to accept that the abandonment objection could potentially be met by supplementing luck egalitarian distributive justice with other values and considerations (and that of meeting needs in particular).

Conclusion

I have conceded in this chapter that a strict application of luck egalitarian justice would leave imprudent patients untreated. But I have then argued that luck egalitarian considerations of justice do not exhaust the array of moral considerations that make up social policy. When coupled with other considerations, such as a concern for meeting basic needs or for autonomy, a full luck egalitarian guide to policy would then recommend treating imprudent patients. This raises an obvious question regarding the theories of justice in health care that I argued against in chapter 2. Daniels's and Anderson's theories failed, when on their own, to justify universal unconditional health care. But the value pluralism proposed with regard to luck egalitarianism, it may be suggested, could equally be implemented with regard to these other two theories and thus salvage their ability to provide a coherent account of health care. To level the playing field, as it were, between all competing accounts of justice in health care, we need to examine how trading off these two responsibility-insensitive theories with other values improves their success in explaining the intuitions we have with regard to justice and health care. I want to close this chapter by responding to that claim.[54] Let me make two points to that effect.

The first point is this. What makes the trade-off with other values so straightforward with regard to luck egalitarianism is the fact that it restricts itself to a narrow slice of morality, namely, egalitarian distributive justice. As such, it allows for a trade-off with other values. Fair equality of opportunity and democratic equality are different in that they take into account other social values besides narrow egalitarian distributive justice (participation in society and politics, opportunity for jobs and life plans). As such, it is difficult to justify trading off such a conception of justice once again with yet more social values.

My second point is simply this. Suppose it is the case that Daniels's and/ or Anderson's account of justice could be coupled with other considerations to produce a less counterintuitive health care policy. And suppose further that they do so in a way that is not inferior to the luck egalitarian rules for regulating health care. In that case Daniels's and Anderson's accounts are not worse than luck egalitarianism in that respect, but neither are they any better. If that is the case, then the end I achieve in this part of the book is slightly more modest than I would have liked. Namely, it would at the very least still show that luck egalitarianism can produce a defensible account of health care, something that was questioned by its critics. The more ambitious goal of demonstrating that luck egalitarianism provides a *superior* account of justice in health and health care compared to other prevailing accounts would then have to await judgment at the end of the book.

The abandonment objection has been troubling luck egalitarians for a while. Without overcoming it, luck egalitarians are unable to justify universal and unconditional health care. I have argued here that the imprudent (e.g., reckless drivers) should not be left to die, but not because of considerations of distributive justice, the only kind of considerations that could potentially undermine luck egalitarianism. Rather, reckless drivers and other individuals who come to require medical treatment due to their own recklessness ought to be treated due to other considerations. These other considerations reflect other moral requirements (including other considerations of justice). One such requirement, I have suggested, is that of meeting basic needs. After putting to rest the abandonment objection by invoking value pluralism, I now turn to explore more carefully how meeting basic needs fits within the luck egalitarian account of universal health care.

5

■

Responsibility-Sensitive Universal Health Care

Introduction

Luck egalitarians, we just saw, are not committed to the view that the imprudent ought to be abandoned. Egalitarian distributive justice is but a narrow slice of morality and thus allows for a plurality of other moral considerations to be coupled and traded off with it. As I said in the previous chapter, one such major concern that is particularly relevant for the matter at hand is that of meeting basic needs, including medical needs. Our positive account of health care thus supplements luck egalitarian distributive justice with a layer of sufficientarian concern for meeting everybody's basic needs regardless of their antecedent health-related conduct. I also said that the moral imperative to meet these medical needs is rooted in their urgency and the interest that individuals have in having their basic needs met. I promised then to say something about how the concern for basic needs fits more fully with my defense of a luck egalitarian conception of universal health care.

I need, first, to say what I mean by "universal" health care. There are two important aspects to the universality of a public service, be it a health care service or any other public service. One aspect of "universality" concerns the opposite of exclusivity. A universal system is one that encompasses everyone and excludes no one. (Let us assume, for the sake of argument, that by "everyone" we mean every permanent resident in the country. I return to that point in section II.) The challenge luck egalitarians face in justifying that aspect of universal health care should now be obvious: how not to exclude imprudent patients. The other important aspect of universality, what I term "in-kind universality," concerns, in a way, the flip side of exclusivity, namely the inability to opt out of the system. A system is universal, not only if it excludes no one, but also if it allows no one to opt out of it. More accurately, a universal system distributes the service in question on the basis of need, without anyone being able to opt out of it and reclaiming its cash equivalent. Think, for example, of parents taking their children out of public schools and asking for cash (or tax breaks) of the equivalent value of the child's public schooling (to which they had no choice but to contribute through tax). A universal health care system is therefore a system that, first, provides treatment to everyone who requires it without excluding anyone, and second, does not allow potential patients to exchange the free medical treatment for which they are entitled for its cash equivalent. Defending the ability of luck egalitarianism to justify health care that is universal in the former aspect of universality is the subject of the first three sections, whereas defending the ability of the theory to justify universality in the latter aspect of the term is the subject of the final section.

Section I, then, seeks to show how the duty to meet basic medical needs fits within the luck egalitarian account of health care. I argue there that no member of the political community is allowed to waive her entitlement to the ensuing health care coverage. For that reason, it is right to shift some of the burden entailed in avoidable medical care to imprudent patients. I also provide reasons that explain why that burden should take the shape of ex-ante taxation rather than ex-post penalties. (Note that while the practical measures my approach recommends are similar to the ones offered by "all-luck egalitarianism," the justification offered is considerably different.) In section II I argue that the inalienable duty to meet medical needs makes basic health care into what I call a normatively nonexcludable public good, and one that applies to all members of the community, whether citizen or resident. In section III I address potential objections to the suggestion that health care confers certain duties on the imprudent: first, the objection that doing so ends up penalizing the poor, since it is they who tend to be disproportionately more imprudent with regard to their health; and second, that I needlessly assume that those who lead unhealthy lifestyles impose a financial burden on the system. In fact, so the objection goes, they actually save it money (by dying early). Finally, section IV addresses the ability of luck egalitarianism to account for the in-kind aspect of universal health care.

I. Meeting Basic Needs

Luck egalitarian health care, I said, is not vulnerable to the abandonment objection because it recognizes a prior duty to meet basic needs, including medical needs. Let me offer two quick points about what I mean by meeting medical needs. First, medical needs are distinct from health deficits. A person may be in need of medical care while not suffering a health deficit (or a departure from normal species functioning). Women in labor require medical care, not least to alleviate their pain, while not suffering any departure from full normal health. (Pain accompanying labor is part and parcel of normal species functioning.) Pregnancy and delivery are not illnesses, but still we commonly think that they constitute medical need and necessitate medical care. (I return to discuss those conditions in chapter 9.) Second, by "meeting" basic medical needs I mean (in addition to alleviating pain, whether or not it is part of an illness) both *curing* illnesses, and also *correcting* and compensating for needs when it is impossible to cure them (eyeglasses, for example, do not cure myopia, they correct it).[1]

In the previous chapter I alluded to Daniels's account of the moral importance of health needs.[2] But my account of basic health needs also differs from his. As we saw in chapter 2, Daniels's concern with health is rooted in his overall concern for securing opportunities for individuals to pursue their respective life plans. Since health itself has a decisive impact on individuals' opportunities to pursue their life plans, it follows that we have a duty to meet these health needs justly. The duty to meet needs is thus rooted, for Daniels, in the contribution that health makes to our opportunities. I criticized that account in chapter 2, saying that it does not provide any justification for providing medical care to individuals who have completed their life plans. But notice now, furthermore, that in my proposed account the importance of health needs is not derived from their contribution to opportunities.[3] The requirement that we meet basic needs, including medical needs, is an independent moral requirement. In particular, it is independent of the contribution of these met needs to the pursuit of equality of opportunity. In fact, Daniels himself, in his allusion to needs, also appeals sometimes to the independent moral force of the urgency of meeting needs (and not just medical needs).[4] His further appeal to the way in which medical needs contribute to opportunities seems to be geared toward justifying a just allocation of health care over and beyond the decent minimum (a move with which I am sympathetic). In other words, the appeal to their contribution to opportunities is offered as a supplement, not as a replacement, to the more fundamental duty to meet basic needs.[5] In sum, Daniels grounds the obligation to meet health needs both in the intrinsic moral urgency of these needs and in their contribution to equality of opportunity, whereas I appeal only to the former. Notice also that on my account there is nothing particularly significant about health needs. Many health needs are basic and as such we are required to meet them, but so are other basic needs that are not medical, such as the basic need for respect, adequate nutrition, education, shelter, and so forth. (I am happy to rely here on the list of capabilities provided by Amartya Sen and Martha Nussbaum as summing up those basic needs.[6]) To put the point differently, on my account there is something special about basic needs, and not necessarily about medical needs.

The concern for basic needs thus overrides luck egalitarian distributive justice and mandates meeting the basic medical needs of the prudent and the imprudent alike. Now, recall the grudge objection of the previous chapter. I said that we often think that if society provides universal coverage for medical treatment, it is then entitled to impose some of the cost of that treatment on those patients who come to require medical assistance out of their own fault. These costs of meeting the health needs of the imprudent may be imposed either ex-post, or ex-ante, in the form of compulsory insurance for certain avoidable reckless activities, such as mountaineering (or even added to the charge of ski passes).

Before I go on to justify making imprudent patients bear at least some of the burden of their treatment, I want to offer three reasons why that burden should take the form of ex-ante taxation (rather than ex-post). First, any just system that transfers some of the costs to the imprudent agent would have to be progressive, in order to avoid allowing the rich to use their superior wealth to buy their way out of recklessness. This gives us one reason to opt for ex-ante compulsory payments, for one means of guaranteeing the progressiveness of the insurance is to impose prior compulsory insurance for reckless activities characterizing the rich (mountaineering, skiing).[7] Another consideration concerns the fact that on any plausible account, medical care necessitates the consent of the patient. We commonly think that it is wrong to force medical treatment on a patient who has not given her consent to it, even when the treatment is without doubt beneficial to her.[8] A conscious reckless patient might be concerned about having the cost of her treatment imposed on her (or on those that will survive her) and thus refuse treatment on financial grounds (whether or not she makes those grounds explicit to the physician who asks for her consent). This is clearly an outcome we would want to avoid, and therefore the possibility that some patients may reason in that way should make us lean in the direction of ex-ante compulsory payments.

Here is a third consideration in favor of ex-ante compulsory insurance instead of charges after the fact. A familiar dilemma with incorporating a concern for personal responsibility in health care is deciding who should be assigned with determining whether or not the patient was culpable. It is clearly problematic to designate that task to doctors and nurses; turning them from caregivers into a policing force would have dire consequences for patients' trust in medical staff and consequently for their willingness to confide in them.[9] Policing in the health care system may cause many needy patients to simply stay at home and avoid receiving badly needed medical attention. It seems to me that there is, or at least should be, universal agreement on refraining from assigning medical staff, including administrative medical staff, the task of investigating the personal responsibility of the patient. The luck egalitarian who is a value pluralist would hold that if the only way to assign personal responsibility is by medical staff then such assignment should never be carried out. It seems that the obvious solution is to tax, ex-ante, certain activities.

It is justified for society, therefore, to make imprudent patients pay some of the cost of their treatment, and it is preferable to do so ex-ante. Notice, however, that I do not suggest that the costs of the treatment be imposed as penalties one incurs for neglecting one's own health. In that sense imposing the costs of treatment on the imprudent is not a paternalistic policy. Rather, according to my proposal those costs are passed on to the imprudent not because they have failed to take good care of themselves as such, but rather because they have avoidably burdened the public health care system. A patient who repeatedly misses her appointments or is not complying with her doctors' orders could be said to be wasting resources (including caregivers' time) that could have been spent on other patients.[10] Society is thus justified in passing on some of the costs of the treatment to the imprudent following their breach of an obligation that they owe to others, *not* for breaching some duty they may owe themselves. The compulsory payment is therefore not paternalistic, and is not based on a presumption of knowing better than the patient in question what is good for her.[11]

But that raises an obvious dilemma. What if the reckless person would prefer forgoing the medical treatment rather than having to pay for its cost? What is the justification for forcing the universal coverage, and its cost, on those who do not ask for it? I want to say in reply that coverage for basic needs is not something a person could waive her right to.[12] The reason stems from the fact that we have a moral duty to meet basic needs. Of course, any person may refuse having her basic needs met at any given time. One cannot be forced to accept a blanket on a cold night in the subway, the same way that one cannot be forced to accept a blood transfusion without consent. But no one may sign away a priori the entitlement to have one's basic needs met. And since we have a duty to meet basic needs, it is right that we make those who avoidably incur these basic needs help cover the expense of discharging our inalienable duties to them. It is because we have a duty to meet basic needs, not because people have a right to have their basic needs met, that one may not waive away one's entitlement to medical care.[13]

II. Health Care as a Public Good

It is possible, then, to think of health care as what we may call *a normatively nonexcludable* good.[14] That is to say, although it is obviously not physically impossible to deny people medical treatment, it may nevertheless be normatively impossible to do so. In saying that something, in this case, medical care, is normatively nonexcludable, we envision society as conveying to each of its individual members a message along the following lines: "It is simply impossible for us as a society to leave any individual to die by the side of the road, however recklessly that individual has acted, and whatever waiver that individual may have issued."[15] Health care (and not just public health) is in that sense a public good, and belongs, along with national security and clean air, in the class of benefits that society provides universally and unconditionally. At the same time, the unconditional entitlement to such provision gives society the license to impose some of the costs of treatment on individuals who avoidably incur medical expenses.

The imprudent may arguably complain, in return, that it is no fault of hers that society "finds it impossible not to treat her." Such squeamishness is not her problem, but society's, she may reasonably say. It is therefore unfair to compel the individual to insure herself, and moreover to penalize her for being reckless with regard to her own health. I concede that that is indeed a weakness of the account. But notice that a similar complaint might be lodged also against any other duty of fair play to support public goods that currently are more widely accepted as such, those of the physically nonexcludable kind (think of clean air or secure borders). Here too it is not the individual's fault or "problem" that society chose to generate or preserve goods that cannot be denied from the individual. Consequently, then, it would be unfair, on that rationale, to ask individuals to contribute toward maintaining clean air and national security. It seems to me that no egalitarian would be attracted by this (typically libertarian) position. However valid the objection is, then, it is no more valid than the familiar libertarian objection to duties of fair play in general, an objection which egalitarians typically do not find appealing.

Notice that nowhere did I restrict the nonexcludability of health care to citizens alone. In that sense health care is similar to the more typical kinds of public goods, mentioned earlier. Being nonexcludable, clean air and safe streets cannot tell citizens from mere residents or tourists. But why ought that to be the case also with regard to health care? Even if health care is a public good (owing to its normative nonexcludability), it may still follow that in difference from physically nonexcludable goods, medical care might still be given to citizens but denied to noncitizens. In other words, the portrayal of health care as a public good is still consistent with denying it to noncitizen residents. For one, since the fact of nonexcludability originates in a sentiment rather than a physical fact, as follows from my line of reasoning above, we may plausibly say that citizens and noncitizens elicit from us different sentiments. We normally do feel a stronger bond of solidarity with fellow citizens than with residents. Why, then, insist on the application of nonexcludability to all residents rather than to citizens alone?

In response, the normative nonexcludability of medical care, we may say, is *spatial* rather than *personal*. That is to say, it is impossible for us to withhold medical treatment from the needy, not because of her identity or membership (a citizen as opposed to noncitizen) but because she happens to be within the political boundaries over which we exert responsibility for meeting basic needs (on the most minimal of accounts; as for expanding this account beyond that minimum, see chapter 11). In other words, it is the space and not the identity of the individual that tracks our obligation here. Think of it this way. We may say, "No family member of mine is going to go to bed hungry," *or* we may say, "In this house, no one is going to go to bed hungry." The latter statement would hold also for guests, friends, relatives, and anyone finding refuge in our home. That latter statement strikes me as closer to the way we normally think about the matter than the first utterance does. We think of meeting health needs, it seems to me, in a very similar way, as generating a spatial, rather than a personal, sense of social responsibility.[16]

I want to emphasize, in closing this section, that my account allows, rather than requires, the imposition of medical costs on the imprudent. The account of health care as a normatively nonexcludable public good does not require punishing individuals who are responsible for their illness. Rather, it legitimizes the imposition of costs when these are deemed necessary for the sake of financing the universal coverage. There is no moral duty here of punishing citizens, then. My account is one concerned with fairness, not with some alleged intrinsic value in holding imprudent patients responsible.[17] The "public good account" of health care is therefore not an account of moral desert or retributive justice: it is not concerned with rewarding for virtuous conduct and penalizing for vices. This is consistent with my account (in chapter 1) of luck egalitarianism as being distinct from the ideal of desert.

III. Some Counter-Objections and Clarifications

I have said that coupling the luck egalitarian distribution of health care with the obligation to meet everyone's medical needs unconditionally allows us to draw a distinction between what people are owed and what judgment we may pass on their imprudent or prudent behavior. As such, the problem of abandoning imprudent patients is avoided. But there still may be some problems with assigning personal responsibility to imprudent patients, and moreover with acting on such judgments, whether in the form of sanctions to the imprudent or in bonuses and rewards to the prudent.[18] I want to mention two rather familiar objections to allowing such considerations of personal responsibility to affect health care entitlement.

One difficulty in incorporating considerations of personal responsibility into health care is that it ends up penalizing those who are already otherwise disadvantaged. The point is often made that it is the poor who tend to be imprudent with regard to their health. It is generally the poor who miss their doctor's appointments, don't take their medication on time, feed on unhealthy food, and avoid exercising. In general, the poorer one is the more difficult it is for one to maintain a healthy lifestyle. To point out a few obvious examples, the poor tend to spend whatever income they have set aside for food on items that are high in calories rather than on the more expensive diet of fresh fruit and vegetables. Their more rigid workday allows them less time for exercise, and when they do find time for exercise they often do not have safe parks (or such places where they could exercise) in the vicinity of their homes. A health care system, even an unconditional one, that penalizes for imprudence would be punishing the victim yet again, it may plausibly be said. What's worse, such a system may be seen as a moralized one, for it punishes people for the vices associated with being poor.[19]

The luck egalitarian would obviously be troubled by such implications of her theory, so let me say three things in response. First, it is worth repeating that it is not exclusively the poor who act recklessly with regard to their health. An example of reckless conduct characterizing the rich mentioned earlier is ski-related fractures.[20] Another example would be leaving childbearing until a later age, something that both increases the risk of breast cancer and results in spending more resources on fertility treatments. Another activity that places a huge financial burden on any health care system is its need to defend itself from malpractice charges, an activity usually associated with wealthier rather than poorer patients. Taxing conduct that places avoidable strain on the health care system is therefore not something that ends up targeting only the poor. Here is a second point to bear in mind. Recall our discussion of Roemer's "pragmatic" solution in the previous chapter. Even if imprudence is linked to a disadvantaged socioeconomic standing, it is still possible to discern what constitutes imprudence *within* a class of individuals similarly situated. Arguably, then, it is not unfair to impose certain costs on an individual who is much more imprudent than her equally situated neighbor.[21] A third and final point to make in this context is that when the state presumes an obligation on the part of the individual to not waste health care resources (e.g., by leading a healthy lifestyle), it thereby also assumes upon itself a corresponding duty to provide the background conditions required for acting in this way. This could imply: constructing and maintaining safe parks and playgrounds in inner city ghettos, making sure that there are cheap available fruits and vegetables in those neighborhoods, and so forth. This is surely a welcome consequence of the policy.

Let me finally deal with perhaps an obvious objection I haven't addressed yet. It is doubtful, one might say, that leading an unhealthy lifestyle does indeed impose burdens (whether unnecessary or not) on the system. This is the well-known point about smokers (and other reckless individuals) who, by dying early, might actually be saving the rest of us money. Prudent individuals, in contrast, present the health care system with many more life years during which they might require treatment. If so, there is no justification to impose on smokers the cost of treatment. In fact, we might even have to reward them for saving us money. Now, arguably a large part of what the smokers are allegedly saving us is in the form of unpaid pensions. People who die before retirement are saving society the pensions that it would otherwise had to pay them. Of course, these very same individuals are also not contributing their income taxes once they die (or contributing in other ways, such as providing child care for their grandchildren). It might be worthwhile distinguishing, then, what smokers who die young save *the medical system*, and what they might be saving us in nonmedical terms. Since my argument is restricted to the former, we may then set aside the savings in pensions (which, in any case, might be offset perhaps by the unpaid income tax and lost working days more generally). Admittedly, even here it seems that smokers are an asset to the system rather than a burden. Some health economists estimate that over their lifetime, smokers cost the medical system some 60,000 Euros *less* than nonsmokers. This is due largely to the prohibitive cost of geriatric care for the latter.[22] But this estimation is disputed. The assumption that underlines it, that geriatric care is more prolonged the older one is, is not an obvious one. The added life years for the prudent could be healthy and thus relatively cost-free, whereas the final life years of the smoker might necessitate geriatric care, whichever age that happens to occur at.[23]

Suppose, however, that it does turn out that smokers save the health care system money, and that those pursuing healthier lifestyles are the ones who burden the system. Would the implications be embarrassing for a luck egalitarian health care system? If smokers are not, in fact, costing us money through reckless conduct that they could have avoided, then there is no need, or justification, to penalize them. The abovementioned empirical finding would therefore actually help luck egalitarians escape whatever remains of the objection that they are harsh on imprudent individuals. Luck egalitarians would therefore be happy to endorse the "smokers save us money" thesis. But wouldn't it equally imply that now luck egalitarians must penalize those leading healthy lifestyles? After all, it would now seem that it is these individuals who are the very ones burdening others with their longer and costlier life years. Fortunately, the implication does not follow. The justification for passing on the costs of treatment to the imprudent was based on the premise that they *unnecessarily* burden the health care system. Pursuing the kind of lifestyle that results in a long and healthy life is precisely what any health care system is supposed to promote. A long and healthy life may represent a financial burden, but it is a necessary, and in fact a welcome, one. (By the same token, the burden imposed by the smoker, even if overall cheaper, is an unnecessary one, and as such detracts from resources that could have been spent elsewhere.[24]) Or to put it differently, the luck egalitarian view of health care justifies imposing on patients the financial burden of their *imprudent* conduct. Since the nonsmokers' conduct is, on all accounts, a prudent one, it follows that the luck egalitarian would be compelled to provide any resulting treatment (geriatric care at old age, say). Thus, no concern for imposing costs on the nonsmoker would arise in the first place.

The point about smokers dying young highlights a difference between the "welfarist" luck egalitarian view of health care and Dworkin's "resourcist" view (more on which in the next section). The latter is premised on the thought that each individual is allotted an equal share of resources, which she is then free to do with as she pleases. If that were the case, I said, we could not have had any complaint against the smoker for "wasting" her share. On the welfarist luck egalitarian view, on the other hand, individuals are not allotted equal shares of health care, but rather are entitled to care for disadvantaging conditions for which they are not responsible. Care for medical conditions that one could have reasonably averted thus constitutes an unnecessary burden on society, whether or not one has exhausted one's equal share of the health care resources. This seems to me a more intuitively appealing way of thinking about health care entitlement, and if so it lends support to the welfarist luck egalitarian and detracts from the appeal of its resourcist counterpart.

IV. In-Kind Health Care

This might be a good time to recap what has been established so far in the first part of the book. In chapters 2 and 3 I examined three attempts to justify universal health care: two responsibility-blind accounts (a fair opportunity account and a democratic equality account), and an account that is extrasensitive to personal responsibility ("all-luck egalitarianism"). We saw that all three had crucial shortcomings that made them unsuitable for that end. In chapter 4 I then examined luck egalitarianism, and how it might respond to the abandonment objection. We saw that the theory can do so by adopting a value pluralist approach to social policy in general and to health care in particular. In this present chapter I then gave a positive account of why a view of justice that distinguishes between the prudent and the imprudent is still committed to meeting the medical needs of the latter, and consequently is committed to universal health care. In this last section of part I, I would like to demonstrate that luck egalitarians are able to justify universal health care also in its other aspect, that of *in-kind* universality. If I succeed, then I will have shown the luck egalitarian account of health care to be superior in this respect to Daniels's account (but, admittedly, not, in this aspect at least, to Anderson's).

I mentioned in the introduction to this chapter the two aspects of universality of public services, the nonexcludability aspect and the non-opting-out aspect (or in-kind aspect). The second of these features of universality is less often discussed in the context of responsibility-catering health care than is the first (i.e., the problem of excluding patients on grounds of imprudence). One reason perhaps why universality of the second kind, in-kind universality, is less discussed is that it appears quite straightforward and something for which it is easy to account. Consider, for example, the democratic equality account against which I argued in chapter 2. Despite its several crucial weaknesses, that account successfully justifies in-kind universality. Democratic egalitarians justify the provision of health care based on its instrumental value for restoring citizens' ability to participate in politics and civil society. Since medical treatment is owed to the individual only insofar as it boosts her participatory capabilities, it follows that the individual is not entitled to the cash equivalent of the treatment. Thus, the capability approach successfully establishes a universal, in-kind, health care system.

In contrast, luck egalitarians, and "ambition-sensitive" (or responsibility-catering) theories of justice more generally, it has been pointed out, might have a harder time justifying in-kind health care. Theories of justice that seek equality in states of mind (of which equality of welfare is a prime example), such as the "welfarist" version of luck egalitarianism that I largely follow in this book, would be vulnerable to the following famous objection. Suppose Roger requires an expensive treatment in order to walk again. According to theories of justice that guarantee equality of capabilities (whether democratic or otherwise) or equality of opportunity (in competition for jobs), society should provide Roger with that treatment (in order to restore him to full democratic capability, or restore his opportunity to compete for jobs). Suppose however that Roger, who is a keen violin player, would be much happier with a Stradivarius than with the treatment (costing roughly the same). In other words, he would rather be in a wheelchair playing the violin of his dreams, than be able to walk and not have the Stradivarius.[25] A capability account of health care, and to some extent also the account focusing on opportunities for jobs, would deny Roger's preference and would insist on the choice between the treatment or nothing. The point of treatment, according to these theories, is to restore to Roger his capabilities, or restore him to normal species functioning so that he can compete as an equal to everyone else. These theories are not concerned with Roger's particular preferences or with his state of mind. In contrast, a theory of justice seeking equality of opportunity for welfare (i.e., "welfarist" luck egalitarianism) is sensitive to the ambition and preferences that individuals have with regard to their lives. Thus, it would arguably be forced to grant him the Stradivarius.[26] If so, it would appear that luck egalitarianism is incapable of justifying universal in-kind health care, and would allow patients to convert health care, to which they are entitled, into other benefits, such as cash. That seems counterintuitive.

There are two points I want to make in reply. First, we may observe that Daniels's (but, as I said, not Anderson's) account is also vulnerable to the Stradivarius objection (and therefore has difficulty justifying in-kind universality).[27] I mentioned in chapter 2 that Daniels expands the dominion of the fair equality of opportunity principle (the principle that regulates the distribution of health care) from jobs and careers to life plans more generally. In other words, he justifies the universal provision of health care on the grounds of providing equal opportunity to pursue one's life plans. But notice that some patients may legitimately claim that these very opportunities (to pursue their life plans) would be better served, in their case, by handing them cash rather than the medical treatment in question—these patients can use that cash to fulfill long-dreamt life plans such as playing a Stradivarius, rather than walking.

My second point is that the luck egalitarian account provided here, contrary to initial appearance, in fact avoids the Stradivarius objection.[28] For one thing, it is pretty obvious that the sufficientarian level of care that targets basic medical needs is immune from the Stradivarius example. We have a duty to meet medical needs, and no duty to give the cash equivalent of treatment for basic needs. Setting that aside, even the full-blown egalitarian care under luck egalitarianism escapes the Stradivarius objection, I want to suggest. The reason is that the account of just health care that it provides does not depend on opportunities, nor on ambition-sensitivity as such. Rather, the account of justice in health care offered here is premised on neutralizing brute luck inequalities. Someone who is ill due to bad luck is entitled thereby to have that bad luck reversed through medical treatment. She does not, in contrast, have an entitlement to the cash equivalent of what it takes to neutralize that bad luck disadvantage. According to luck egalitarians, an individual only gains entitlement to the cash equivalent of that disadvantage (in this case, a health deficit) when the bad luck in question cannot be directly reversed. Only then do individuals become entitled to a monetary compensation. (We will return to this point in chapter 9.) Thus, if there exists a medical treatment that could restore to Roger the ability to walk (supposing he lost it as a consequence of bad brute luck) then the entitlement Roger has is to that treatment and not to the equally priced Stradivarius. To put the matter in other words, welfarist luck egalitarians are committed to restoring Roger's equal *opportunity* for welfare compared to others; not to restoring his level of welfare to that of others. Thus, they recommend providing him with the means that would restore that opportunity (namely, the wheelchair), and not providing him with whatever means would boost his welfare. In sum, luck egalitarianism (of the "welfarist" kind) justifies health care in kind, and does not allow for it to be substituted with cash benefits.

Conclusion

I have sought in this chapter to demonstrate how luck egalitarians are able to provide a coherent account of universal yet luck-sensitive health care. I have argued that they are able to do so with regard to both aspects of universality. First, luck egalitarians can justify health care that does not exclude imprudent patients. They do so by conceiving of health care as a normatively nonexcludable public good, on account of our inalienable duty to meet basic needs, including basic medical needs. This way, they justify both society's obligation to treat reckless patients, and those patients' liability to pay the cost of their reckless conduct. On the other, second, aspect of universality, luck egalitarians justify in-kind medical coverage based on the requirement to reverse brute luck disadvantages. Thus, patients are only entitled to have their (unfortunate loss of) health restored; they are not entitled to the cash value of that restoration (unless that restoration proves medically impossible).

This concludes my defense of the luck egalitarian view of health care. I proceed, in the next part of the book, to discuss how that theory offers an account of justice in the distribution of health itself.

Part II

Health

6

■

Why Justice in Health?

Introduction

This part of the book shifts the focus of discussion from health care to health. In this chapter I outline the reasons for doing so, and consequently, for the need for a luck egalitarian theory of justice in health. In the three chapters to follow I shall attempt to fill in the details of such an account. Chapter 7 will attempt to justify a luck-sensitive distribution of health. Chapter 8 will further develop the account of justice in health by inquiring whether we ought to pursue equality or rather priority (to the worse off) in health. Chapter 9 will then extend that discussion from inequalities in deficits to health into inequalities in enhancement of health beyond the normal species functioning.

Our expansion of the discussion of health care to include health itself raises (at least) two (related) fundamental issues. First, why the need to speak of health in addition to health care? And second, once we have broadened our focus from the isolated sphere of health care, why stop at health? Why, that is, do we need a separate theory of justice in health rather than a general theory of justice (regulating, say, levels of welfare or primary goods)? I shall address these issues in turn.

I. Is Health Care (Still) Special?

Until quite recently, discussions of justice and health have focused on health care. Whenever justice and health were discussed it was assumed that what was called for was a just distribution of health care. Two assumptions, I speculate, drove this line of thinking, one empirical and the other normative. First, it was assumed that health care is the sole or at least a major determinant of our health. How good our health is depends, so the assumption went, on the quality of the medical care we receive. The second, normative, assumption was that a just allocation of health could only be stipulated in terms of health care. In other words, there is nothing else, normatively speaking, that we ought to be distributing in the realm of health (whether or not, factually speaking, there are other factors that may affect it). Health care was thus conceived as the only good that is pertinent for the distribution of health, both factually and normatively speaking.

Recently, the centrality of health care in discussions about health has been revisited. Empirically speaking, the more recent understanding is that health care has quite a limited impact on it, and that other goods are perhaps more important in determining our health.[1] As a growing body of empirical literature reveals, difference in access to health care accounts for a rather small percentage of the difference between individuals' health outcomes. Dan Brock makes the point most forcefully:

> [But] health care's impact on both health and health inequalities is quite limited; for example, medical care is estimated to account for only about one fifth of life expectancy gains in the twentieth century. More important, inequalities in health among individuals and groups that are within human and social control are not primarily the result of inequalities in access to or use of health care. This is not to deny, of course, that medical care is often of great importance for the life and well-being of individual patients. But differences in access to and use of health care have only a negligible effect on health inequalities among social groups, in particular individuals of different socioeconomic classes. The crucial point is that differences in the incidence of illness and injury from social causes swamp the effects on health of differences in access to and use of medical care to treat that illness and injury.[2]

Indeed, the current understanding in epidemiology is that differences in health are determined primarily by factors other than health care, and most significantly, by socioeconomic factors (as well as, obviously, natural factors, and chiefly one's genetic makeup). To be clear: by "socioeconomic factors" it is meant socioeconomic factors that affect health *directly*, independently and apart from socioeconomic factors that affect access to health *care*.[3] Although there is some disagreement concerning the exact impact health care has on life expectancy,[4] and on health more generally, it is more or less universally accepted that socioeconomic factors are predominant in determining our health. It ought to be pointed out, however, that most studies on the social determinants of health were conducted in developed countries, and thus the validity of the thesis for developing countries is yet unproven.[5] Bearing this qualification in mind, there is still a strong indication that health care is not nearly as significant in determining our health as was once thought. As Richard Wilkinson and Michael Marmot conclude: "While medical care can prolong survival and improve prognosis after some serious diseases, *more* important for the health of the population as a whole are the social and economic conditions that make people ill and in need of medical care in the first place."[6] The point is echoed by Daniels, Kennedy, and Kawachi:

> Health is produced not just by having access to medical prevention and treatment but, to a measurably *greater* extent, by the cumulative experience of social conditions across the life course. In other words, by the time a 60-year-old presents to the emergency room with a heart attack to receive medical treatment, that encounter represents the result of bodily insults that accumulated over a life time. Medical care is, figuratively speaking, "the ambulance waiting at the bottom of the cliff." Much of the contemporary discussion about increasing access to medical care as a means of reducing health inequalities misses the point. An emphasis on intersectoral reform will recognize the primacy of social conditions, such as access to basic education, levels of material deprivation, a healthy workplace environment, and equality of political participation in determining the health achievement of societies. A focus on intersectoral reform does not imply that we should ignore medical services and health sector reform because other steps have a bigger pay-off. [...] What sort of policies should governments pursue in order to reduce health inequalities? Certainly, the menu of options should include equalizing access to medical care, but it should also include a broader set of policies aimed at equalizing individual life opportunities, such as investment in basic education, affordable housing, income security, and other forms of antipoverty policy.[7]

Now, "health care" can be understood to comprise not only clinical care but also public health policy. "Public health" means nonclinical procedures that are aimed directly at improving the health of the population. These include water and food safety, anti-pollution regulation, workplace safety, nutrition programs for infants and children, and health education.[8] In downplaying the role of health care in determining our health, aren't we overlooking the importance of public health measures? Or, in other words, isn't health care sill significant in determining our health when it is understood to include also measures of public health? I mentioned earlier that when epidemiologists speak of the social determinants of health, they are not speaking about the social determinants of *access* to clinical care. Nor, I wish to stress now, are they speaking about the effects of nonclinical health policy such as public health. Instead, the bulk of the social determinants of health established in the past two decades or so are ones that cannot normally be captured under "public health policy," however broadly the latter are currently construed. These social determinants include the effects of familial nurture in early life, social exclusion, unemployment, work (not work safety, but rather the effects of stress and workplace hierarchy),[9] the availability of social networks, substance addiction, diet (again: quality, as distinct from safety, of food), and transport.[10] To illustrate: public health measures (at least the way we conventionally understand the term) remove unsafe food from supermarket shelves; "public health" is *not* normally responsible for keeping grocery stores that sell fresh fruits and vegetables, at affordable price, inside urban ghettos. Public health measures tell us to wear helmets in constructions sites; public health policy does *not* instruct us to redesign jobs so that our work environment can become less hierarchical (something that we have a good reason to believe will help curb the incidence of cardiovascular disease). It appears, then, that the social determinants of health are predominantly ones that cannot be cast as measures of public health, at least not as the term has been conventionally understood so far.

Health care, then, even when understood in its broadest sense (i.e., as including public health), has only a limited impact on our health. If we seek justice in the way in which health is distributed in society we ought to broaden the scope of our concern, and rather than look at health care exclusively, start thinking also about the just distribution of health proper. Fortunately, this is coming to be the accepted view of both philosophers and policy makers.[11] How to distribute health justly is therefore the subject of this second part of the book, which attempts to examine this problem through the luck egalitarian prism.

II. Why a Separate Theory of Justice in Health?

If our (largely) empirical discussion in the last section is sound, it may raise at least two difficulties for the project undertaken in this book. First, if health care is no longer "special," and if we need to focus our attention on health, then why bother providing a theory of justice in health care, as we have over the preceding four chapters? The second, perhaps more challenging, question is the one indicated in the title of this section, and is of obvious significance for the remainder of the book. If health care is no longer morally special, then why limit a discussion of justice to the sphere of health in the first place? Why, in other words, should we not discard the attempt to provide a theory of justice in a narrow sphere and rather revert back to a comprehensive theory of justice, one that is not restricted to one type of good or one particular sphere of public policy? I shall address these two issues in turn.

First, then, why the need for a theory of justice in health care, given its limited impact on health? This dilemma is obviously not particular to a luck egalitarian account of justice. Rather, it is a challenge to any attempt to provide a separate theory of justice to health care (and also to health, for that matter). In fact, it may actually be the case that the "social determinants of health" thesis is more troubling for Daniels's account than it is for mine. For, if health care accounts for so little of our health, then a concern for the way that health shapes our opportunities to pursue our life plans may actually lead us to divert all the resources we spend on health care and shift them onto the other determinants of health (education, housing, employment).[12] This is worth repeating. If what we care about is health, and the way that good health helps us equalize people's opportunities to achieve their life plans, then we might do well to scrap health *care* altogether. In contrast, the "social determinants of health" thesis poses no such difficulty to the luck egalitarian account I provided in part I. The reason is this. Nowhere did I claim, as Daniels does,[13] that health care is special. Neither of the two patterns of distribution that my account stipulates (a sufficientarian provision of care to meet basic needs, and a luck egalitarian provision of all other medical care) is dependent on the putative specialness of health care. As I pointed out in chapter 5, section I, basic medical needs should not be seen as more special than all other basic needs. And as for the second pattern my account stipulates —an egalitarian provision of care to address brute luck disadvantages—here again there was nothing peculiar to these disadvantages to distinguish them from non–health-related disadvantages. Thus, my luck egalitarian account of justice in health care is not contingent on how decisive health care turns out to be in determining our health.

There are a couple of other, more general, points about the need for a theory of justice in health care. One general reason is one that may seem as mere sophistry but underlies an important truth, I believe. Someone providing a theory of justice in X does not necessarily need to justify that X is a proper subject of justice. Rather, she may say that "insofar as X is an appropriate subject of justice, here is what I believe to be the correct theory of justice that applies to it." Think, for example, of genetic enhancements, which we shall discuss in chapter 9. Such enhancements were not conceivable until recently, and so, needless to say, there was no need for concern for justice in the distribution of those enhancements. With the advent of medical research more of us have come to believe that there is a need for a theory of justice to regulate the distribution of those genetic enhancements. Whether or not there is an agreement on the need for such a theory, there is certainly no harm in having one at hand.

The other point is more specific to health care. Very simply, as long as there is health care there is a need for principles of justice to regulate its distribution. Health care systems, including public health care systems, are, thankfully, still with us for the foreseeable future. And as long as these function as public services there is a need to figure out a theory for the just allocation of these goods. Such a theory would include, among other things, principles for determining the entitlement for care of those who have contributed to their own illness. As such, there is a need not only for a separate theory of justice in health care, but one where luck egalitarianism has a distinctive input.

Justifying the need for a separate theory of justice in health (as opposed to health care) may be trickier. The dominant account of justice in health care, namely Daniels's, was premised, as we saw, on the recognition of the specialness of that sphere. If that specialness no longer obtains, then what point is there in theorizing separately about health to begin with?[14] We could, however, think of some mundane and practical reasons that make it a worthwhile goal identifying what justice in health requires. The World Health Organization, for example, might be seen to require guidelines for the pursuit of a just distribution of global health. In that case, philosophers are called upon to help ascertain what such a policy would be. WHO is probably not concerned with the just allocation of all conceivable goods but rather in the just allocation of health alone. Rather than turning their noses up at such a challenge, philosophers, it seems to me, ought to embrace it and respond to it. The need to respond to a policy challenge of providing a theory of justice specifically for health explains perhaps why several philosophers have already engaged that question.[15]

But the fact that policy makers, whether on the domestic or global level, require a theory of justice that isolates health from other goods and aspects of well-being does not of course allow philosophers to ignore the larger picture. While providing a theory of justice in health, we still need to keep an eye on how that theory fits within a more general theory of justice. If a theory of justice in health leads to prescriptions that undermine overall justice (in welfare, say), those prescriptions would be something to worry about. Again, this is a challenge facing all those theorizing about justice in health, not only luck egalitarians. Admittedly, Daniels might have an easier time in facing that question than would others. Let me explain. Recall that in theorizing about justice and health care Daniels focused on the instrumental value of health care to one's opportunities for life plans. Shifting from health care to health, Daniels can still maintain, and in fact does, that health itself is an even greater determinant of our opportunities in life, and so is even more worthy of a separate theory of justice.[16] The Rawlsian concern with opportunities for life plans thus justifies the special focus on health. But notice that the luck egalitarian line provides a result that is in a way quite similar. Luck egalitarians are typically concerned with opportunities for welfare, a concern that is obviously broader than opportunities for life plans. If health is significant for our opportunities for life plans, then it is surely even more significant for our opportunities for welfare more generally. In that sense, the luck egalitarian account is not inferior to Daniels's. In fact, it is superior, for, recalling the point I made in chapter 2, it provides a better account of our intuition that health is also important when it serves individuals who have completed their life plans.

For that very reason, it seems to me, luck egalitarianism also provides a superior answer to Daniels's with regard to the question, "Why a separate theory of justice in health?" We said that for luck egalitarians, the currency of distributive justice is generally taken to be opportunity for welfare or the related "access to advantage." Now, as Amartya Sen has pointed out, it would not be too much off the mark to suggest that health underlies much of our welfare.[17] Much of how well our lives go depends on our health status.[18] If health underlies much of our welfare, then it would follow that a theory of justice in health would not deviate much from a more comprehensive theory of the just distribution of (opportunity for) welfare. Or, at the very least, it might be suggested that the pursuit of justice in health would not clash with or undermine the general quest for distributive justice.[19] In responding to the challenge by policy makers to provide them with principles of justice that are specific to health, the philosopher need not worry too much that she is pursuing an end that conflicts with overall distributive justice—with at least one obvious exception. As we shall see in the next chapter, a theory of justice in the isolated sphere of health might lead us to give priority to men, whose life expectancy is almost universally lower than that of women. Surely on a more comprehensive view of justice, this advantage of women is more than offset by their disadvantage in many other spheres of life (income, opportunities for self-fulfillment, political power). This, then, is one major circumstance where a theory of justice in health as a separate sphere may lead to the opposite result than would a more comprehensive theory of justice. This seems to me a weighty consideration, and it ought to compel us to bear in mind that in pursuing justice in health we are, at the end of the day, still pursuing *partial* justice. At the same time, though, philosophers ought to remember that they might be called upon to provide a theory of justice in health that is applicable to an ideal world, one that is gender-free. Presumably, we would still want to know then what justice in health would look like.

Here is one final reason for developing a theory of justice in health, a reason I hinted at in my introductory chapter. It is the thought that the focus on health might actually teach us something about the nature of justice itself. As Sen has put it: "there are some special considerations related to health that need to come forcefully into the assessment of overall justice. In doing this exercise, the idea of health equity motivates certain questions and some specific perspectives, which enrich the more abstract notion of equity in general."[20] If we can be vigilant about trading off the theory of justice in health with considerations of overall justice, there is a lot to be gained, and nothing to lose, from searching for a new such theory.

Conclusion

Health care is a relatively minor determinant of our health, and consequently of our well-being. Anyone interested in justice ought, therefore, include health itself, and not merely health care, in a frame of discussion. This need not spell the end of ethical theorizing about health care, for as long as that remains a sphere of public policy there would be a need to stipulate the appropriate principles of justice for regulating it. Here, luck egalitarians have a challenge on their hands (the abandonment objection), but potentially, we saw in part I, also a satisfactory response. The non-specialness of health care, I also argued, should not lead us to jettison ethical theorizing about health proper in favor of a comprehensive theory of justice whose currency is welfare. I reasoned that, first, as political philosophers we might still be called upon to provide principles of justice to regulate health policies (in addition to health care policies). As such, we would be failing our professional responsibility if we abstained from theorizing about justice in health. And second, I said, theorizing about justice in health might teach us something about justice itself. In any event, while theorizing about justice in health we must bear in mind the interplay of that aspect of our well-being with other such aspects.

Over the course of the next three chapters, then, I shall try and explore what luck egalitarianism might have to say about justice in health. Let me preface the discussion by drawing attention to one particular (and perhaps rather obvious) difference between distributing health care and distributing health proper. Health is a natural good, while health care is a social good. We all have some level of health. (That level of health ranges, let us say, from zero for death, to one hundred for full health of the highest currently possible life span, and beyond a hundred for enhanced functioning beyond the full normal species functioning.) Health care, in contrast, is something that none of us has unless it is allocated to us by social institutions. One implication of this is that since health care is a social good, we are able to approach its distribution with a clean slate, and stipulate how much is to be allocated to each individual. The case with health is obviously different. Since individuals already posses varying degrees of health, when discussing justice in the distribution of health we inevitably discuss existing *inequalities* in health. The relevant currency is therefore the inequalities in health that we already witness around us. Pursuing justice in health therefore proceeds through identifying which inequalities are to count as just and which as unjust.

Here is one final technical remark. I shall speak, throughout the next three chapters, about "healthy life expectancy." Healthy life expectancy is an accepted measure of inequalities in health.[21] It takes into account not only the length but also the (health) quality of one's life. Healthy life expectancy can be measured either in "quality-adjusted life years" (QALY) or in "disability-adjusted life years" (DALY).[22] (The difference between these two measurements is irrelevant for the purposes of my discussion.) I should also say that I use "health equity," "just health," and "justice in health" interchangeably throughout this part of the book.

7

■

Luck Egalitarian Justice in Health

Introduction

When, then, are inequalities in health unjust? An initial response may be—"always." From an egalitarian perspective, it may be argued, it is always unacceptable that individuals do not enjoy the same level of health or that different social groups do not have the same healthy life expectancy. If so, it would follow that justice requires making everyone's health as equal as possible.[1] Let us term this view *outcome equality* in health.[2]

Critics often observe the following two problems with outcome equality in health:[3] First, some inequalities in health originate in individuals' freely chosen lifestyle. The ideal of outcome equality in health would mean that society is committed, as a matter of distributive justice, to equalizing the health of the chain smoker and that of the diligent jogger.[4] Note that equalizing the health of the smoker and the jogger is a far more demanding requirement than simply equalizing their access to health *care* (which is in itself controversial, as we saw in the first part of the book). Rather, the ideal of outcome equality says that there is something *unjust* about the inequality in health between the jogger and the smoker even when that inequality is the direct result of their voluntary and informed choices. This seems quite problematic. We may think it is right to grant the jogger and the smoker equal access to health care, and we may even attempt to curb the health inequality between them through some preventive measure (a ban on smoking in public places, subsidies for gym membership). But it seems implausible that there is something "unjust" about the way that health happens to be distributed between the two, when that inequality is owed in its entirety (as stipulated) to their respective voluntary actions. Call this the *smoker/jogger* objection to outcome equality in health.[5]

Here is the second common objection to outcome equality in health (and to the suggestion that health inequalities are always unjust). In almost any contemporary society men have shorter healthy life expectancy than women. But it is often pointed out that inequalities in life expectancy between men and women are not normally considered unjust.[6] If this view is correct (I return to examine this assertion later on, but will accept it for now for the sake of argument), then it cannot be true that health inequalities are *always* unjust. Call this the *inequality between the sexes* objection to outcome equality in health.[7]

Part of what I seek to do in this part of the book, then, is to advance the egalitarian discussion of health equity beyond these two familiar objections.[8] To do so, I offer two competing egalitarian principles to try and cope with these initial objections. The two principles represent, respectively, a luck egalitarian approach and an approach based on Rawls's *fair equality of opportunity principle* (with which we are familiar from chapter 2). Here are the two principles:

1. *Equality of opportunity for health*: It is unfair for an individual to end up less healthy than another if she invested at least as much effort in looking after her health.

2. Fair *equality of opportunity for health*: It is unfair for an individual to end up less healthy than another if she invested at least as much effort in looking after her health, *provided she has at least as good a genetic disposition as that other person.*

The first principle, it is easy to see, makes a stronger demand than does the second principle. I will argue that the first principle better corresponds with our intuitions about health inequalities than does the second principle, and consequently, that the luck egalitarian approach to health equity is superior to this Rawlsian approach. The argument unfolds as follows. Section I presents the abovementioned two competing egalitarian principles of health equity—the luck egalitarian "equality of opportunity for health" and the Rawlsian "*fair* equality of opportunity *(FEO)* for health"—and shows how they cope with the smoker/jogger objection and the inequality between the sexes objection. FEO for health, it turns out, copes better with the latter objection than does the luck egalitarian principle. In section II, though, I present two decisive objections to adopting FEO for health. Having rejected the Rawlsian approach, I return in section III to examine in detail how the luck egalitarian approach copes with the inequality between the sexes objection. Effectively, I demonstrate there that, despite its prominence in the literature, that objection is misplaced. I thus conclude that luck egalitarianism offers a better account of justice in health than does the Rawlsian conception of justice.

I. Rawlsian vs. Luck Egalitarian Justice in Health

Let me, then, sketch the two competing egalitarian principles of health equity and the different approaches that underpin them. Here is the first principle mentioned:

1. *Equality of Opportunity for Health*: It is unfair for an individual to end up less healthy than another if she invested at least as much effort[9] in looking after her health.

Now, it is easy to see how the principle just stated avoids the smoker/jogger objection. According to this principle it is *not* unfair for the smoker to end up less healthy than the jogger, for she did not invest as much effort in looking after her health as did the jogger.[10] What makes this approach to justice in health a luck egalitarian one is that it seeks to equalize opportunities for health rather than health itself.[11] This idea, that people are entitled to an equal opportunity to be healthy, has an immediate appeal. It not only avoids the smoker/jogger objection but appears, in general, less paternalistic than equalizing health as such. For society, according to the ideal of equal opportunity for health, only seeks to allow individuals to be as healthy as they themselves choose to be.[12]

Notice, however, that this approach is still vulnerable to the "inequalities between the sexes" objection. For it is a medical fact that even at birth (and arguably even before)[13] men and women do not enjoy an equal opportunity for health. Pursuing equal opportunity to be healthy would require, then, equalizing opportunities for health between men and women. "Equal opportunity for health" is therefore still vulnerable to the inequality between the sexes objection. Let me now elaborate on the alternative approach, which, as I hope to show, easily avoids *both* objections to outcome equality in health.

The alternative egalitarian principle, FEO for health, is able to move around the inequality between the sexes objection by switching from the general notion of equal opportunity to the more specific Rawlsian "fair equality of opportunity" principle (FEOP). Rawls's FEOP, recall our discussion in chapter 2, says that equally talented individuals who exercise an equal level of effort in honing their talents should have equal access to jobs and careers. In contrast to *formal* equality of opportunity, the FEOP thus seeks to neutralize all social impediments to individuals reaping the fruits of their talent and effort.[14] Here is what, I said, FEO *for health* would look like:

2. *Fair Equality of Opportunity for Health*: It is unfair for an individual to end up less healthy than another if she invested at least as much effort in looking after her health, provided she has at least as good a genetic disposition as that other person.

Notice that in adopting the FEOP as the principle of justice regulating inequalities in health we would be treating health in the same way we treat jobs: normally, we do not object to some people having better jobs than others, but we do object when equally qualified individuals do not have an equal shot at those better jobs. I have mentioned that FEOP in Rawls's scheme holds between individuals of equal talents and skills. That is why, I propose, we could perhaps fit genetic differences between the sexes into the category of "talents and skills." Thereby, FEO for health would mandate that society guarantee individuals of equal genetic disposition (as pointed out, men compared to men, and women compared to women, but also many other instances)[15] an equal shot at being healthy.[16] In that way, FEO for health avoids the inequality between the sexes objection.[17]

FEO for health also easily avoids the jogger/smoker objection. Rawls's FEOP, I have said, requires equal access (to jobs and positions) to hold not only between individuals who possess equal talent, but also between those who in addition exercise equal *effort*. Individuals who possess equal natural talent, and who invest an equal measure of effort in honing these natural talents and developing those skills, ought to have an equal chance in the competition for jobs.[18] As mentioned, in the application to health we may say that leading a healthy life is, in a way, like exerting effort in the Rawlsian sense.[19] Applying the FEOP to health would therefore mean that people of equal genetic disposition who invest the same effort in looking after their health ought to have the same health prospects.[20] In this way, we see, the FEOP allows us to escape the counterintuitive conclusion that the jogger and the smoker are entitled to an identical health outcome.

II. Two Problems with Fair Equality of Opportunity for Health

Although initially attractive, there are nevertheless some undesirable consequences to using the FEOP to regulate justice in health. If I am correct, the two problems I am about to outline ought to lead us to reject FEO for health (and endorse, rather, the luck egalitarian approach).

My first objection to using the FEOP as a principle of health equity is, perhaps, rather straightforward. FEOP, we have said, mandates equal opportunity for health between individuals of equal genetic disposition. It is a principle that stresses a societal obligation to remove social obstacles to good health. Removing social obstacles to good health is, admittedly, an attractive feature of FEOP, since, in effect, it mandates that group membership, and social background more generally, should not determine one's prospects of attaining the goods and positions in question (in this case, health). And indeed, health disparities caused by socioeconomic and racial background are precisely the type of health disparities that many commentators see as especially warranting the attention of justice.[21] Furthermore, a societal obligation to remove only social obstacles to good health might also seem desirable given that doing so sidesteps the (arguably) undesirable outcome of equalizing life expectancy between men and women. At the same time, note, to pursue equal opportunity for health between individuals of equal "natural" disposition is to imply that justice requires us to attend *only* to the social causes of ill health. That means that justice does not require treating medical conditions that result from genetic factors. But that would be highly implausible, as we commonly think that a just health policy is one that attends to bad health also when it has natural (genetic) causes.[22]

To illustrate the point, consider the following case. Andrea and Beatrice have an identical genetic disposition. Clarissa and Dina also have an identical genetic disposition to one another, but one that is weaker compared to Andrea and Beatrice. Suppose, for the sake of simplicity, that all four individuals exert an identical effort in trying to maintain a healthy lifestyle. FEO for health says that it is unfair for Andrea to end up with worse health than Beatrice (the same applies between Clarissa and Dina). FEO for health also says that it is *not* unfair for Andrea and Beatrice to end up having better health than Clarissa and Dina. The following situation is therefore not unfair: A: (75, 55), where the numbers represent the healthy life expectancy of the two pairs. Imagine now that we could invest enough resources, medical and otherwise, in Clarissa and Dina such that they end up having a level of health closer to that enjoyed by Andrea and Beatrice. Note that this investment in Clarissa and Dina may entail that Andrea and Beatrice now enjoy a somewhat lower level of health than they could otherwise have had. Suppose the new situation is (B): (70, 65). Egalitarians would clearly favor policy B over A. That otherwise desirable policy, however, is not recommended by FEO for health, for according to that principle it is not a requirement of justice that we give those of weaker genetic disposition (Clarissa and Dina) an equal (or at least, more equal than previously) opportunity for health compared to that enjoyed by those of better genetic disposition. This is, it seems to me, a distinctive weakness of FEOP in its application to health.

Now, it may be objected that I needlessly assume that, on the Rawlsian account, the FEOP is the only principle of justice regulating health inequalities. Instead, one might argue, it is possible to complement FEO for health with other principles, ones that would take care of naturally caused illness. It is possible, for example, to complement FEO for health with a principle that maximizes the health of the worse off, along the lines of the difference principle (the difference principle or DP, recall, says that inequalities are justified so long as they benefit the worse off).[23] The difference principle would then be taking care of the remainder of health deficits, including, importantly, those owed to natural causes, thus, apparently, avoiding my objection. Note that that response in effect amounts to saying that (the good of) health should be regulated *twice* in a Rawlsian scheme: first by the FEOP, and then again by the DP. Rawls himself, it should be noted, does not allow for anything of this sort. While it is the case, admittedly, that each of his three principles of justice[24] *constrains* the operation of the principles that are lexically inferior to it, it is also the case that liberties, opportunities, and the other primary goods are *distributed* only by one of the three principles of justice in Rawls's scheme. There is a good reason for that, and it is the same reason that explains why the counter-objection under review has no force here: it is impossible to distribute the same good, namely health, according to two different patterning principles, one stipulating strict equality and the other stipulating maximin.[25]

Consider, for example, what it would be like to distribute access to jobs and careers both by the FEOP and by the DP. The FEOP requires strictly equal access (between individuals of equal talent). The lexically inferior DP tells us to distribute the same good in a way that would most benefit the worse off. The DP may thus recommend an end-state whereby individuals who have the same talent do not have an equal opportunity for a particular job. This may happen, for example, if unequal opportunity would somehow make everyone, including the worse off, have better access to jobs than they previously had. (Suppose that in exchange for having a greater opportunity for certain jobs, the well-off promise to create more jobs for other, less well-off individuals. More on this issue shortly.) The two principles may therefore recommend conflicting policies. The same would happen if we tried to regulate health both by the FEOP and by the DP. Either opportunity for health ought to be strictly equal between those of equal natural disposition, or, alternatively, opportunities for health are allowed to be unequal between those of equal natural disposition (provided everyone is made better off). We cannot have both.

Here is my second objection to FEO for health. Rawls, it is worth remembering, stipulated that opportunities for jobs should be equalized even if to do otherwise would somehow generate more jobs for everyone. Allowing for this effect (known as "leveling down") is perhaps the main difference between the FEOP and the DP, and is also the reason why the FEOP is, in the first place, lexically prior to the DP in the Rawlsian scheme. Rawls thought that the "waste" involved in leveling down is an appropriate price to pay here, the reason being that when it comes to jobs, he maintained, it is important to guarantee a truly equal (rather than merely a Pareto optimal) access, and for a variety of reasons.[26] Note, then, that FEO for health would mean equalizing people's opportunities for health, even when having unequal opportunities would somehow improve everyone's health. Suppose, for example, that some medical procedure could improve public health, but would make those who are already healthier even more relatively healthy than others. In other words, suppose the procedure in question could improve everyone's health, *while* aggravating already existing health disparities. Note that as a matter of fact this sort of thing happens quite often. It is generally the case that individuals who are better off (health-wise and otherwise, the two are almost universally correlated) are more likely to benefit more (than those who are already worse off than they are) from any given medical intervention. (This phenomenon is owed to a whole host of factors, such as the better off having superior education and a more flexible working day. These factors contribute both to individuals' ability to secure better medical care for themselves, and to their ability to better comply with medical advice.) In fact, it has been observed that only a minority of medical procedures improve population health *without* deepening already existing inequalities in health.[27] To avoid increasing inequalities in health, we would have to deny medical treatment to individuals who would otherwise benefit from it, which hardly seems like a desirable policy. Equalizing opportunities for health appears, then, to mandate leveling down potential absolute levels of health.[28] And that seems like a distinctively undesirable consequence of FEO for health.[29]

A proponent of FEO for health might remind us that it is no accident that Rawls's FEOP forbids leveling down in the first place. Rawls's reason for rejecting unequal access to jobs even when that would improve everyone's access to jobs is based on considerations of self-respect. His concern was that Pareto optimal access might undermine the self-respect of those who end up having lesser access.[30] A similar reasoning might be employed in order to counter my argument here. Namely, it might be said that to give some individuals lesser opportunity for health compared to others, in order to avoid leveling down, is disrespectful. But (borrowing on Arneson's discussion of FEO for jobs)[31] it is not obvious that allowing inequalities in health that improve the position of those whose health is worse off would be disrespectful. If due publicity is given to the fact that an equalizing policy would have inevitably resulted in significant loss of health to the worse off, then it is far from obvious that such a policy would be perceived as disrespectful.

It might still be objected that the consequence of leveling down does not yet demonstrate that FEOP is defective as a principle of *justice* in health. There are other ethical considerations besides those of justice that a health policy ought to take into account, such as a concern for maximizing utility (in this case, health; see my discussion in section II of the next chapter). FEO for health might not be desirable *all things considered*, the critic might say, but that does not mean that FEO for health is *unjust*. Notice that my objection was not that the FEO for health leads to unjust results by virtue of its leveling down, but rather that it leads to undesirable results. To escape those consequences, the FEOP does not need merely to be traded off with other principles and values, but must actually be overridden. Recall that the FEOP does not merely *permit* leveling down. So coupling the FEOP with the DP in order to escape leveling down in fact implies overriding its (FEOP's) requirements. Consider how different that is from the trade-off we undertook with regard to luck egalitarianism in part I. I said there that luck egalitarian justice proves indeterminate (in that it views treating the imprudent as neither fair nor unfair). Coupled with other values it then yields a desirable policy that is not necessarily required by justice. But we were never asked there to override or breach the requirements of justice in order to escape the abandonment objection. In that respect, the trade-off I undertook in part I is of significantly different nature than the one required of the Rawlsian approach to health if it is to escape the leveling down objection.

Let us take stock of what has been said so far in this chapter. In the introduction I outlined two common objections to outcome equality in health, namely, the jogger/smoker objection and the inequality between the sexes objection. FEO for health, we saw in the previous section, overcomes both these objections. But, as I have demonstrated in this section, FEO for health has at least two decisive weaknesses, and so, despite its initial attractiveness, it now proves not so attractive as an account of justice in health.

III. Health Inequalities between the Sexes Revisited

By rejecting FEO for health we now fall back to the luck egalitarian account of health equity. However, that principle, recall, did not cope so well with the inequality between the sexes objection (or in any case, it did not cope with that objection as well as the FEOP did). Furthermore, on the face of it, the luck egalitarian principle is also likely to be as vulnerable (as the FEOP) to the leveling down objection (the latter of the objections presented in the previous section). In the rest of this chapter and in the next one, then, I defend the luck egalitarian approach from these two objections (and in the process modify it). I begin that endeavor, in this section, by addressing the inequality between the sexes objection.

The FEOP, recall, avoided the inequality between the sexes objection by advocating equalizing opportunities for health between individuals *of equal genetic disposition*. The luck egalitarian principle does not contain a proviso of that kind. It is therefore vulnerable to the "inequalities between the sexes" objection because pursuing equal opportunity to be healthy would require equalizing the opportunity for health between men and women.[32] Recalling the example we used earlier, equal opportunity for health would not only recommend narrowing the gap in life expectancy between Andrea and Clarissa; it would also recommend doing so between Andrea and Christopher, say. Many people find that suggestion to be counterintuitive.[33] Indeed, it has been suggested that the view that we ought to attempt to equalize the opportunity for health between men and women is "absurd."[34] Any luck egalitarian account of health equity, then, would have to overcome this obstacle. I want to suggest that a luck egalitarian account of health equity in fact bites the bullet and asserts, against widespread (but ultimately misguided) intuition, that inequalities in health between the sexes *are* a concern for justice. To do so, I examine first the assumptions that underlie the popular view that health inequalities between the sexes are not unjust.

1. *Inequalities in life expectancy between men and women are, in effect, inequalities between very old people. And whether someone lives to be 78 instead of 75 should be very low indeed on our list of priorities given that there is so much life-saving and health-improving to be done for other, younger patients.*

This is a common misconception that overlooks the fact that the term "life expectancy" represents a statistical average that normally takes into account deaths of both younger and older individuals. In fact, then, we are dealing here with differences in mortality between men and women of *all* ages. Moreover, suppose we do accept the suggestion that inequalities in life expectancy between men and women are not of moral concern since they only amount to negligible differences in life years late in life. On that rationale, note, the frequently invoked disparities between socioeconomic classes could turn out to be even *less* worthy of moral concern. For example, in Britain differences in life expectancy between men and women are *greater* than the much-talked-about differences in life expectancy between social classes.[35]

2. *There is nothing unjust about health inequalities between the sexes because differences in life expectancy between men and women are due to natural factors alone. Women's genetic makeup simply allows them to live longer, and there is, therefore, no concern for justice here to begin with.*

Setting aside for a moment the controversial normative premise at the base of this view, the factual premise here turns out not to be true. Health disparities between men and women are in fact owed to both genetic *and* social factors. Concerning genetics, the most influential factor seems to be the effect of estrogen, which prolongs women's resistance to cardiovascular diseases by more or less a decade. The *social* factors that cause women to live longer seem to be that men "smoke more, drink more, engage in risky behavior more often and are exposed to more occupational hazards."[36] In fact, we know that genetic factors contribute to only about half of the difference in life expectancy between men and women[37] (and according to some studies, even less).[38] The perception that the inequality in life expectancy between the sexes is owed to natural factors alone is therefore mistaken, and cannot be the reason why inequalities in life expectancy between the sexes should be considered just (or not unjust). Returning to the normative premise, the claim about natural inequalities not being unjust is also not convincing. As Tsuchiya and Williams have already noted, many believe that the inequality between the handicapped and the nonhandicapped is unjust even when it is owed to natural factors alone.[39] Therefore, the fact that they are natural does not show the inequalities between the sexes to be just.

3. *The social factors just mentioned are also not unjust because they are risk factors, things that men assume voluntarily (e.g., smoking, drinking, and occupational hazards).*

One problem with that view is that it assumes a measure of voluntariness in the way that men lead their lives that is somewhat implausible. Many of the risk factors that men take upon themselves are of the type the avoidance of which would exact a considerable cost. For instance, few men, especially in developing countries, can afford quitting work in hazardous workplaces.[40] More generally, we may say that some of the risk-taking that causes men to have shorter lives is precisely the product of gender. That is to say, these higher risk factors are the consequence of the allocation of risks between male and female family members. (Although here we should probably assume that the inequality in risk factors between men and women decreases as we move from traditional to more developed societies.) It therefore does not seem fair that a theory of justice in health, especially one that stresses gender,[41] would overlook the gendered origins of men's unhealthy lifestyle. That, again, seems especially to be the case with regard to occupational hazard. And, occupational hazard, it turns out, is a much stronger determinant of disparities in life expectancy between men and women than other risk factors such as smoking or drinking.[42]

Someone might still insist that the inequality in life expectancy between men and women is not unjust because, perhaps, she thinks the following:

4. *Differences in life expectancy happen to work to women's advantage. Women are generally worse off than men in almost all other aspects of well-being. Inequalities in health are therefore like some sort of "cosmic affirmative action," and are thus an acceptable, and even desirable, incidence of inequality.*

In response, let us suppose, counterfactually, that the inequality in health were to work to men's advantage. We would probably not think then that inequalities in health between the sexes are acceptable. If this is so, then, it cannot be the case that current inequalities in health between the sexes are themselves just; rather, they are, at best, unjust inequalities that are countervailed by other considerations of justice. Similarly, observe, current health disparities between socioeconomic classes *are* commonly perceived to be a concern for justice. And, the fact that, hypothetically, the correlation between socioeconomic status and health could have gone the other way does not change that initial judgment. In other words, if it were the case that the richer one was, the less healthy one tended to be, we would probably be less alarmed by health disparities between the classes.[43] But that would hardly be an indication of health disparities between the classes being irrelevant to justice. The concern that a given state of affairs raises is not a conclusive measure for the justice or injustice of that state of affairs, since, as we saw, countervailing forces may be at work and explain our intuitions.[44]

Consider, finally,

5. *Even if health inequalities between men and women are unjust, there is simply nothing we can do about those inequalities. For men to complain about the "unfairness" of having a shorter life expectancy would be like their complaining about the "unfairness" of not having the ability to get pregnant and give birth. There is simply no concern for justice here.*

In reply note, first, that the fact that nothing can be done directly to rectify a state of affairs is no judgment about the justice of that state of affairs. We often encounter cases where we can do little for people born with natural handicaps. The fact that we can do little to cure their handicaps does not undermine the injustice of their worse-off position. If nothing else, it is always possible to grant monetary compensation to such a person who is unjustly worse off. If the inability to become pregnant and give birth is truly seen as a disadvantage (the way having a shorter life commonly is), then there may be a case to compensate those who suffer that disadvantage. (I revisit this point in chapter 9.) But even that point aside, it is simply false that nothing can be done to reduce inequalities in life expectancy between men and women. Having shorter life expectancy is different, in that respect, from not having the capability to be pregnant.[45] It is possible, among other things, to invest more resources in morbidity and mortality causes of men than in those that afflict women.[46] For example, we could, if we deemed it necessary (and I by no mean say we should), invest more in research for cardiovascular treatment and less on breast, ovarian, and cervical cancer.

There is no reason, it seems, to think that inequalities in life expectancy between men and women, at least in an otherwise ideal world, are acceptable.[47]

If health disparities between men and women are a concern for justice, then that would seem to put these inequalities on a par with interclass and interracial health disparities. But many people think that this is problematic, since, very understandably, they find the latter much more objectionable than the former. It seems to me that it is correct to think that there is something deeply disturbing about health disparities between classes and between races. And I also do not dispute that these health disparities are more troubling than, say, health disparities between the sexes. Health disparities between social groups tell us that there is some systematic disadvantage that generates these patterns of health disparities, and thus, in these cases, work as a "sensitive barometer of the fairness of the underlying social order."[48] That in itself does not yet demonstrate, however, that those health inequalities are in themselves unjust. Such health disparities point out the injustice of the background conditions that generate those disparities, and not necessarily the injustice of the disparities themselves.[49] Instead, I propose, the reason these health disparities *are unjust* in and of themselves, independently of the unjust social background that exacerbated them, is that it is *always* unjust for one person to be less healthy than another through no fault of her own. That, in a nutshell, is the input that luck egalitarianism brings to discussions of health equity.[50] It therefore does not matter, on the luck egalitarian view, whether health inequalities stem from natural or social factors. Accordingly, health disparities between men and women are as unjust as those between social classes, even though they might be less alarming or less repugnant.

Let me mention a qualification in conclusion of this long section. Amartya Sen writes that giving priority in clinical care to men (due to their being worse off in terms of healthy life expectancy) is wrong because to do so would violate the principle of "nondiscrimination in certain vital fields of life, including the need for medical care for treatable ailments."[51] Nothing of what I have said so far contradicts that assertion. In particular, my argument so far is compatible with the suggestion that disregarding inequalities between the sexes in clinical care might be the most desirable policy, *all things considered*. Having said that, it is worth noticing that the kind of reasoning employed by Sen here would apply equally to prioritizing other statistical groups that happen to be worse off in terms of health, such as the poor, or African-Americans, say.[52] There is, therefore, nothing in Sen's objection to differentiate inequalities between the sexes from inequalities between classes or races. Furthermore, it should be obvious that we can bypass that aversion to discrimination in clinical care by giving men priority in nonclinical interventions such as public health measures or, more likely, medical research. In other words, to avoid discrimination we may give the worse off (men, African-

Americans, the poor) priority in the way that health care systems are *set up* rather than in the way that health care is *delivered*.

Conclusion

I have sought in this chapter to defend a luck egalitarian account of justice in health. I began by considering two familiar objections to outcome equality in health, the smoker/jogger objection and the inequality between the sexes objection. I presented two alternative principles that can overcome those objections, namely the luck egalitarian principle of equal opportunity for health and the Rawlsian principle of fair equality of opportunity (FEO) for health. I then showed why the latter does not give an adequate account of justice in health. First, FEO for health does not address health inequalities that are owed to natural factors. And second, it recommends the distinctively undesirable policy of leveling down health inequalities. The main weakness of the luck egalitarian account of health equity, in turn, appeared to be its vulnerability to the inequality between the sexes objection. Yet, that objection, I argued, in fact makes a moot point. I thus concluded that the luck egalitarian view offers a superior account of justice in health compared to its Rawlsian counterpart.

In the next chapter I move on to examine how luck egalitarian justice in health copes with the leveling down objection to which the Rawlsian approach proved vulnerable.

8

■

Equality or Priority in Health?

He did not retain for long the spiteful desire for his brother to lose his health—
that far he could not go as an envier, since his brother losing his health would
not result in his regaining his own. Nothing could restore his health, his youth,
or invigorate his talent. He could, nonetheless, in a frenzied mood, almost
reach a point where he could believe that Howie's good health was responsible
for his own compromised health, even though he knew better, even though he
was not without a civilized person's tolerant understanding of the puzzle of
inequality and misfortune.

—Philip Roth, Everyman[1]

Introduction

In this second part of the book I set out to defend a luck egalitarian account
of justice in health proper. The previous chapter contrasted that luck egalitarian
approach with a Rawlsian approach (fair equality of opportunity for
health). I argued that the Rawlsian approach is vulnerable to two crucial objections
and that this ought to lead us to dismiss it as an account of justice in
health. But how does the luck egalitarian account cope with the objections
that have led us to reject FEO for health? In particular, luck egalitarianism,
I have already conceded, is as vulnerable to the leveling down objection
(mentioned in section II of the previous chapter) as is the FEOP. Luck egalitarian
health equity, recall, says that "it is unfair for an individual to end up
less healthy than another if she invested at least as much effort (compared to
that other person) in looking after her health." Crucially, that principle could
potentially be satisfied by making the healthier person as sick as the other
person, or indeed by letting both of them die. Both individuals would have
equal health, namely none. For that reason, I want to suggest that luck egalitarians
can and should sidestep the problem of leveling down by adopting a
position that is "a plausible close cousin of luck egalitarianism,"[2] namely luck
prioritarianism. Consequently, I argue that a revised version of the luck egalitarian
principle, namely, a luck prioritarian one, avoids all three objections to
outcome equality in health reviewed in the previous chapter (smoker/jogger,

inequality between the sexes, and leveling down), and as such presents the most attractive account of justice in health. Here is that principle:

> *Prioritizing the opportunity for health of the worse off*: Fairness requires giving priority to improving the health of an individual if she has invested more rather than less effort in looking after her health, and of any two individuals who have invested equal amounts of effort, giving priority to those who are worse off (health-wise).

In order to establish that luck prioritarian principle as the proper ethical guide to health, I wish to argue, in section I, that it is permissible to give up on pursuing equality in health (and to pursue, rather, priority to the worse off). I justify doing so by arguing that equality in health has only a negligible instrumental value and it is therefore priority to the worse off that ought to be pursued in the sphere of health. Section II responds to some potential objections to the prioritarian case in health and offers some qualifications. Section III sums up the luck prioritarian approach to health equity.

I. The Value of Equality in Health

As Derek Parfit famously argued, the commitment to equality leads to leveling down, and therefore the egalitarian sentiment is more accurately captured by assigning priority to the worse off.[3] When applied to health, this ideal of prioritarianism tells us to, other things equal, assign priority to those who are at a lower absolute level in terms of their health.[4] Unlike the ideal of health equality, prioritarianism does *not* recommend leveling down potential gains in health or life expectancy.[5] Now, even agreeing that, in practice, priority to the worse off is the fairest principle to pursue, can we not at least say that when it comes to health, equality does have an important value? Larry Temkin, for example, writes that "the concern for equality is an important aspect of our concern about fairness. Correspondingly, national and international organizations must not lose sight of the value of equality in structuring health care systems."[6] The luck *egalitarian* position I adopt here concurs with Temkin in that equality is a constant feature in our concern for fairness, including fairness in health. But at the same time, I want to argue that equality in health does not have an instrumental value. If I am right about that, then it would mean that it is *permissible* to abandon the quest for equality in health in favor of priority to the worse off. If that is the case then the luck prioritarian approach I advance here can avert the leveling down objection (to which the Rawlsian FEOP is vulnerable).

Now some people think that Parfit and Temkin are mistaken to think that there is any meaningful distinction between equality and priority, or between egalitarians and prioritarians for that matter. Most egalitarians, the argument goes, recognize that leveling down is wasteful and thus would not recommend it, all things considered. Egalitarians, in other words, also care about things other than equality, such as a concern for aggregate well-being (recall our discussion in chapter 4, section II). Thus, while egalitarians and prioritarians might have different reasons for caring about equality, their practical judgments tend to be identical.[7] Others disagree.[8] I need not take a stand on that debate here. Rather, I want to argue that while an equal distribution of health is intrinsically valuable, it is at the same time *permissible* from the standpoint of justice, and thus *mandatory*, all things considered, to abandon equality in favor of priority to the worse off in health policy. Given that other things equal justice would have favored equality in health, and given that all things considered it is permissible to allow inequalities in health, it might also be a requirement of justice to compensate those whose health is worse than others' by the means of non-health benefits (e.g., income).[9]

Let me begin, then, by noting that crucial to Parfit's discussion of the leveling down objection is the distinction between the instrumental value and the intrinsic value of equality.[10] The intrinsic value of equality is whatever value equality in itself has, whereas the instrumental value of equality denotes those instances where the fact of equality (or inequality) itself affects individuals' well-being.[11] Throughout his discussion Parfit sets aside (for reasons that are relevant for the scope of his inquiry) potential accounts of the instrumental value of equality, and rather focuses on investigating what, if anything, is the intrinsic value of equality.[12] Parfit concludes that (inasmuch as it is vulnerable to the leveling down objection) equality has no intrinsic value, and therefore any (intrinsic) value "egalitarianism" might have rests in the priority it assigns to improving the well-being of the worse off. In other words, since there is "no respect" in which leveling down can be said to be (intrinsically) good, the only intrinsic value of egalitarianism rests with the priority it assigns to the worse off. Notice that Parfit allows for the possibility that in circumstances where equality does have some *instrumental* value, it may be preferred to merely giving priority to the worse off. In other words, in cases where equality would tend to have an instrumental value, it might be right to allow for (some measure of) leveling down. We need to examine, then, the instrumental value of equality in health. I have said that equality is said to have an instrumental value when the fact of equality (or inequality) itself affects individuals' well-being. Such instrumental value (of equality) includes avoiding unacceptable forms of power and control, preventing stigma through differences in status, preventing harm to individuals' self-esteem, removing impediments to community and fraternity, and facilitating and maintaining democratic institutions.[13] When such instrumental value of equality is likely to obtain, we ought to prefer equality to priority (i.e., to allow for some measure of leveling down). Conversely, it is permissible to revert to prioritarianism (that is, forsake the quest for equality) in instances where equality is likely to have little or no instrumental value.

How does health fare in that respect? It seems to me that health is one of those goods in relation to which equality has only a negligible instrumental value. Unlike income, there is only a negligible respect in which leveling down health inequalities can be said to be better. Let me explain why. It is generally agreed that to level down income would be better in at least some respects: equality of income brings (to some individuals, at least) many of the benefits mentioned above, of which, conversely, *in*equality of income would deprive them. Income inequality may, for example, undermine a sense of community (by allowing the crystallization of durable and visible social classes). Having less income than others may also harm a person's sense of self-esteem and self-respect. Income inequality may also generate relations of unequal power, which in itself risks the prospect of one class of individuals being in a position to exploit another. Such unequal relations of power have the further instrumental disvalue of weakening democratic institutions.[14] Finally, income inequality has the distinctive disvalue of lowering overall levels of health.[15]

Now, bad health, not to mention death itself, is, to be sure, an obvious disutility and a major impediment to our well-being. But does health *inequality* present a disutility (or disvalue)? In other words, does the way in which health deficits are *distributed*, independently of the absolute amount of health deficits suffered by individuals, affect a person's well-being? Consider for a moment the question as it pertains to health *care* rather than health proper. Many people (present author included) think that inequality in health care does have that effect. As I pointed out in chapter 2, having less access than others to health care may very well harm a person's sense of self-respect,[16] and consequently may also weaken society's sense of community and solidarity. But in contrast with inequalities in health care, not to mention inequalities in income and wealth, inequalities in health themselves do not seem to harm individuals' self-respect or self-esteem in any meaningful way.[17] Nor do health inequalities seem to prohibit individuals from socializing with one another in the way that income inequalities notoriously do. To be sure, being confined to a hospital bed drastically reduces one's chances of socializing with others. But it is the fact of the health deficit, not the way in which health is distributed, that reduces one's opportunity to socialize. One's chances of socializing would not improve if others were also to become bedridden. (To use Parfit's terminology, what is bad in the story described is that the person is less healthy than she could be, not that she is less healthy than others.) Nor does inequality in health, for that matter, appear to pose a risk to democratic institutions. One's inability to be up and about, attending political rallies and strolling to the polling booth, represents a serious limit to one's contribution to preserving and strengthening democratic institutions in one's society (assuming, of course, that all measures of accommodating infirmity, such as the use of postal ballots, have been exhausted). But if others were to be reduced to the same state of poor health, the cause of democracy would gain very little, if at all. So whereas income inequality (and, to some extent, inequality in access to health *care*) has a strong instrumental disvalue, health inequality does not appear to have an equivalent disvalue.[18]

Prioritizing the health of the worse off seems like a desirable policy, then. It avoids the leveling down objection, and avoiding leveling down is particularly appealing given that equality in health does not seem to have any meaningful instrumental value.

II. Some Potential Objections and Qualifications

Some people may think that inequalities in health do matter. Consider the following three examples. First, it may very well matter for a deaf person, for example, if there are more rather than fewer deaf people around. Having other deaf individuals in her community would make that deaf person's life easier in the sense that she would have more people with whom she would be able to communicate in sign language. Furthermore, any stigma that might be associated with being deaf would be reduced if more people in her vicinity were deaf.[19] A second example is that of bad teeth. Bad teeth are not only a disadvantage in themselves, but are also commonly a source of stigma and consequently of discrimination, particularly in hiring for jobs. Moreover, the stigma attached to bad teeth is much worse than that associated with deafness, for unlike deafness, bad teeth happen to be correlated with low socioeconomic status.[20] Third, if you are not the only person to have lost a leg in an accident then you may benefit from having more people who readily empathize with your condition and understand what it is like to have lost a leg. Don't the effects of greater scope for communication, reduced stigma, and wider empathy count as a positive value, one to be taken into account when evaluating inequalities in health?

In assessing that suggestion we should be mindful not to conflate equality with sameness (or similarity). These are two separate issues: how many other people enjoy the same *level* of (overall) health as you, and how many other individuals are suffering from a particular medical condition that you yourself suffer from. Two individuals enjoying exactly the same level of health (whichever way it is measured) might not be suffering from the same combination of ailments. Furthermore, it is possible for the most well-off person in society (health-wise) to suffer from some minor medical condition not shared by anyone else. And correspondingly, it is possible for the worst-off (health-wise) people in society to be so due to some medical condition afflicting millions (AIDS, say). The answer to the question "How many people are sharing your level of health?" is therefore independent of the question "How many people share the same medical condition as you?" This point turns, as I said, on the straightforward observation that equality does not imply similarity, and greater inequality, in turn, does not always imply greater dissimilarity. That observation bears on the matter of leveling down. To see how, imagine two paraplegics, one of whom also suffers from diabetes (call her Susan, and call the other person Tom). Suppose that the paraplegia in question is curable, whereas diabetes is not. The only way to reduce the inequality in health between Tom and Susan is therefore to cure Susan of her paraplegia. The new, more equal, state of affairs is one where Tom suffers paraplegia and Susan suffers diabetes. Thus, inequality has been reduced, but at the cost of denying Tom the benefits stemming from having a fellow paraplegic person (empathy, having potential fellow campaigners for the rights of the disabled, etc.). It is therefore the case that arguments concerning the benefits of having other people suffering from one's particular medical condition are not always relevant in evaluating the instrumental disvalue of health inequalities (as opposed to "dissimilarities").[21]

Here is another potential objection to my conclusion that equality in health has no instrumental value. Inequalities in health between salient social groups, say blacks and whites in the United States, disprove the claim that health equality has little to no instrumental value, so the objection goes. It is obvious that awareness of such inequalities most probably generates a sense of stigma and resentment in those who suffer inferior health. As such, it might be said that inequalities in health do have an instrumental disvalue. Note, in response, that the source of the disvalue, according to that objection, stems not from the inequalities themselves but from what is perceived to lurk behind them. As noted at the end of the previous chapter, it is the suspicion that inferior health is caused by some *other* systematic disadvantage that generates the sense of resentment in question. It is, incidentally, for that reason that the inequality in life expectancy between men and women is not normally seen as having an instrumental disvalue.[22] So whatever deleterious effect inequalities in health between salient social groups might have is owed not to the health inequalities themselves but to other, prior, inequalities that the health disparity may reflect. It is those prior inequalities (e.g., income, education) that have instrumental disvalue, not the health disparities themselves.

Consider a further objection. Inequalities in health inevitably result in other inequalities. Bad health limits the range of opportunities open to us (which is why health disparities are of such moral concern to begin with).[23] Health disparities, then, aggravate inequality in opportunities, which in turn aggravates income inequality (and income inequality, in turn, aggravates health disparities). Can we not say, on that account, that inequalities in health have a strong instrumental disvalue?[24] And, must we not, consequently, admit that leveling down health would be commendable at least in one respect, that of reducing inequality of opportunity? To be sure, leveling down health does help in reducing inequality of opportunity (whether for welfare or for the pursuit of life plans). Indeed, as I indicated earlier, one way of achieving equality of opportunities between a healthy person and a less healthy person is to undermine the health of the former. If both individuals are equally ill (or, indeed, dead), they then enjoy equal opportunities.[25] It is the case, then, that concern for the opportunities of worse-off individuals (say, to pursue their life plans) ought to lead us to prioritize the health of these worse-off individuals, not to level down health. A concern for opportunities thus favors priority in health, not equality.

Let me now raise two further caveats and qualifications concerning prioritarianism in health. First, I wish to stress that the prioritarian view adopted here is of the egalitarian, as opposed to the sufficientarian, family.[26] It is the view that the concern for equality, properly understood, implies assigning priority to the worse off. Prioritarianism, it follows, says that we should give priority to the worse off *regardless* of how well these individuals are doing. In other words, even if the worse-off individuals are doing quite well, and are above some perceived threshold of decent living, the prioritarian view says that we still ought to distribute the next available benefit to them. The priority view adopted here is therefore not to be confused with a sufficientarian view.[27]

Second, it is often pointed out that giving priority to the worse off is vulnerable to the "bottomless pit" objection: the concern that this might result in impoverishing the lives of everyone else in society.[28] Let me make three points in response to that objection. First, the "bottomless pit" objection is not peculiar to prioritarianism but also affects egalitarianism, and in fact, even more so. A commitment to strict equality, we said, may lead to leveling down. But strict equality would also require, note, piling all available resources onto those who are the worse off, until they are brought to par with others. It is therefore the case that prioritarianism in fact represents an improvement over egalitarianism in terms of addressing the bottomless pit objection (since it does not force us to level down, which implies piling even more resources on the worse off). The second point I want to make is that prioritarians do not necessarily give absolute priority to the worse off. *Non-absolutist* prioritarian-ism says that improvements are more valuable the worse off the person in question is.[29] It is easy to see that the latter version escapes the accusation that prioritarianism ignores the condition of those who are just above the worst-off persons, even if they themselves happen to be doing quite badly. Non-absolutist prioritarianism thus avoids the bottomless pit objection. The third point is this. It should be clear that priority to the worse off and fairness more generally are not the only ethical consideration when contemplating the dis-tribution of health. Another important ethical consideration is the concern for average utility, or in the case of health, average healthy life expectancy. Notice that even though prioritarianism already does give some weight to aggregate well-being (as my first point indicates), it only does so within the limits permitted to it by fairness. But of course, all things considered it might sometimes be right to override the requirements of fairness in favor of more weight to aggregate well-being. It is easy to see that giving due consideration to maximizing average life expectancy answers the bottomless pit objection, for it implies that benefiting the worse off is not the sole consideration in re-distributing health. As such, maximizing average utility is an important com-ponent of any ethical guide to health distribution. The two considerations, priority (and fairness more generally) and average utility, will obviously clash frequently. Often it is the priority principle that should most likely triumph, but we can also think of cases where the concern for maximal utility should come out on top. For example, (2, 10) appears distinctly better than (2.01, 5) (when the numbers represent QALYs).[30] My discussion here, and in the book more generally, does not bear on how one should settle these trade-offs be-tween fairness and utility.[31]

III. Luck Prioritarian Justice in Health

The upshot of my discussion in this chapter is that health equity instructs us to give priority to individuals the worse off (health-wise) they are. But how does the prioritarian account combine with the luck egalitarian account (of the previous chapter) to provide a coherent guide to health equity? In other words, what, exactly, does a *luck* prioritarian approach to justice in health look like? To answer that we need, first, a clear view of what luck prioritarian-ism as such is.

Luck prioritarianism seeks to capture the sentiment "that one ought as a matter of justice to aid the unfortunate, and the more badly off someone is, the more urgent is the moral imperative to aid."[32] The ideal consists, obviously, of two premises: luck egalitarianism (or "luckism") and prioritarianism. The first premise is that "it is morally bad if some are badly off through no fault or choice of their own."[33] The second premise is that "the moral value of obtaining a benefit for a person is greater [...] the lower the person's life time expectation of well-being prior to receipt of the benefit."[34] Luck prioritarianism has, therefore, two goals: to neutralize brute luck disadvantage, and to give priority to the worse off. It thus stipulates: improve the situation of those who are badly off through no fault of their own, and of those, give priority to a person the more worse off she is.

Luck prioritarian health equity, in turn, requires aiding those who are not responsible for their health deficit, and among those, giving higher priority to individuals the less healthy they are. We could formulate the principle of luck prioritarian health equity as follows:

> *Prioritizing the opportunity for health of the worse off*: Fairness requires assigning priority to improving the health of an individual if she has invested more rather than less effort in looking after her health, and of any two individuals who have invested equal amounts of effort, giving priority to those who are worse off (health-wise).

One immediate objection to luck prioritarian health equity so formulated is that its policy implications may appear harsh and counterintuitive. Contrary to common sense, it does *not* tell us to, first off, look out for those who are worse off, and only then compare levels of effort (or, prudence in looking after one's health). Rather, the luck prioritarian ideal tells us to compare levels of prudence first, and use the severity of the medical condition only as a tie-breaker between those who were equally prudent in looking after their health. That appears not only harsh but also impractical. Would it not make more sense, at the very least, to switch the order of the principle's two components?[35] Notice that as an operative principle that suggestion would make far more sense. For, surely it is best to look at the severity of the medical condition of individuals before comparing anything else, let alone degrees of prudence.[36] But a principle of justice in health, notice, is not a triage principle. It is not intended as a set of guidelines for clinicians. Instead, *prioritizing the opportunity for health of the worse off* is a principle of justice. It tells us how to evaluate the justice of a distribution, not how to go about delivering medical care in the ER. And, as a principle of justice, luck prioritarianism tells us to neutralize bad brute luck first, which (according to the luck egalitarian reading) is the point of egalitarian justice. Only then, luck prioritarianism tells us, should we distribute benefits in the order of their moral weight, which, given the principle's prioritarian tilt, implies distributing these benefits according to how much worse off individuals are. Notice also that the principle first tells us to treat all those who are not responsible at all for their ill health, and among those give priority to those whose health is the worst. So in fact once we have identified the prudent, the principle, even in its pure form, tells us to simply give priority (among prudent patients) to the worse off. At least in that respect, it does seem to conform to common practice.

Let us see, finally, how prioritizing the opportunity for health of the worse off sidesteps the objections to outcome equality and Rawlsian justice in health discussed in the previous chapter. It is easy to see how the principle avoids the smoker/jogger objection. Luck prioritarian health equity gives priority to improving the health of an individual if she has invested more rather than less effort in looking after her health. It thus says that the smoker has a weaker claim to full health than the jogger does. The luck prioritarian approach to health equity also sidesteps the two particular problems observed in the application of Rawls's FEO for health. The first problem with FEO for health was that it justifies treatment of only social, and not natural (genetic), causes of ill health. Luck prioritarian health equity avoids that problem. Luck prioritarians (and luck egalitarians more generally) treat *all* involuntary inequalities in health, whether social or natural, as of concern for justice. The second weakness of FEO for health concerned its vulnerability to leveling down absolute levels of health. By virtue of its prioritarianism, the approach offered here sidesteps the problem of leveling down. Luck prioritarian health equity allows for unequal levels of health between individuals even when they have invested equal amounts of effort in looking after their health, provided that inequality improves the health of the least healthy person. The luck prioritarian approach to health equity thus avoids the two problems that afflict FEO for health.

Conclusion

My aim in this chapter has been to demonstrate how a revised version of luck egalitarian health equity, namely prioritizing the worse off's opportunities for health, copes well with the various objections to the Rawlsian FEO for health. I therefore hope to have demonstrated in the course of the past two chapters that a concern for justice in health does not imply directly *equalizing health*, nor does it imply equalizing *fair opportunity* for health, or equalizing *opportunity* for health. Rather, justice in health requires prioritizing the opportunity for health of the worse off. I therefore conclude that luck prioritarianism is the best guide to justice in health. In the next chapter I shall attempt to extend that "luckist" account of justice beyond full normal health.

9

■

Distributing Human Enhancements

Introduction

As a result of the success of the human genome project and other recent advances in biomedicine, new opportunities for so-called human enhancement are becoming conceivable. Understandably, these opportunities are only now beginning to be fully assessed from an ethical perspective. To be sure, in recent years, there has been much inquiry into the *permissibility* of human enhancements (mostly through genetic means). Philosophers have discussed, for example, whether parents should be allowed to genetically improve their offspring, or whether athletes should be allowed to artificially enhance their performance.[1] Considerably less attention has been given by philosophers to fairness in the distribution of such enhancements.[2] Even less attention has been given to the interplay of fairness and luck in the distribution of human enhancements, which is the focus here. In this chapter, then, I seek to defend a luck egalitarian account of the distribution of biomedical human enhancements.

Whatever other merit it may have, the luck egalitarian view on biomedical human enhancement is distinct for its simplicity. According to luck egalitarianism, all preventable disadvantageous conditions that are unchosen ought to be eliminated. It does not matter, on that reading, whether these unchosen and unwanted conditions are owed to social circumstances or to natural ones. Both kinds ought to be eliminated. And, in case of *non*preventable unchosen conditions, the luck egalitarian view recommends compensation. Thus, luck egalitarianism specifies that society ought to fund any biomedical intervention that allows us to rid individuals of unchosen and disadvantageous bodily traits, whether doing so would constitute treatment of illness or enhancement of normal human functioning.

My aim in this closing chapter of part II is to argue that a comprehensive theory of justice in health is one that incorporates this luck egalitarian stance on enhancement. In other words, justice in health requires correcting unchosen bodily traits even when the latter are not pathologies. In defending the luck egalitarian stance on enhancement I oppose Norman Daniels's Rawlsian approach according to which society is obligated to fund only treatment to illness and not enhancement of normal functioning.

In the first section I explain what I mean by "biomedical human enhancement," and what distinguishes it from ordinary medical treatment. I attempt to show there, actually in support of Daniels, that it *is* intelligible to draw a distinction between treatment and enhancement. In section II, I present Daniels's Rawlsian view, in which the distinction between treatment and enhancement plays an explicit and important ethical role. I contrast Daniels's emphasis on that distinction with the luck egalitarian view, according to which the treatment/enhancement distinction has no bearing on determining which biomedical procedures society ought to provide and fund. Section III then examines and rebuts several potential responses to the luck egalitarian dismissal of the relevance of the treatment/enhancement distinction for justice. After establishing the *currency*, as it were, of justice in the distribution of enhancements, the final section (IV) turns to a discussion of the exact *pattern* recommended by luck egalitarianism. Specifically, it tackles the dilemma that may (and often does) arise when it turns out to be impossible to offer the same extent of enhancement to all members of society. I argue there, in apparent discord with my position in the previous chapter, that we have reasons to be egalitarians, as opposed to prioritarians, with regard to the distribution of biomedical human enhancement.

I. What Is Human Enhancement?

Let me begin with the term "biomedical" with which I qualified "human enhancement" earlier. Aggressive piano lessons and a diet rich in potassium could lead to the enhancement of normal human capabilities and features, but they are not biomedical means. The qualifier "biomedical" thus signifies that I restrict my discussion to enhancement of human capabilities through biomedical means only. These include genetic, surgical (I include here surgery to implant *mechanical* devices, say a silicon chip), and chemotherapeutic means. I bracket the discussion in this way not because luck egalitarians see some morally relevant difference between biomedical and nonbiomedical means of enhancement (they don't), but simply for the purposes of keeping the discussion within the more strict confines of health policy.

What, then, is "human enhancement"? The use of this term assumes, not without controversy,[3] that it is possible to identify a level of perfectly healthy biological functioning of the human body (or any other organism for that matter). We may follow Daniels (and others) and term this level as "normal species functioning."[4] That level of functioning represents what it is for humans to be perfectly (that is, 100 percent) healthy. To function below that level of health—to posses less than 100 percent of health, as it were—is to have a health deficit (or a pathology). To function any better than that level of full health as a result of deliberate intervention would count as being enhanced. Obviously, what precisely constitutes that level of 100 percent of health is debatable even among physicians and biologists. But for our purposes the term itself should be clear enough.

Let me offer five points of clarification on "normal species functioning" and on "human enhancement" in an attempt to establish the coherence of the treatment/enhancement distinction and set the stage for the discussion on justice in the sections to follow. First, "normal species functioning" does not represent some *average* human health. Instead, the term signifies what it is for the human body, and for each of its organs and faculties, to function properly, that is, without illness or trauma. Note, for example, that it is all too normal for any organism, including the human organism, to age and die. Thus, normal, non-premature aging is not a health deficit on this reading.

Second, "normal species functioning," and thus "being healthy," refers to health narrowly understood, and not to the broader notion of "physical condition." Two individuals may both be 100 percent healthy, yet one of them may be in a better shape than the other, for whatever reason (perhaps because she exercises more, maintains an even better diet, or simply has better genes).

Third, whether or not an intervention counts as enhancement would depend on what it does to the particular individual in question. This point has two main implications. First, it is not a necessary condition of enhancement that it produce features or functionings that other, unenhanced human beings do not possess. Being extended from 7 feet to 9 feet in height constitutes an enhancement, but so is, under certain conditions, being extended from 6 feet to 7 feet. If my growth is perfectly healthy and normal, an intervention that extends me from 6 feet to 7 feet would count as an enhancement. Thus, a necessary condition for enhancement is that prior to it the particular body in question functions normally, and, in the example above, that none of the corporal components responsible for growth are malfunctioning. The second implication of the person-relativity of enhancement is this. A certain intervention can under some circumstances count as treatment, but under different circumstances count as enhancement. An often used example in this context is Ritalin, which can be used to treat, but can also be used on normally functioning individuals to enhance their cognitive capacities and improve their concentration during exams, say.[5]

Fourth, I distinguished human enhancement as a procedure that is aimed at enhancing normal features from one that aims at treating a health deficit.

But of course, it may well happen that a certain medical procedure aims at treating a health deficit and yet ends up being so effective that it not only eliminates that individual's health deficit, but also boosts that particular faculty beyond the level of normal species functioning.[6] Thus, the explicit intention to enhance is not a necessary condition here. Nevertheless, in my discussion below I shall restrict myself to intentional enhancement only.

Finally, it ought to be plain enough that having a health deficit is not, strictly speaking, the same as "being ill" or "requiring medical attention." A person suffering from hemophilia, say, may not, as such, be in need of medical attention so long as he never bleeds. But even if he succeeds in avoiding bleeding throughout his life, we would not want to say that he enjoys normal species functioning, or has no health deficit. Instead, "health deficit" ought to be interpreted to include also "abnormal susceptibility to illness." Obvious examples include immune deficiency diseases and allergies. In all these cases the individual has a particular condition that makes her susceptible, in rates significantly higher than normal, to incur some loss of functioning. So cases of susceptibility to illnesses that are not part of normal functioning, say AIDS, are clear cases of health deficits. In contrast, many other cases of susceptibility to illnesses *are* part of normal functioning (currently, at least). Think, for example, of the susceptibility to catch a cold, or to get a burn if you put your hand in the fire. These susceptibilities for illness and injury cannot be characterized as "health deficits," for they do not represent departures from normal species functioning. (To stress, having a cold *is* a health deficit; having the susceptibility to catch a cold is not. Correspondingly, having a cold is not part of normal species functioning, and so is, crucially, having *immunity* from colds.) Accordingly, vaccinations for common colds or, on the other hand, some future genetic treatment that would allow you to put your naked hand in the fire and not get burned are clear cases of enhancements.[7]

Having clarified what I mean by human enhancement, let me now turn to sketch the Rawlsian position on human enhancement as it is put forward by Daniels.

II. The Treatment vs. Enhancement Distinction

Daniels's "Normal Function" View

In chapter 2 I questioned the ability of Rawls's fair equality of opportunity principle (FEOP), as developed by Daniels, to provide an account of the just distribution of health care. The "just distribution of health care" was short, of course, for the "just distribution of treatment of deficits to full health." Now we turn to Daniels's approach to enhancement of full health,[8] an approach that is modeled on that same principle, and compare it with the way in which the luck egalitarian approach of leveling brute luck inequalities handles the issue. The main difference between the two approaches, we shall shortly see, is that Daniels's restricts society's obligation to fund treatment of deficits to full health, and argues that there is no obligation to fund enhancement of normal human functioning. For luck egalitarians, on the other hand, the distinction between treatment and enhancement is, for the most part, morally irrelevant (with an exception to be discussed in section IV). More accurately, perhaps, for luck egalitarians the treatment/enhancement distinction does not bear on the *currency* of justice in health (whereas it might bear on its *pattern*). In short, while on the luck egalitarian view a just health policy ought to cover both treatments and enhancements, on Daniels's account society's obligation is, by and large,[9] restricted to the former.

Daniels's position on enhancement is based on his "normal function" view. We ought to be familiar with that view from our discussion in chapter 2. On that view, it is a requirement of justice that society guarantee its members' ability to compete as equals "in all spheres of social life,"[10] and for jobs and careers in particular. To equalize individuals' starting points in the pursuit of their respective life plans, society is obligated to keep its members functioning as close to full health as possible. Thus, the commitment to equal opportunities implies restoring individuals to full health (as much as is medically possible), so that they can compete for jobs and careers from a level playing field (at least so far as their health is concerned). Daniels thus concludes that society is obligated to bring individuals only up to the level of normal species functioning, or in other words, to full health.[11]

Daniels, thus, rejects extending society's duties of justice from treatment to enhancement, and holds that the treatment/enhancement distinction has important implications for our duties with regard to just health. Notice that on Daniels's view the treatment/enhancement distinction has implications for our duties of justice because of the instrumental effect that normal functioning has for equality of opportunity. It is therefore important not to impute to Daniels the much stronger view according to which the treatment/enhancement divide has some intrinsic, metaphysical importance as representing the difference between what is "normal" and what is not. Such a view may yield an opposition to enhancement as such, based on the grounds that it is an affront to human dignity,[12] that it undermines social solidarity,[13] or that it undermines individual autonomy.[14] This opposition to enhancement as such is not Daniels's position. He opposes public funding for enhancement not because he thinks it is wrong to enhance, but because he thinks there is no duty of justice for society to provide its members with the benefits of enhancement. On the other hand, and as I mentioned earlier, it is possible to reject Daniels's position by rejecting the plausibility of the very distinction between treatments and enhancements.[15] That is not my view either. Rather, I accept Daniels's premise (against John Harris) that there is a valid distinction between treatment and enhancement, and I also agree with him that this distinction does not carry a metaphysical significance that ought to prevent us from allowing enhancements. My disagreement with him is therefore limited to the issue of whether or not society has an obligation to fund enhancements.

Let me first offer an internal critique of Daniels's position before moving on to contrast it with the luck egalitarian position. The point is this. It is not clear how the commitment to equality of opportunity leads, in Daniels's account, to affirming the relevance of the treatment/enhancement distinction to distributive justice. Suppose members of a certain segment (perhaps an affluent one) of the population obtain for themselves and their offspring, through their own financial means, some benefits of genetic enhancement, say IQ enhancement. This, we said, is not something that Daniels would oppose on some independent moral grounds (solidarity, autonomy). Now such a development would surely undermine equality of opportunity in that society, even on a Rawlsian account. The rich, and now also intelligent, would now have better qualifications with which to compete in the job market. Surely an account devoted to equality of opportunity for careers would require correcting that turn of events. It is therefore unclear how committed a Rawlsian needs to be to the treatment/enhancement distinction. Rawlsians would typically respond by saying that society's obligation is to bring all individuals up to full health, so as to allow them to compete as equals. But given recent advancements in biotechnology, it is easy to see that this is far from sufficient in guaranteeing an equal starting point in the competition for jobs and careers. One thing Rawlsians could say here is that just as in sports artificial enhancers such as steroids are banned in the name of equality of opportunity, so in life more generally enhancements ought to be banned. But given the various benefits of enhancement, both medical (a future vaccination for cancer) and nonmedical (enhanced memory), it is unlikely that Rawlsians would opt for this strategy of banning all enhancements. Once Rawlsians reject the policy of banning enhancements wholesale, it is difficult to see how they can avoid public funding for enhancements for those who cannot otherwise afford them, given their commitment to equality of opportunity.

Rawls's concern for equality of opportunity (as distinct from whatever other concerns Daniels might have) need not commit one, then, to affirming the treatment/enhancement distinction. Setting that internal critique aside, let me now present the luck egalitarian view on enhancement, and try and demonstrate how it is superior to the "normal function" view just reviewed.

The Luck Egalitarian View

We already said that in difference to Daniels's position, the luck egalitarian concern with regard to health policy is not exhausted by the instrumental impact of medical treatment on people's ability to compete for jobs (or even to pursue their life plans more broadly understood). To remind ourselves, luck egalitarians speak of a justice-based duty to eliminate (and alternatively, compensate for) disadvantaging conditions for which individuals are not responsible. A just health policy, according to the luck egalitarian view, requires society to try and rectify any health-related disadvantaging condition that the individual could not have reasonably avoided. Thus, according to the luck egalitarian view, society ought to fund biomedical treatment for any condition that:

1. is disadvantageous;
2. could be fixed by biomedical intervention;
3. it would be unreasonable to expect the individual to avoid.

It is clear from this formulation that on the luck egalitarian account it does not matter whether that particular medical condition is characterized as a health deficit, i.e., a pathology, or as an enhancement of normal human capabilities. Consider the following often-used example. Suppose we are presented with two individuals of equally short stature. For one the shortness is the result of having short parents, whereas the other individual's shortness is the result of a deficient growth hormone.[16] On Daniels's own admission, his "normal function" view has difficulty in coping with cases of this sort.[17] His position restricts us to offering treatment only to the latter person (which is the case of treatment of health deficit), but not to the *equally short* person whose shortness is the result of having short parents (i.e., the case of genetic enhancement).[18] This clearly seems arbitrary and problematic.

Now it might be suggested that there is nothing counterintuitive in the way the "normal function" view interprets this case. For, arguably, the reason Daniels would treat these two individuals differently is simply the fact that they suffer two different conditions. In the latter case what we treat is shortness as such, whereas in the former case what we treat is the growth hormone deficiency (and not shortness as such). It is therefore unproblematic to treat these two different cases differently.[19] While there is something true in that observation, the point ultimately only has a rhetorical effect. To see this, it is useful noting that the reason the first patient has approached us is *not* her suffering the hormone deficiency. For, if the deficiency had not caused the short stature (or any other disadvantageous trait for that matter), she would not have approached us for intervention in the first place. Nor, I think, would there be any justification for treating the growth hormone deficiency (even on Daniels's opportunity view) had it not resulted in the short stature or any other disadvantageous feature or loss of function.

Consider, in contrast, how the luck egalitarian view approaches such a case. If short stature is a disadvantageous feature in one's particular society,[20] luck egalitarians would intervene and correct for shortness, whatever its cause might be (assuming, of course, that the shortness wasn't in some way the individual's fault). Thus, the luck egalitarian view recommends treating the two short individuals in exactly the same way, regardless of the fact that for one the intervention would constitute enhancement whereas for the other it would constitute treatment. The luck egalitarian position, at least on this occasion, appears to yield a result that is more plausible, it seems to me.[21]

The luck egalitarian view of the moral irrelevance of the treatment/ enhancement distinction copes well not only with exceptional cases (such as the short stature example) but also with more mundane ones. We may point out that health care systems ordinarily do treat medical conditions that cannot be properly categorized as deficits to normal human functioning, that is, as pathologies. Pregnancy, labor, and menstruation, for example, are not illnesses but rather part of the normal functioning of the (female) body. (Notice that someone subscribing to Daniels's view [but not, I think, Daniels himself] might object already at this point, saying that all these conditions are *not* part of the normal functioning of the *species*, for they only afflict women. But of course, saying so would also commit him to the implausible view that ovarian or testicular cancer is also not a departure from normal species functioning.[22]) Yet, we normally do monitor women during their pregnancy, we offer women who are in labor the choice of being hospitalized, and we provide painkillers during menstruation. Now admittedly, part of the reason for doing so, especially in the cases of pregnancy and labor, is the concern to prevent complications that could be quite dangerous for both mother and child. Yet, as the case of menstruation demonstrates, I think, we would have offered medical care to women during pregnancy and labor even if it weren't for those complications. Some aspects of these conditions are simply unpleasant and painful even though they do not constitute pathologies.[23] Thus, intuitively, we should offer medical care in all those cases, as we normally actually do.

Now, on the luck egalitarian view, observe, all of the unpleasant and painful aspects of these conditions are clearly undesirable and disadvantageous conditions that the person, at least in the case of menstruation, is not responsible for. (As for pregnancy and labor, admittedly in most cases women *are* responsible for getting pregnant and giving birth. Arguably, then, luck egalitarians are committed to the absurd view that women who intentionally get pregnant do not deserve medical care. But as I argued in chapter 1 and in my formulation earlier in this section, the luck egalitarian principle speaks of neutralizing undesirable conditions that it would be *unreasonable to expect the individual to avoid*. It seems to me that most of us would agree that it is unreasonable, to say the least, to expect women as a rule to not get pregnant.) The luck egalitarian reading, then, seems to conform to our intuition that certain conditions call for publicly funded medical assistance, even though these conditions cannot be characterized as deficits to full normal human functioning.[24]

Of course, Daniels could always (and probably would) justify medical care in the cases of pregnancy, labor, and menstruation on grounds other than his "normal function" view, and thus other than justice. He could justify the coverage of such treatment by referring to the value of compassion and ridding individuals of unnecessary pain. As such, he is in no weaker position than is the luck egalitarian who justifies treating the imprudent patient on similar grounds (recall our reference to basic needs in chapters 4 and 5).[25] There is still a difference between the two cases, however: Daniels's denial of justice-based treatment on these occasions (pregnancy, labor, and menstruation) appears arbitrary (and thus counterintuitive), whereas the luck egalitarian denial of justice-based treatment for imprudent patients does not. Denying free treatment to the imprudent may be harsh, but it is not necessarily unjust. In contrast, denying free treatment to women in labor merely because their condition does not count as a health deficit is not only harsh but also unjust.

Here is another "mundane" example that Daniels's "normal function" view has a hard time explaining. Vaccination for polio, measles, mumps, rubella, and common colds are all intended to boost our immune system and protect us from conditions that it is part of our normal function to be susceptible to. As I said in the previous section, suffering from polio *is* a departure from normal species functioning, but being susceptible to it is not. It is, in fact, *being immune* to polio that represents a departure from normal species functioning. Vaccination against polio thus constitutes enhancement. Daniels's "normal function" view therefore fails to provide society with a justice-based reason to provide the individual with such vaccinations.[26] Recently, Daniels has attempted a reply to this criticism, saying that such vaccinations do, after all, constitute treatment rather than enhancement because "anything to do with maintaining normal function falls under the scope of 'treatment' as opposed to enhancement."[27] But it ought to be plain enough by now that this response is of not much use here. For, on that understanding of "treatment," the futuristic genetic intervention I described earlier, the one that would allow us to roast our hands in the fire without ever getting a burn, would fall under the category of treatment rather than enhancement. But that seems false.

Compared with Daniels's "normal function" view, the luck egalitarian position on the treatment/enhancement distinction seems to yield judgments that cohere better with our intuitions about justice in health. Still, the luck egalitarian approach to the distribution of enhancements has certain aspects that may seem problematic, and that I wish to address now.

III. "Fair" Skin and Other Potential Objections

Let me present some counterexamples whereby the luck egalitarian disregard for the treatment/enhancement distinction seems, at least initially, counterintuitive. Take the following example, put forward by Daniels. Many health care systems cover reconstructive breast surgery following mastectomy. At the same time, we do not normally think that health care systems ought to cover plastic surgery for women who feel that their life would improve if their breasts were made larger or smaller.[28] The former is a clear case of treating a deficit to full health, whereas the latter is a case of enhancement of normal human functioning (or features, for that matter). Daniels's normal function view copes well with such an example. It says that we ought to cover the restoration of normal functioning and provide reconstructive plastic surgery, but that we do not have an obligation to cover surgery in the latter case, for there is no deficit to normal functioning involved. The luck egalitarian view, on the other hand, does not cohere so well with our intuitions here. Both conditions are a matter of bad brute luck: women are (generally) no more responsible for breast cancer than they are for the size of their breasts.[29] Thus, the luck egalitarian view recommends covering plastic surgery in both cases. On this particular occasion, then, the luck egalitarian view appears, at least initially, to commit us to a somewhat less plausible result (compared to Daniels's view).

Notice however that it is becoming less and less rare for public health care systems to include, or to contemplate including, surgery for breast reduction (admittedly, not yet for enlargement) in their public coverage. If the size of one's breasts is truly a source of physical pain, but also, crucially, of embarrassment and low self-esteem, and is, moreover, not something the person is responsible for, it does not seem implausible that a public health care system should cover this procedure.[30] To be sure, we may still feel more strongly in favor of reconstructive surgery than we do about breast reduction. But the luck egalitarian may yet be able to provide an explanation that would successfully account for the different intuitions we have regarding these two cases. We may reasonably say, for example, that the difference between the two cases consists primarily in the fact that the loss of a breast is almost always much worse than having intact breasts that are either "too small" or "too large." Another difference between the two cases concerns moral hazard. Cases of mastectomy or loss of a breast due to trauma are not simply rarer than those of women's dissatisfaction with the size of their breasts. Rather, it is plausible to assume that if surgery were to be available to all free of charge, then many more women would opt to change the size of their breasts who would otherwise not have, compared to the percentage of victims of mastectomy who would not apply for surgery if it were not free. In short, there are many more gray areas with regard to requests for breast enlargement or reduction than there are with regard to reconstructive surgery, and thus the former is more susceptible to moral hazard than is the latter.[31] (By "moral hazard" I simply mean changing of one's preferences due to the availability of free coverage.) In sum, on the luck egalitarian reading, both cases, having lost a breast and having breasts of the "wrong" size, are a matter of bad brute luck. As such, society has an obligation to fund surgery in both cases. Yet, luck egalitarians can also identify important differences between the cases, differences that make treating the former case, for both practical and moral reasons, a more urgent matter. Thus, given budgetary constraints in health policy as well as in other areas of policy, it is likely that on the luck egalitarian reading reconstructive surgery would have priority over cosmetic surgery.[32]

One could think of other, perhaps even more challenging, counterexamples for the luck egalitarian view. Skin color, one's sex, and even (as mentioned in chapter 7) the inability of men to become pregnant and give birth are all a matter of brute luck. These conditions could also be described as a matter of *bad* brute luck. Consider, first, dark skin, which is obviously a matter of brute luck.[33] If it is also a disadvantageous feature, then on the luck egalitarian reading, society ought to fund operations to lighten skin color for any dark-skinned individual who asks for it. Likewise, the luck egalitarian view recommends funding sex change operations for anyone who thinks the male or female body they were born with is an unfortunate mistake on the part of God or Nature; it constitutes a disadvantage to have a body of the wrong sex when most other people are able to enjoy a body of the correct sex. And, if some men really wanted to, we ought to make it possible for them to get pregnant, or alternatively compensate them for their inability to do so.[34]

All of these conditions could be characterized as matters of bad brute luck. As such, the luck egalitarian view seems to recommend publicly funded medical care for all these conditions, which may seem counterintuitive.

In reply, notice that luck egalitarian justice calls for leveling brute luck inequalities. *Eliminating* the condition that constitutes bad brute luck is not necessarily the most effective way of leveling the inequality in question. Sometimes the best way to level brute luck inequalities is to alter certain aspects of the social structure so that the condition no longer represents a disadvantage. In the example of dark skin it is probably the case that the best means of reversing the bad luck in question is to make sure that dark-skinned individuals can enjoy life prospects and opportunities as good as those of fair-skinned individuals. That seems like the obvious way of rectifying the bad brute luck faced by African-Americans, say, and would therefore be the course of action recommended by luck egalitarians. Perhaps more importantly, changing the stigma rather than the skin color would be fairer for those blacks who actually prefer to retain their original skin color, with which their identity might be bound up. If there were a wholesale policy of converting the majority of blacks into whites (rather than getting rid of the stigma), then the position of these minority blacks would probably become more precarious. The luck egalitarian would therefore not opt automatically for operating on people's skin color.

But suppose that even after we altered society and made it color-blind, individuals still had reasonable grounds to prefer a skin color different than their own. Presumably, the luck egalitarian would still be committed then to funding the operation. But would that be so counterintuitive? John Harris discusses, in a different context, an example that may be of use here. Suppose it turned out to be the case that due to rising levels of UV radiation, courtesy of our depleting ozone layer, dark skin proved better in reducing the risk of skin cancer. And suppose that skin change operations proved medically possible, safe, and inexpensive. Surely then we would have a good reason to publicly fund that enhancement and surgically darken skin color for those who want it.[35] If this seems plausible, then it is the case that there is nothing wrong with public funding for skin-color change as such. And if that is the case, the luck egalitarian recommendation for funding operations for those with disadvantageous skin color ceases to appear so counterintuitive. The same is true for sex change. If that condition is genuinely undesirable, a complete theory of justice in enhancement would recommend funding sex-change operations (as Cuba has in fact recently done).[36] And, it is not so difficult to imagine the same being implemented with regard to male pregnancy should that prove medically possible, safe, and inexpensive. Again, given budgetary constraints these medical procedures may not be very high on our health agenda, but that does not mean that funding them is not a requirement of justice.

IV. Equality or Priority in Enhancement?

My aim in this chapter so far has been to extend the currency of justice in health from health deficits to enhanced health. Or, in other words, I sought to establish society's obligation to provide and fund biomedical enhancement for its members. But what ought we to do when it is not possible to offer the same extent of enhancement to everyone in society? Suppose that enhancement can benefit some more than others. Or suppose that due to limited resources it is only possible to enhance some but not others. Ought we to allow, and moreover fund, enhancement nevertheless? Is it right to enhance some individuals at the cost of exacerbating inequality in health—inequality, that is, between the health of the enhanced and the health of the unenhanced?

To get a hold of the dilemma presented by these questions, recall our discussion of health inequalities in the previous chapter. Philosophers almost unanimously agree that to level down health is wrong. On the other hand, few other philosophers (e.g., Larry Temkin) think that while it is wrong, all things considered, to level down health, it is nevertheless good at least *in one respect*.[37] In the previous chapter I tried to distinguish the discussion of the intrinsic value of equality in health from the one about its instrumental value, and I said that equality in health has little to no instrumental value. The conclusion I drew there was that inequality in health deficits is permissible. The case before us now is to examine whether the same judgment is true with regard to inequality in the distribution of enhanced health.[38]

It seems to me that there *is* indeed an important difference between inequalities in enhanced health (or enhancements) and inequalities in health deficits, and that, consequently, the distribution of enhancements *can* sometimes be instrumentally bad. To see why, suppose there exists a medical procedure that could extend the human life span of half of a given population to 200 years (or even beyond, to immortality). One need not subscribe to some of the recent doomsday scenarios about the "clash of civilizations" that would ensue between such superhumans (or "post-humans") and "the garden variety humans"[39] to see that the resulting inequality may have an instrumental disvalue. One consideration (although by no means a decisive one) against pursuing that medical procedure is that it might create a social division between what amounts to humans and superhumans. As such it would deprive members of both groups of the goods that stem from a sense of community and solidarity, as well as potentially harming the self-respect of those whose life span remained unenhanced. In other words, inequality in the distribution of human enhancement might have a negative instrumental value precisely because it potentially differentiates between "ordinary" humans and super-humans. Contrast this with medical interventions to restore normal life span and normal healthy functioning. Illness and disability are regular and famil-iar human features, and correspondingly, inequalities in health deficits do not normally amount to differences between humans and *sub*humans.[40] In the example above, I spoke of a population half of which has an enhanced life expectancy double the normal human life expectancy (say, 200 years). But in fact, as Harris points out, we have already reached a similar situation of such "parallel populations,"[41] where those living in Andorra live to be 83 whereas those in Zambia live only to 40. Whatever else is wrong in that story (and a lot in it *is* wrong, something about which I will say more in chapter 11), it does not seem that this disparity leads us to consider Andorrans to be super-humans and Zambians as subhumans. It seems therefore that there is a real difference in perception between inequalities in health deficits and inequali-ties in enhanced health. It is therefore the case that inequalities in the distri-bution of enhancements could potentially have a much stronger disvalue than do inequalities in health deficits. Consequently, while inequalities in the distribution of health deficits are not as such bad, inequalities in the distribu-tion of enhancements potentially could be.

Consider now a slightly more complicated case. Suppose the scenario presented to policy makers was one whereby genetic enhancements were of-fered, in the first phase, to those who could afford them, with the promise that within twenty years, say, those interventions that proved successful would become available to all. Surely, it would then be in everyone's interest to ac-cept such a course of action, even at the cost of the temporary inequality it would inevitably carry.[42] One thing to note here is that the unfairness of al-lowing the better off to use their superior wealth to purchase the benefits of enhancement might be offset with their bearing a disproportionally larger burden of acting as guinea pigs for these procedures. But in general, it seems to me that the just course of action, in this case, would depend on the balance between the harm represented in the temporary inequality, and the harm in waiting the twenty years (say) that it might take for the rest of society to catch up on that enhancement.[43] In any case, the injustice of the temporary in-equality would be much reduced if the identity of those who received the enhancement now would be determined by lot rather than by ability to pay.

What I have just said about the instrumental disvalue of inequality in enhancements may seem to contradict my earlier statement about the luck egalitarian disregard for the treatment/enhancement distinction. Earlier in this chapter I said that, as opposed to Rawlsians, luck egalitarians do not attach moral significance to the treatment/enhancement distinction, and are committed to funding both. But my point in this section regarding the justice in leveling down enhancements but not in leveling down normal health seems to suggest that the normal life span *does* have some moral significance. The key to resolving that apparent inconsistency lies in the different role the treatment/enhancement distinction is called upon to perform here. In the previous two sections I inquired whether that distinction ought to play a role in determining the *currency* of justice in health, and have ruled against it. In this current section, in contrast, I examined the potential role the distinction might play in the *pattern* of justice in health. And upon reflection it becomes clear that the treatment/enhancement distinction performs different work in the two respective arguments. The reason we ought to attach moral significance to the current[44] level of normal species functioning (as it pertains to the pattern of distribution) is that it is a fact of life that affects people's perception of themselves and others. What we perceive to be the normal species functioning and the normal life span may affect how we form and maintain our self-respect, and as such carries certain moral consequences. In other words, the fact that the normal life span is morally arbitrary does not prevent it from generating expectations, self-perceptions, and value judgments. There is nothing unusual about that. It is arbitrary, from a moral point of view, whether or not certain clothes are part of normal appearance in one's society. Yet the answer to that arbitrary question may carry moral implications: in Adam Smith's example that was mentioned earlier, if in our society one is not to be seen in public without a linen shirt, then the fact that I cannot afford to buy one is a fact that carries moral implications.[45] Morally arbitrary facts thus often do have important moral implications.[46] Now, when speaking about the value of equality in health I said that our self-respect is not normally harmed when some people are healthier than we are. But, crucially, our self-respect *may* be harmed, and our sense of community may weaken, when some people enjoy (some types of) enhanced human functionings that we do not. Normal species functioning, or at least the perception of it, acts as a ceiling that has some moral consequences. That is why it is not only permissible but actually mandatory to take the level of normal species functioning into account when evaluating the instrumental value of equality in the distribution of enhancements. Our earlier discussion of justifying public funding for enhancement, on the other hand, concerned the intrinsic value of equality, not its instrumental value. Thus, expectations about normal species functioning played no role in our evaluation of the fairness of public funding for enhancement.

Conclusion

A luck egalitarian account of justice in health does not stop at regulating the distribution of deficits to full normal health. Since that theory of justice is concerned with rectifying unchosen disadvantageous conditions, it sees no difference between treatment of deficits to normal health and enhancement of normal human functioning. Any medical condition that can reasonably be seen as a matter of bad brute luck is of concern to a luck-sensitive account of justice. The luck egalitarian account of justice in health offered in chapter 7 is thus extended here from the distribution of deficits to full health to the distribution of the benefits of enhancement of normal human functioning. That extension of the theory is done with one notable exception, though; while in the case of health deficits I offered (in chapter 8) a prioritarian approach, here I have defended an egalitarian one.

This concludes my account of luck egalitarian justice in health, and thus part II of the book. In the next and final part of the book I apply various aspects of the theory offered in the first two parts to the realm of social policy, and more particularly, to the issue of political borders. I want to inquire how luck egalitarian justice in health and health care applies within and beyond the traditional boundaries of the nation-state.

Part III

Health without Borders

10

■

Devolution of Health Care Services

Introduction

The first two parts of this book attempted to delineate a luck egalitarian account of justice in health care and then in health. In this last part of the book I intend to apply lessons from that account to the issue of political boundaries. In a world which, paradoxically, is increasingly both more globalized and more localized, political boundaries have important normative implications for almost any area of policy. Accordingly, this chapter deals with subnational boundaries, whereas the next and final chapter goes beyond national boundaries. In addition, mirroring the order of the first two parts of the book, the first of these last two chapters deals with health care, whereas the other deals with health.

This last part of the book, then, deals with the intersection of health and health care with the notion of political boundaries. To that intersection we should add a third ingredient, that of luck egalitarianism. That triple intersection would hopefully yield two interesting aspects of the theory of health, luck, and justice. The first aspect is that of communal responsibility for medical tastes and habits. It might be interesting to see what a luck-sensitive account of justice in health care has to offer on that matter. The second principled point to anticipate is this. Recall that in chapter 1 we characterized Rawlsian justice as political, and luck egalitarian justice as natural or "cosmic." That distinguishing feature of luck egalitarianism might have interesting implications for the way in which the theory conceives of our obligations toward the health of people who reside outside our state. First, though, let us examine the issue of health care delivered on a subnational level.

In chapter 5 we faced the challenge of providing a luck egalitarian defense of universal medical care. The discussion mentioned two aspects of universality, universality as the opposite of exclusivity, and universality as the inability to opt out (in-kind universality). A further, related, aspect of a public service worth mentioning in this respect is whether or not it is a unified one. In a unified system the same service is offered to everyone. Yet, unity is not a necessary condition of universality. A public service may be universal in its coverage, in both aspects of universality discussed above, and yet be fragmented. The quality of the service is the same across the citizenry, yet different subpopulations get different packages of service. In this chapter I want to argue that according to the account of justice developed here we ought to favor a unified system over one that is devolved.[1]

To understand the appeal of a devolved, yet still arguably universal, system, it may be useful to consider the following illustration. Suppose that Israeli Jews consume a greater share of the national health care budget than their proportion of the population (and proportionally more than the 20 percent-strong Arab minority in Israel). Suppose also, for the sake of argument, that the sole reason for this discrepancy in consumption of medical goods is that Jewish prospective parents ask for more fetal screenings per pregnancy than do their Arab counterparts. (Suppose these screenings are extra tests for intelligence and Down syndrome.) Supposing that the unequal demand is the product of choice alone, rather than of bad luck (i.e., a greater genetic susceptibility to Down syndrome),[2] this unequal consumption represents an unfair state of affairs.[3] What, then, should be done to rectify this apparent unfairness? How ought we to respond to the inequality in consumption of health care brought about by one group's expensive taste?

Broadly speaking, it seems that one of two strategies must be applied if the unfairness in question is to be tackled. One strategy is to allow one group to continue to consume a greater share of the medical resources while making its members pay the actual cost of their expensive taste. The other strategy is for the state to impose uniformity in the consumption of health care resources. (In our example, this would imply both actively encouraging Arabs to have as many screenings as Jews do [or at least increase their awareness of their entitlement to do so], and, more realistically, to restrict the Jewish population's access to these expensive screenings [or otherwise strike some balance between the two groups].) The former strategy could be carried out by allowing distinct linguistic or cultural communities to develop their own separate health care systems (on the condition, of course, that these communities constitute coherent geographical entities, admittedly a complicating factor in the Israeli context). The latter strategy could be carried out simply by denying some of citizens' medical preferences.

A prominent political philosopher, Philippe Van Parijs, has suggested recently that we ought to support the first strategy, and for two reasons.[4] First, to make individuals (and by derivation, the groups they belong to) pay the true cost of their choices is part of what justice requires.[5] Splitting the health care system along cultural lines would require each community to bear alone the burden of its members' medical preferences. I already rejected that "desert egalitarian" view in chapter 3, so will not address it again here. The second reason offered is the argument that this chapter is primarily concerned with.

Breaking up the system along group lines (be it cultural, linguistic, ethnic, or national)[6] would create subsystems, each of which serves its clients' needs more accurately. And, the more accurately a health care system (or subsystem) responds to medical needs, the more just it is (a premise I do not dispute). The assumption seems to be also that, in any event, dividing the health care system along group lines would not lead to a system that is any *less* just (than an existing unified one). It would be no less just because an identical transfer of resources across the communities would still take place, as each health care budget would still be funded through the federal (rather than a regional) tax basis.[7] This reform amounts to devolution of health care services. By "devolution" I mean a policy that keeps the responsibility of levying taxes with the national (or federal) government, while placing in the hands of regional government the authority to devise and administer services.[8] The crucial feature of this policy, for the purposes of our discussion, is that each region receives a per capita health care budget.

I wish, therefore, to examine whether or not justice requires, or even permits, the devolution of health care. More specifically, I ask whether it is the proper way for dealing with unequal consumption (across communities) of medical resources. Since my concern is with the impact of devolution on justice in health care (the next chapter will deal with health proper), I will bracket the following issues. First, for the sake of simplification, I will assume that to allocate health care resources justly is to allocate them according to medical need. Second, I shall also assume, for the sake of argument, that the more accurately the health care system responds to the medical needs of the population it serves, the more just it is. Third, I shall set aside considerations of global justice and assume, again for the sake of argument, that the relevant unit for evaluation of distributive justice is that of the nation-state (an assumption I shall then question in the next chapter). Finally, my concern with devolving health care services is restricted to issues of distributive justice. I therefore set aside reasons for devolution that are independent of distributive justice (such as considerations of cultural recognition, or considerations of efficiency, which are admittedly relevant ones).

I. The Case for Devolution

Devolution of public services means giving homogeneous communities greater control over the management of local affairs. Since homogeneous societies have relatively similar needs and tastes, it is easier in such societies to arrive at a more generous social insurance program.[9] Such a program insures against eventualities that most members of the community would agree are real risks, and it attends to needs that most would agree are genuine. The underlying thought here is that in homogeneous communities it is easier to arrive at a shared understanding of what constitutes a need. That is why it is sometimes thought that such societies are more likely to create and maintain generous systems of health care.[10] It is thus suggested that in culturally divided societies, health care systems should be broken up along regional lines (again, whenever cultural and geographic lines coincide). Van Parijs, a proponent of this position, states that the main justification for this reform is that

> keeping culturally different parts of a society together blocks the just institutionalization of more generous health care systems, while splitting a society along cultural lines would enable each part to justly develop its own distinct and more generous system. Yet, this shrinking of the health care package does not translate into a corresponding shrinking of the overall level of redistribution, as whatever is no longer redistributed in a targeted form is now to be redistributed to all, while whatever was redistributed in kind must now be redistributed in cash.[11]

According to this view, then, devolving health care systems along communal lines does not entail each community funding its own system. For, each system would still be funded through the federal budget, and hence the same extent of redistribution is maintained.[12] Given this assurance, and given that a devolved system serves needs more accurately than a unified system, distributive justice appears to be furthered by devolution.

This would seem to be a plausible solution to the problem of unequal cross-communal consumption.[13] Still, I would like to offer a counter-view. I would like to suggest that the alternative policy that the luck egalitarian reading of distributive justice recommends, namely, imposing a uniform pattern of consumption (of medical services) across society, might yet be more just. Such a policy may seem harsh and perhaps even authoritarian at first glance. Nevertheless, I want to suggest that distributive justice is better served by enforcing a unitary pattern of consumption across the citizenry, and keeping a unified health care system.

Let me quickly qualify that claim. I do not wish to make the case for a unified health care system at all costs. That would clearly not be advisable in cases where trust between the two (or more) communities breaks down irreparably. In other words, I do not inquire, in this chapter, after what Don Horowitz has termed "severely divided societies."[14] (I make here the plausible, if not entirely uncontroversial, assumption that Belgium and Israel [two of the countries I use as examples here], despite their respective intercommunal difficulties, do not count as *severely* divided, or as divided beyond repair.) It does not seem a good idea to try and impose, in such societies, a unitary health care system, and it is probably better to allow the different communities to separate (through devolution or even secession). In this, devolution acts just like any other form of divorce.[15] And just like divorce, devolution is not something to be encouraged or actively sought. Communities, like individuals, should, no doubt, be allowed to divorce each other. But other things being equal, there is no reason to encourage them to do so.[16] The argument below is restricted, therefore, to what we may call a functioning plurinational society.

II. How Devolution Upsets Distributive Justice

Bearing in mind, then, that our discussion is restricted to healthy, functioning, yet plurinational societies, I wish to outline several undesirable impacts that devolution of health care services has on distributive justice, and why we ought to retain a unified health care service. Let me begin by examining the assertion that a devolved system is at least as egalitarian as a unitary system. Those making this claim seem to assume that if funding for the devolved system remains federal, and that if taxes are still raised in a progressive way (i.e., graduated according to income) across the nation, then the system remains as egalitarian as a unitary health care system. But of course, how egalitarian a distributive scheme is is relative not only to how funds are raised, but also to how they are spent or distributed.[17] In a unitary health care system health care resources allocation is carried out (ideally) according to need. Under devolution, in contrast, allocation between regions is (merely) equal. That is to say, compared with fellow citizens who are members of the other ("rival") community (or communities), each citizen is, other things being equal, entitled to an equal share of the health care budget, compared to a needs-adjusted share under a unitary system. Let us see what that means.

A unitary health care system distributes goods and services across society according to medical need. That is, health care resources are distributed across the nation in accordance with the requirements of each local hospital, with equal weight given to the medical needs of all.[18] A hospital that, say, serves an area with an unusually high occurrence of kidney deficiency would accordingly get more dialysis machines. Devolution of the system means that within communities the need principle still reigns, but across communities (e.g., between Flanders and Wallonia), distribution will take place in accordance with the principle of *equal shares*. That is, the previously centralized health care budget is divided up and each regional health care authority receives a budget proportional to the size of its population. That distribution (of equal shares) is obviously less egalitarian than distribution according to need.[19]

To illustrate the anti-egalitarian effect of that reform, suppose a society of 10 individuals that is made up of two communities (A and B), each consisting of 5 individuals. Suppose each member of A has a medical need of 20 units per year, whereas each member of B has an annual need of only 10 units. The total health care budget of the society in question is 120 units. Under a unitary system, with resources distributed in proportion to need, members of A would receive 16 units (ending up at −4), whereas each member of B would receive 8 units (ending up at −2). Each citizen, independently of community membership, thus has ⅘ of her medical needs covered.[20] Under devolution, each community receives a budget proportional to its population, which in our simplified example translates into 60 units. If each community continues to distribute health care in proportion to need, each citizen would end up with 12 units. But now each member of A has only ⅗ of her annual needs met (compared to ⅘ under the unified system), whereas in group B, members now have all their needs met (with a spare budget, available, let us say, for other medical purposes).[21] A society that aims at equalizing needs (or the proportion of unmet needs) is therefore less egalitarian after devolution than before the reform, even when taxation remains in federal hands.[22]

Of course, distribution after such a reform would be more egalitarian than one under a more radical reform, that of entirely separate subsystems, funded by the separate tax base of each community[23] (assuming the two communities have nonidentical tax bases). Yet, the reform still makes for a system that is potentially less egalitarian than a unitary system, contrary to what its proponents may claim.

III. Ignoring Cultural Preferences in Health Care

Having shown how devolution upsets distributive justice, let me defend a proposal according to which it is better to ignore, rather than respond to, culturally driven differences in consumption of medical resources. I indicated earlier my agreement with the claim that the more accurate and authentic the perception of medical needs employed by the health care system in serving its population, the more just the health care system is (indeed I just used this very premise to show why a devolved system is less egalitarian than a unified one). But here we must be careful to distinguish *needs* from *preferences* (recall our discussion in chapter 4).[24] Accordingly, it is essential to ascertain when health care caters to needs and when it caters to preferences.

There is no reason to dispute that different social circumstances (including cultural circumstances) breed different medical needs.[25] For instance, a mining community is likely to have a slightly different set of medical needs than a fishing community. More to our immediate concern, culture itself may also breed different medical needs. Catholics and Protestants, for example, may have different medical needs following different patterns of socializing. The typical Catholic way of socializing may be centered on dining, while Protestants cannot begin socializing if no drinking (alcohol) takes place.[26] This cultural difference may have an important effect on the respective medical needs of the communities, with the latter requiring greater resources to deal with the effects of alcohol abuse, say.[27] But there may be further ways in which culture affects medical needs and, conversely, preferences. We may observe, then, the following differences in cases of demands for medical care that are affected by cultural membership:

1. Culturally *driven* medical needs—These are recognized medical needs, which individuals are at a greater likelihood to contract due to their cultural membership (e.g., alcohol abuse in a protestant society).

2. Culturally *aggravated needs*—In this case, the (recognized) medical condition is not necessarily induced by the cultural membership, but rather, represents a greater impairment due to cultural membership. In Nigeria, for example, speech impediment is considered more acute among Ibos because of the special importance of oratory skills in that culture.

3. Culturally *determined* needs—These are procedures that do not respond to a medical condition but that are considered necessary in that community, and are best performed by medical staff (e.g., male circumcision, female genital cutting, and certain types of cosmetic plastic surgery).

4. Culturally aggravated *preferences*—These are culturally driven uses of recognized medical procedures or services (e.g., preference for nursing care at home based on the cultural pattern of caring for one's parents, or preference for more fetal screenings based on the cultural significance of breeding "successful" offspring[28]).[29]

Consider the case of culturally driven medical needs (type I). Suppose our luck egalitarian health care system does not categorize alcohol abuse as purely voluntary and would thus treat such cases. Or suppose our hypothetical system treats alcohol abuse at least for those who are below the Roemerian mean for their social class.[30] Assuming that it would be undesirable to ask individuals to give up their cultural membership, ignoring the request for medical care here would then seem unfair.

It would also be unfair (assuming the same premise) to ignore the request for medical care in the case of culturally aggravated needs (type II).

Note that in this second case, the needs in question qualify as needs not, or not merely, because *members* recognize them as such (or recognize them as more *acute* needs), but because an outside observer is able to recognize them as such. Objectively speaking, unless these needs are met one would be unable to fully integrate into one's community. To elaborate the example mentioned earlier, due to the dominance of oratory skills in their culture,[31] Ibo members suffering from a speech impediment have a more urgent *need* for speech therapy, for the impediment hinders their inclusion in their community (to a higher-than-normal extent). Thus, these impediments represent a greater *disadvantage* when afflicting an Ibo than when afflicting other Nigerians. (In the same way, dyslexia may represent a lesser need, and therefore a lesser disadvantage, in an illiterate society.[32]) In this second category of culturally aggravated needs I also include cases where the aggravation refers to the type and, consequently, the cost of the treatment required. To illustrate, suppose a Jewish patient requires a heart valve, and suppose a pig's valve is both cheaper and safer to implant than that of a cow.[33] Here cultural membership leads to a choice of treatment (for a condition that represents an equal need cross-culturally) that is more expensive. On my account it would be unfair in this case to ask the patient to pay the cost of her cultural membership.

Types I and II represent cases of how culture determines differences in the severity of one's medical need (or in the urgency and cost of medical needs), and therefore, on my account, ought to be catered for.[34]

Third, consider the case of culturally *determined* needs. As we seek to judge all cases here on grounds of distributive justice alone, we must therefore set aside any non–distributive-based aversion we might have toward procedures such as female genital cutting. Suppose, then, a homogeneous society in which male circumcision (to use a less contentious practice) is an established practice throughout the society. It is plausible that in that community it would be difficult (for any male member) to lead an inclusive life without having been circumcised. Thus, although the procedure does not respond to a medical need,[35] it would still be *reasonable* to include circumcision in the publicly funded health care services. Although public funding in this case would be reasonable (assuming everyone in that society has an interest in that procedure, and assuming it is best performed by medical staff), it is nevertheless not a requirement of justice if it does not meet the pre-requirement of qualifying as a medical need. It is one thing for a homogeneous community to collectively provide a nonmedical treatment within its health care system. It is quite another to expect a health care system to attend to a nonmedical condition when it is not shared by all (or even all households, in the case of male circumcision). So although a homogeneous society may include these procedures in its public health plan, there is no requirement of justice that a health care system in a plurinational society do so. Crucially, the unitary health care system is not any less just for excluding this procedure, as it is not a medical one to begin with. We can therefore set aside cases of culturally driven needs that are not, in fact, *medical* needs.

Type IV demonstrates that a difference in culture can also breed different medical preferences that may only appear as needs. Recall the example we opened the discussion with, that of Jewish culture's emphasis on breeding successful offspring. This cultural emphasis does not generate a need for more fetal screenings, but simply a stronger (and in this case more expensive) preference. Consider the difference between the second and fourth types (that of culturally aggravated *needs* as opposed to culturally aggravated *preferences*). I noted earlier that culturally determined needs qualify as such not simply because members recognize them as needs, but because unless they are met one would be unable to fully integrate into one's own community. The relevant criterion for determining what counts as a need, then, is what an outside observer would identify as constituting a decent life in a certain community, and not (or not necessarily) what members of that community consider to constitute a decent life.[36] The subjective perception (even if shared by many) that one *needs* additional fetal screenings does not then qualify as a medical need. Rather, it is a medical taste (or preference). Whatever obligation there is to meet preferences, it is, in any case, a much weaker one compared with the obligation we have to meet medical needs.[37]

The account of justice in health care offered here thus holds individuals responsible for their culturally aggravated medical *preferences*, but not for their culturally determined medical *needs*. While it may be right to hold individuals responsible for certain aspects of their own culture, it is at the same time unfair to ask them to pay the full price of their cultural membership. The crucial distinction, I proposed, is between aspects of the culture that determine what constitutes a decent life in that community, and aspects of the culture that affect *what the individual may see* as constituting a decent life in that community. Just health care, at least on the luck egalitarian reading, ought to cater only for the former.

I should say that Daniels's account also successfully explains the intuition that just health care ought to cater for culturally aggravated needs. Daniels allows for health care to be socially relative because his account is based on the impact of health needs on one's range of opportunities. A certain medical condition may have a different impact on one's opportunities depending on the type of society one lives in (think again of dyslexia in an illiterate society). A national health care system catering for two communities, one of which is more literary than the other, would, on Daniels's as well as on my account, reflect this difference and not ignore it. But notice the difference between my account and Daniels's. His account is socially relative in how culture impacts *opportunity*, and derivatively, medical care. My account is socially relative in how culture impacts *disadvantage*, and derivatively, medical care. The account offered here is thus broader than Daniels's. To use an example mentioned earlier, the luck egalitarian would be sensitive to the fact that the Ibo person's speech impediment is graver given her particular society and culture even when that cultural difference does not affect her opportunity to pursue her life plan but merely disadvantages her, say in terms of socializing opportunities.

IV. How Devolution Weakens Social Solidarity

It follows from the preceding discussion that ignoring cultural differences in medical preferences is not as harsh as it initially appears, and so, it follows, is maintaining a unified health care system in a plurinational society.[38] I now want to establish some further reasons for pursuing the latter policy, and for imposing uniformity in the way that health care goods are to be consumed across society. If I am right, it would follow that health care providers should give the same treatment (that is, when the medical need is equal) to patients with expensive cultural preferences and to those with cheaper cultural preferences (or at least, ignore a discrepancy in preferences), and resist calls for devolution, even when these patients form two (or more) coherent geographic communities.

Besides the direct impact on distributive justice discussed in the past two sections, we may have two further reasons for retaining a unified health care system rather than opting for a devolved one. First, separating the systems, even while funding them from the common federal budget, would mean that from now on the wealthier community (say, the Flemish in the case of Belgium) has nothing to gain from an increase in the poorer community's health care budget; it (the wealthier community) can only lose from such an increase. This breaking up of the unitary system leaves each community to scrap for its own health care budget, and leaves the poorer community more exposed to future budget slashing.[39] As a consequence of devolution, then, the more affluent (and, as it often happens, the healthier) community has an interest in reducing the federal health care budget.

A second reason for resisting devolution addresses its potentially harmful effects on social, intercommunal solidarity. I discussed earlier how devolution implies a move from distribution according to medical need to distribution of equal shares. The previously needs-based national health care budget becomes, at the intercommunal level, a per capita budget, based on the principle of equal shares. We know from experiments in social psychology that a shift from distribution according to need to distribution of equal shares weakens solidarity in the group in question.[40] Devolution of health care is a shift from allocating according to need to allocating equal bundles of resources (in disregard of unequal need). As such, devolution potentially undermines solidarity across society. Since social solidarity is considered to be significant in the pursuit of distributive justice,[41] weakening social solidarity across communities would appear detrimental to the pursuit of distributive justice across society.

Consider the following two potential objections to this solidarity argument for resisting devolution.[42] First, it may be argued that devolution does not, in fact, imply switching to equal distribution between regions. There is no reason to suppose that in devolving the health care system, so the objection runs, the discrepancy in needs between communities would be excluded when drawing up the devolved national health care budget. The need principle, in other words, can be enshrined in the very structure of the devolved system. Suppose it is acknowledged that one community has greater medical needs than the other (as is the case in Belgium).[43] It could be decided then that, upon devolution, for every Euro spent on a Flemish hospital, for example, a Walloon hospital would receive 1.05 Euros.[44] Conceivably then, the disparity of health needs between communities could be recognized and mirrored in the respective regional health budgets even *after* devolution. I see two problems here, though: a practical one and one of principle. First, the practical problem (quite apart from the inflexibility of adopting such a formula)[45] is that the wealthier community would have an incentive to slash the disparity of funding in the future, and bring the situation back to equal per capita funding. Acting on such an incentive is a well-documented phenomenon in social policy,[46] and there is no reason to think that it would not occur also between rich and poor communities post-devolution. Second, and perhaps more importantly, a devolved health care system that reflects unequal needs would defeat one of the purposes of devolution, namely dealing with the resentment by members of the wealthy community of what they regard as the "expensive taste" cultivated by members of the poorer one. Why adopt the reform if it enshrines the "unfairness" of the old system? It appears that distribution according to need *across* communities is unlikely after devolution, or at the very least, is unlikely to be stable.[47]

A second potential objection to the suggestion that devolution undermines social solidarity is that a unified health care system in a plurinational society does not, in fact, distribute goods according to the need principle, the reason being that it is difficult, to begin with, to assess what counts as a medical need in such a society (since individuals belonging to different communities have such different conceptions of need). It would follow, then, that the non-devolved (i.e., retained) health care system allocates according to a *flawed* conception of need (or at least, according to a conception of need that does not adequately represent needs *in the whole of* society). Given this account, devolution is the only way to arrive at a genuine distribution according to need. If the claim is correct, then devolution does preserve social solidarity, contrary to what I have established so far. In response, suppose it is true that in plurinational societies it is impossible to arrive at an agreement on what counts as a need.[48] Even in such a case, the central authority still distributes according to the need principle, albeit while having, arguably, a flawed idea of what those needs really are. What is crucial here, as far as the effect on solidarity is concerned, is that members of society perceive the allocation to be conducted according to the principle of need, regardless of what the conception of need actually encompasses.[49] And, a shift from distribution according to need—even when everyone agrees that the particular picture of needs is distorted—to distributing equal shares results in weakened solidarity.

V. Imposing a Uniform Pattern of Consumption

I have argued in the last section that devolution weakens social solidarity across communities, which in turn is detrimental to distributive justice across society. Supporters of devolution, however, may question whether what I have established so far ought to count against devolution. They may argue that distributive justice *across* the communities should be traded off for greater distributive justice (and greater solidarity) *within* those communities. It is not clear, however, that greater justice across the communities comes at the expense of justice within the communities. It may be true that the health care system could be made somewhat more generous if it is allowed to devolve. And it is also plausible to assume that the more generous a system is,[50] the more likely it is to be just. Yet, the correlation between generosity and justness is not a direct one. The extent of redistribution achieved by a generous distributive scheme depends on the extent of the initial inequality. The more equal the starting point (and in other words, the more socioeconomically homogeneous, the society is), the weaker the distributive effect of the system's generosity. And, since the point of devolution is to search for evermore homogeneous communities, the effect of devolution on justice, even *within* those communities, is therefore rather limited.

Recall that our starting point was the suggestion that the more culturally diverse a society is, the more meager the agreed-upon health care package.[51] Yet things may now be put in perspective. Even allowing for the differing preferences that supporters of devolution may mistake for needs, the overall estimated contribution of the reform they propose is negligible. Consider this. Let us term the health care package to which everyone is entitled in a devolved system (regardless of cultural membership) as the "thin" package, and refer to the culturally specific health care package as a "thick" one. The size of the "thin" health care package is overwhelmingly (and confusingly)[52] "thicker" (in range of services, but mainly in its overall cost) than the "thick" package. The thin package includes all those services and medical treatments that most citizens consider to be basic (everything from mental counseling to cancer treatment). The "thick" package, in contrast, consists, by definition, of all those differing preferences that people may find it difficult to agree on as requiring public funding (anything from rhinoplasty to additional fetal screenings). One can easily see that the cost of any "thick" package is likely to be negligible compared to that of any "thin" package. If that is the case, the argument for devolution loses much of its urgency (though admittedly not its coherence).[53]

Whereas the benefit of devolution to intra-communal distributive justice is rather limited, the cost to short-term and long-term intercommunal distributive justice is potentially substantial. In the short-term, distribution, we saw, becomes less egalitarian (moving from "to each according to her needs" to "to each an equal share"). And in the long term, the upset to distributive justice is likely to be no less substantial. First, devolution risks a consequent shrinkage of the overall health care budget (due to "un-packing" the better-off and worse-off communities from one another).[54] Second, devolution weakens cross-communal solidarity, which in turn undermines the prospects of cross-communal distributive justice.

Devolution thus upsets distributive justice on two accounts. In the short term it shifts the principle of distribution from need to equality, and in the long term it undermines social solidarity across the communities. This conclusion points us back to the strategy of ignoring culturally driven medical preferences, and imposing a more or less uniform pattern of consumption of medical services. But would that strategy be justified all things considered? We may be more willing to accept that it is if we think of the just operation of a health care system as depending not only on the actions of the providers (or in other words, on the pattern of distribution), but also on those of its consumers. Citizens ought to be encouraged to realize that the justness of a health care system depends also on their own manner of consumption.[55] In particular, patients need to be encouraged to act in a non-wasteful manner and to re-frain from cultivating expensive medical preferences.[56] That (as I showed in chapter 5) is something luck egalitarian health care might be particularly adept in.

Conclusion

I have argued that there are justice-based reasons for favoring a unified health care system over a devolved system. A devolved system is less egalitarian in the immediate term, and risks undermining social solidarity, which is crucial for the attainment of distributive justice in the longer term. These reasons, it seems to me, are sufficient in rejecting devolution of health care services and in imposing uniformity of consumption of medical services. It is not harsh (or disrespectful of cultural difference) to ask citizens to drop expensive cul-tural medical preferences. It is, in fact, obligatory to do so when it serves distributive justice.

11

■

Global Justice and National Responsibility for Health

Introduction

The moral issues concerning intercommunal differences in health pale in comparison to those concerning international disparities. It hardly needs pointing out that the inequality in the health of nations is vast: for example, people living in Zambia have an average life expectancy of 40.5 years, whereas those living in Japan can enjoy more than double the life expectancy of 82.3 years.[1] This inequality is no doubt disturbing. But the important question for us is whether it is also unjust. I want to employ the luck egalitarian perspective and inquire when, if ever, it is unjust for a population of one nation to have a lower healthy life expectancy than that of another. I hope to conclude with a set of necessary conditions under which global inequalities in health are *not* unjust. It will emerge that in today's world these conditions are far from being met, and therefore that we have grounds to consider much of global disparity in health to be unjust.

Obviously, there are a number of factors that underlie the huge discrepancy in the health of nations. Within those factors that are socially controllable, the epidemiological literature distinguishes socioeconomic factors from the more direct health factors, but no doubt there is a strong link between the two. Probably the most significant factor behind the disparity in the distribution of the global burden of disease is a nation's economic status. Health status seems for the most part to correlate with wealth (I shall point out a qualification later on). Nations that have some of the lowest healthy life expectancy (mostly sub-Saharan ones) tend also to be among the poorest nations on the globe. Low economic standing is of course also linked to push factors for emigration, which causes brain drain of medical staff in these countries, which in turn worsens the health of the population.[2] The socioeconomic factor also affects the more direct health factors explaining the disparity in health between North and South. Poor nations do not have the financial means to conduct medical research, and "Big Pharma" is less keen to conduct research on diseases afflicting the poor. This is evident from the fact that 90% of the global expenditures on medical research are on diseases that cause only 10% of the global burden of disease. This bias in medical research is also evident from the fact that out of 1,223 drugs developed between 1975 and 1997, only 13 were for tropical diseases.[3] Another direct factor accounting for the so much worse-off health state of developing countries is of course the prevalence of armed conflicts. Wars account for poor health in a variety of ways: they increase domestic spending on arms at the expense of public health, they bring on poverty, and of course they directly inflict death and injury on combatants and noncombatants alike. Finally, we could mention that poorer nations are likelier to resort to older technologies and industries, leading to greater risk of pollution and water contamination. There seems, therefore, to be a multitude of socially controllable factors, some global, some domestic, that affect a nation's health. Bearing this background in mind, I want to ask when, if ever, it is unjust for one nation to suffer lower healthy life expectancy than another.

Building on our discussion in chapter 7, a luck egalitarian would want to say that individuals should have an equal opportunity to achieve the highest possible healthy life expectancy, irrespective of their nationality. One's national membership is as morally arbitrary, luck egalitarians and cosmopolitans typically argue, as one's race or sex, and as such should not affect one's health prospects. This aim of equalizing individuals' health cross-nationally is vulnerable, however, to the following prominent objection. Suppose one nation (call it Prudentistan) actively pursues measures of public health (say, banning smoking in public places) while its neighbor (call it Imprudentia) does not. In that case, the resulting inequality in life expectancy between the two nations is owed, at least partly, to domestic policies. Arguably then, on the luck egalitarian reading, these inequalities in health (or at least some of them) are not unjust. It would therefore be wrong to make the citizens of Prudentistan subsidize their neighbors' expensive taste, as it were, and force them to contribute toward improving the health of their neighbors. Correspondingly, it is unfair for the WHO (or for any hypothetical global distributive mechanism) to allocate the same (let alone greater) medical aid to the citizens of Imprudentia compared with the citizens of Prudentistan.

This "national responsibility" objection to global egalitarianism (whether in health or in welfare more generally), formulated by John Rawls and further developed by David Miller,[4] has a strong intuitive appeal. The focus on responsibility also makes this objection of particular concern to cosmopolitans who are of luck egalitarian persuasion. This chapter is therefore mostly concerned with addressing this "national responsibility" objection to global egalitarianism (as it applies to health). I defend the view that justice requires redistributing wealth and other determinants of health across nations in order to address health inequalities. In other words, I shall try to defend here a cosmopolitan account of global health, one that sees national membership as a morally arbitrary fact, and thus seeks to equalize individuals' healthy life expectancy irrespective of national borders. (More accurately, and in line with our conclusions from chapter 8, I in fact endorse the position of prioritizing the health of those who are worse off health-wise, and not that of equalizing health as such, but for simplicity's sake I shall talk about global egalitarianism in health.)

I shall begin by addressing the claim that the national responsibility objection shows luck egalitarian cosmopolitanism to be guilty of a *double* double standard: one that occurs between the domestic and the global scene, and a second double standard that arguably occurs between its approach to developed and developing nations. In section II I shall point out the problem of holding citizens of nondemocratic nations responsible for their health, and moreover, doing so under the global economic order as it exists today. From then on, in the rest of the chapter, I shall assume, for the sake of argument, a background of democratic nations operating under a just global economic order. There are at least two problems with holding nations responsible for their health that persist even in those idealized conditions. In section III I discuss the problem of holding dissenting minorities responsible for national health policies that they actually did not support. And in section IV I discuss the problem of holding children and, more generally, successive generations responsible for health policies they could not (and did not) choose. Then, in the next two sections I move to examine some residual non-responsibility-based objections to global egalitarianism in health. Section V discusses the objection that what is troubling in the distribution of the global burden of disease is not the fact of its inequality, but rather the fact that some populations needlessly fall below some decent minimal level of health. Finally, in section VI I address the claim that the discovery of intelligent life on other planets would show global egalitarianism in general, and in health in particular, to be counterintuitive.

I. Justice, Responsibility, and Double Standards

When, then, are global inequalities in the burden of disease not unjust? Answers to that question would most likely track attitudes to the more general issue of global justice. Broadly speaking, it is possible to explain the obligation to transfer resources from wealthier nations to poorer ones either on cosmopolitan grounds or on humanitarian grounds. Cosmopolitans generally do not see a principled difference between distributive justice at home and abroad. If we are egalitarians domestically, then so should we be globally. Thus, on the cosmopolitan (and egalitarian) reading, affluent nations ought to transfer resources to poorer nations, and as a matter of egalitarian distributive justice.[5] Those holding the more restricted humanitarian conception of global justice, in contrast, argue that, for various reasons, principles of distributive justice are restricted to the state. Consequently, obligations of distributive justice, and certainly comprehensive obligations of social justice, do not apply globally.[6] That does not, of course, mean that affluent nations have no obligations toward poor nations. Rather, the "global humanitarian" typically believes that global justice consists of a number of important, but minimal, obligations: affluent nations ought to observe the basic human rights of people in less developed nations; they ought to avoid exploiting them; and they ought to make sure that no nation is left to suffer destitution.[7] In sum, while cosmopolitans deny the key relevance of compatriotism in curbing global inequality, including inequality in the global burden of disease,[8] humanitarians affirm it.

Within the cosmopolitan camp it is possible to draw some further distinctions. One distinction we could draw is between "interactionist" cosmopolitans and non-interactionist cosmopolitans (or Rawlsians—as distinct of course, from Rawls himself, who was not a cosmopolitan—and non-Rawlsians).[9] For the former, global distributive justice depends either on the prevalence of some global basic structure,[10] or on economic interaction across nations,[11] whereas for the latter it depends on neither.[12] And within the non-interactionist cosmopolitan camp we may distinguish between those who are *resource* egalitarians and those who are *opportunity* (or luck) egalitarians.[13] For the former, who are largely left-libertarians, global egalitarianism consists in a fair redistribution of global natural resources.[14] The latter, the cosmopolitan luck egalitarian position, says that "[s]ince one's place of birth is morally arbitrary, it should not affect one's life prospects or one's access to opportunities."[15] In this chapter I shall largely attempt to defend that latter position (in its application to health) from the national responsibility objection.[16]

One of the things that the national responsibility objection purportedly shows is that cosmopolitan luck egalitarianism is guilty of inconsistency. I shall address, in this section, that more general claim, before moving in subsequent sections to the more specific objection about national responsibility for health. The broader claim then is that while luck egalitarians are quick to apply a responsibility-sensitive account of distributive justice at home, they seem to shy away from such considerations when thinking about global justice.[17] Luck egalitarian cosmopolitans seem to expect affluent nations to assist poorer nations without examining, as they normally would domestically, whether the worse-off nation was perhaps responsible for its worse-off condition. In short, cosmopolitans seem to favor global transfers even when the worse-off nation suffers what appears to be, strictly speaking, bad option luck.[18] Cosmopolitans are guilty, it is moreover suggested, of yet another form of double standard. While they are reluctant to hold citizens of developing nations responsible for their destitution, they are quick to hold citizens of affluent nations collectively responsible for all sorts of things. Cosmopolitans tend to do so, for example, with regard to certain historical injustices. Nowadays it is not uncommon to hear about this or that government issuing an apology and taking responsibility (and accordingly offering reparations) for their colonial past, for slavery, for maltreatment of their aboriginal populations, and the like. Cosmopolitans are typically happy to attribute such collective responsibility to the affluent, but are quite reluctant to apply the same standard of collective responsibility to developing nations, and hold them collectively responsible for their own reckless policies.[19] One might add that this alleged double standard on the part of cosmopolitans shows not only inconsistency but also disrespect for the moral agency of members of developing nations.

Let us look first at the latter of the accusations of double standard mentioned, namely the case of reparations for historical injustices perpetrated against other peoples (e.g., colonialism, slavery).[20] It would clearly be absurd for a current American president, say, to take *personal* responsibility for the slavery that ended almost a century before she was born. Equally, it would be nonsensical for her to assume collective responsibility, on behalf of her *generation*, for such historical wrongs. Instead, reparations in such a case express the fact that the current generation may still benefit from the fruits of historical wrongs (e.g., social wealth accumulated through slavery and colonialism). It is that personal and communal benefit from past injustices that generates the duty to apologize and compensate; it is not some alleged personal responsibility for perpetrating the injustices. All of this is by now pretty familiar stuff in the literature on reparations and historical injustices.[21] The important point for us to take is that cosmopolitans do not blindly attribute moral responsibility to citizens of affluent countries. Rather, in cases of historical injustices, they may join in identifying a responsibility to compensate for an injustice that one has not perpetrated but nevertheless benefits from. To refrain from applying a double standard, then, we are required to hold citizens of developing nations liable for policies from which they benefit, even if they are not morally responsible for enacting them. (We shall revisit that lesson in section III.)

Let us turn now to the other charge of double standard, that of holding agents responsible domestically but not globally (namely in the case of imprudent developing nations). The first thing to notice here is that the charge of double standards could be leveled also in the opposite direction. It would be equally correct, it seems to me, to say that those who are quick to hold nations responsible on the global level are *not* so quick to adopt considerations of personal responsibility at home. Leading philosophers who are reluctant to apply distributive justice internationally for (partly) reasons of national responsibility happen to be the same philosophers who shy away from applying considerations of personal responsibility to domestic social justice. The charge of double standards can thus be leveled in both directions.

One reply opponents of global egalitarianism (I shall henceforth refer to them as "global humanitarians") may have, though, is to reject the parallel to which my reversed charge alludes. For what distinguishes the global humanitarian position is precisely the fact that it sees a certain discontinuity between the domestic and the global scene. Thus, falling for the alleged double standard is not something humanitarians are embarrassed about but, rather, is the very point that they are trying to make. It is therefore right to hold such a double standard and hold nations responsible in the global context but not hold individuals responsible while pursuing social justice. But the charge of a double standard does not, it seems to me, turn on humanitarians' explicit stance on the discontinuity of justice between the domestic and the global. Rather, what is at stake is humanitarians' employment of the logic of "the ant and the grasshopper" (a reference that both Rawls and Miller use).[22] The intuitive appeal of that fable is supposed to carry the argumentative force of their critique of global egalitarianism. But if one is supposed to be convinced by the force of that fable when it concerns global egalitarianism, it is difficult to see why one should reject the same logic when applied domestically, the discontinuity of the domestic and the global notwithstanding.[23]

None of what I have so far said, of course, gets luck egalitarian cosmopolitans off the hook (yet), but it does point out the fact that key humanitarians such as Rawls and Miller may face an equally important challenge of inconsistency of their own. Furthermore, if anything (and as some of those global humanitarians have themselves conceded),[24] it ought to be less controversial to adopt a responsibility-sensitive approach to justice domestically than it is globally. For it is surely much less contentious to hold an individual responsible for her own actions than it is to hold her morally responsible for the actions of a group as large as her nation.[25] Accordingly, it is one thing to hold a citizen responsible for her unhealthy lifestyle, it is quite another to hold her responsible for the health policy (and the other determinants of health) adopted by her nation.

II. "The Health of Nations" and the Global Economic Order

How then, should, luck egalitarian cosmopolitans respond to the "national responsibility for health" objection? That objection, as illustrated in the example of Prudentistan and Imprudentia, is compelling. In fact, recent evidence in epidemiology seems to corroborate the view of developing nations as being responsible for their low health status. Let me explain. We said in the introduction to this chapter that much of the discrepancy in the global burden of disease is correlated with inequalities in the wealth of nations. And it is often pointed out by cosmopolitans that the wealth of nations should not be seen as the sole responsibility of each state, given the legacy of colonialism and given how the current economic world order further harms the world's poor.[26] But on the other hand, recent findings may suggest that the health of nations is not primarily determined by their standing in the global economy. We know, for example, that above a certain threshold of GDP per capita (U.S.\$6–8,000) an increase in wealth makes little contribution to population health.[27] Instead, it now appears that much of population health is owed to domestic policies, both in health and in other areas of policy that affect health. This is evidenced in the so-called "high achievers": nations that enjoy a life expectancy that is above global average despite having below-average GDPPC: China, Cuba, Vietnam, Sri Lanka, Costa Rica, and the Indian state of Kerala. Most epidemiologists now believe that equality between the sexes, culturally induced diet (e.g., vegetarianism in Kerala), aggressive recruitment of public health workers (notably in Cuba), and egalitarian policy more generally, are strong determinants of the health of nations.[28] Other nations, it may be argued, have simply failed to follow suit. All these findings seem to lend support to the view that the health of nations is primarily the responsibility of domestic institutions. If so, citizens of developed nations at most owe a humanitarian duty of medical aid to those in developing and less healthy nations. They do not owe them the (much stronger) duty of egalitarian distributive justice, or so the claim goes.

It is important to notice, though, as Thomas Pogge and others have stressed, that domestic policy in developing countries, often undemocratic, incompetent, and corrupt, is not forged in a vacuum. We know that the current economic global order often encourages and supports such a conduct.[29] It would therefore be wrong to lay the responsibility for corruption and mismanagement exclusively at the door of developing nations. For very similar reasons, it would be wrong to expect all developing nations to match up to the phenomenal achievements (in the case of health) of Cuba, Kerala, and Costa Rica.[30] As mentioned, a successful public health policy depends on spending a considerable part of one's national resources on the recruitment of health care workers,[31] on investing in the prevention of disease, on equality between the sexes, and on women's literacy and education.[32] The global economic order is nowhere near neutral toward these policies. Owing to the policies of the IMF and the World Bank it is quite difficult for developing nations to pursue extensive public spending, let alone egalitarian public spending.[33] The blame rests not just with international institutions but also with wealthy nation-states that lure doctors and nurses away from their native (developing) nations, thereby seriously undermining the health of the population there.[34] The "high-achieving" nations have managed to perform very well on many of the criteria mentioned above, but they have done so *despite* the global economic order, not because of it (and indeed, as the Cuban case demonstrates, doing so may come at a considerable cost in other aspects of the life of the nation). Correspondingly, it would be unfair to expect other nations to achieve the same phenomenal results. Principles of justice should assume normal, not heroic, agency. It would therefore be wrong to assume that the blame for low health prospects in developing nations rests with domestic institutions, at least not the way the current global economic order is structured.

In order to critically examine the principled objection entailed in the national responsibility claim, we need to set aside the real-life cases of nations whose health status is poor due largely to the nondemocratic regimes that rule them,[35] and largely due to the adverse economic world order in which they operate. What, then, about fully democratic nations, operating within the hypothetical ideal background condition of a just economic world order? Surely, the humanitarian might argue, global inequalities in health would not then be unjust. In the rest of the chapter, therefore, I shall adopt these two simplifying assumptions in order to examine whether we should, even in principle, hold nations responsible for their health.

III. Holding Nations Responsible for Their Health

Suppose, then, we limit our discussion to democratic nations, operating within a just global economic order. The latter implies, among other things, a rough equality of resources, no pressure from such international bodies as the IMF and World Bank to pursue policies that are bad for population health, and no systematic luring of health care workers from one nation to another. Surely, the thought may arise, egalitarian justice does not then require equalizing the health prospects of the two nations, given that at least part of the discrepancy in health between them is owed to the different policy they each democratically and voluntarily adopted. Yet, two familiar problems still remain. First (recalling the example with which we started), what if a sizeable minority of the population of Imprudentia did vote for the ban on smoking? Is it still right to hold this minority, along with the rest of their fellow citizens, accountable for a policy they actually opposed? On the face of it, at least, this would be inappropriate, given that they have made only prudent choices, both personally and politically. Second, suppose the lax smoking policy of

Imprudentia has stunted the growth of children who were exposed to smoking in public places (let us assume, for the sake of argument, that their parents could not have avoided taking them to some of these places). On the face of it, at least, these children should not be denied global compensation, since they made no imprudent choices. These are of course two general and familiar problems with the national responsibility argument.[36] Notable among humanitarians' attempts to deflect these objections is David Miller's important new (and some older) work on global justice and national responsibility.[37] I want, then, to examine these responses to the two objections mentioned, starting with the case of dissenters in this section, and then moving to that of holding children responsible in the next section.

One thing it might be possible to say in support of making the dissenters in Imprudentia, those who lost out the vote on the ban on smoking, bear the liability for that policy is that they are in no different position than any other unsuccessful democratic minority. Their position is unfortunate perhaps (in that they have lost a democratic vote), but crucially, no injustice has been perpetrated against them.[38] They may not be responsible for their nation's policy, but they nevertheless should be held liable for it.[39] Correspondingly, they may not be responsible for their nation's poor health, but it is still right to hold them liable for it. This claim deserves careful examination. It is certainly right to expect the "losers," as it were, of a democratic vote to comply with the consequent majority rule. After all, that is what democracy is all about. But having to comply with a policy one did not favor is one type of price (expected from a dissenting minority); being held liable for your nation's choice of that particular policy, quite another. Consider this. The term "ministerial responsibility" implies that when a decision is adopted by cabinet in a majority vote, those in the cabinet who voted against it are still held collectively liable for the policy chosen and for its outcomes. If these dissenting ministers wish not to be held liable for that particular policy, then, they are free to resign from the cabinet. In contrast, a dissenting minority in a democracy does not normally have the option of "resigning." Barring extreme circumstances (the perpetration of crimes against humanity, say), it would be unreasonable to expect a dissenting minority to pack up and leave in order to escape moral liability.[40] Moreover, democratic minorities should be expected to follow the policy adopted even if they opposed it. This is the price that is legitimately expected from dissenters. The dissenters of Imprudentia may therefore be expected to endure the policy of smoking in public places. But to then deny them (what we may call) the "global health dividend" on account of the policy to which they actually objected is to inflict a further unjustified harm on them. It is, indeed, a case of double jeopardy.

We have, however, discussed only part of the picture. Consider the following example. Suppose we are faced with the policy choice between trying to conserve our national energy resources, and using as much energy in the present as we want at the expense of available energy for future generations. Suppose I vote for the former, but lose. In that case my preferred policy got defeated but, as a consequence of the policy adopted, I get to enjoy using up as much cheap energy today as I wish. It seems plausible that in this case, although one cannot be held morally responsible for the policy adopted, it is nevertheless right that one be held liable for a policy that, although one did not choose, one nevertheless got to benefit from.[41] This tells us, I think, that where dissenters are still likely to benefit from the policy they opposed, moral responsibility and liability may come apart. Notice the similarity between this latter case and the case mentioned in section I regarding benefiting from historical injustices that one did not perpetrate. In both cases one is not morally responsible for the policy and yet is expected to bear (at least some of) the liability for it. In such cases, dissenters ought not to expect compensation from a global distributive justice scheme.

It does not seem, however, that much of the current inequality in the global burden of disease fits the scenario just described. Those bearing the greater share of the global burden of disease seldom otherwise benefit from the policies that have led to their poor health status. In other words, the poor health of developing nations is not generally owed to policies from which the individual is otherwise likely to benefit. Rather, that low health status is owed to policies, both domestic and international, that appear to yield very little if any non-health benefit for the majority of the members of that nation. It does not seem to be the case, for example, that Zambians have a low life expectancy because the Zambian government chose to invest in magnificent football stadiums or in generous tax breaks for the middle and lower classes rather than in hospitals and literacy programs. In other words, the policies that lead to Zambians' poor health status are not ones from which they benefit otherwise.

In principle, though, it *is* sometimes right to hold dissenting minorities liable for their national policies, including ones that were bad for population health. The proviso that justifies doing so is that they stand to benefit from those policies, which they opposed. At the same time we note that this proviso does not generally seem to hold for developing countries in the case of health-related policies.

IV. National Responsibility and Future Generations

Even when it is right to hold dissenters liable for health policies they opposed (because they otherwise benefit from them), humanitarians would still run into the other familiar problem mentioned: namely, they would end up allowing children to suffer from policies they could not, and did not, choose. This problem of holding children responsible has been well recognized as the Achilles' heel of the national responsibility argument. In the case of health, it would imply denying the current citizens of Imprudentia a global transfer of a health dividend if their low health status is a result of imprudent health policy by previous generations. That seems wrong. But, again, the picture might be more complex than that. It is possible to think of various reasons why it might *not* be unfair for children to suffer a disadvantage bestowed on them by their parents, including the disadvantage of having a low life expectancy. I will argue, however, that ultimately none of these reasons are persuasive, and that consequently we should, at the very least, equalize health prospects for each generation so that children would not suffer from policies over which they had no control.

Here is one argument for allowing children to suffer the consequences of health policies enacted by their parents. David Miller has argued that it is right to hold a child liable for the policies enacted by her parents' generation because it is likely that the child would grow up to develop similar tastes to those of the dominant culture in her society (e.g., consumerism and frivolous spending as opposed to thrift). After all, people normally acquire their habits by emulating their parents and other individuals in their immediate surroundings. Thus, continuity in preferences between generations is very likely, and therefore it would (turn out to) be right to hold younger generations liable for decisions made by their predecessors.[42] But there are at least two, quite obvious, problems with this argument. First, it is unclear what relevance there is, in the current context, to how the child *will* act in the future. The question is not (or not only) what that child will be entitled to as a grown-up person, but rather what that child is entitled to *now*. Does a Zambian child deserve to have a much smaller chance of reaching the age of five than her Norwegian counterpart as a consequence of policies over which she had no control? The question of distributive justice thus arises in the present and in the immediate future and not merely in the distant future. It is therefore irrelevant, for the present inquiry, to speculate how that child would behave as an adult. Second, what humanitarians are required to address here is not a point about the *likelihood* of continuity between generations, but rather the question of responsibility of the child for the decisions that were made before she assumed moral agency. If the response that humanitarians provide is that in any case the child, once grown-up, would come to adopt similar attitudes, then they seem to leave no room for autonomous agency. This is even more so if the reason why it is thought that the child would develop those similar attitudes is because she is likely to adhere to her local culture rather than because she went through an independent reflective process. Miller's rationale would equally justify incarcerating someone, as a sort of preemptive measure, simply because he happens to come from the neighborhood that typically breeds criminals.[43]

Another argument for denying redistribution from descendants of Prudentistan to descendants of Imprudentia is this. Suppose we accept that the children of Imprudentia are worse off than they should be (due to their parents' reckless health policies). Why should it then be the duty of their neighbors to help them out? After all, it is not the fault of Prudentistanians, current and previous generation alike, that the people of Imprudentia are in the sorry mess that they are in. Indeed, it is not the case, in our example, that the current generation of Prudentistan is responsible for the bad fortune that has befallen their neighbors in Imprudentia. But neither is it the case, notice, that Prudentistanians are responsible for their own *good* fortune. That good fortune was bestowed on them by someone else, namely their parents, without their doing anything themselves to become entitled to it. If the advantage that they have is in fact unmerited, then it is not obvious why it would be wrong to require them to help improve the position of the citizens of Imprudentia, especially given that the latter have suffered what we agree is bad brute luck.[44]

Another possible response to the "future generations" objection is that equalizing the life chances of children of all nationalities inevitably implies that prudent parents, those who have saved for their children, would be subsidizing the selfish and imprudent conduct of other parents. Global egalitarianism toward children thus comes at the price of treating prudent adults unfairly.[45] But why exactly would that be the case? In what way can the elders of Prudentistan be said to be wronged as a consequence of global egalitarianism? If we stipulate that the health subsidy or dividend is to be taken from the current generation of Prudentistan and not from its elders, then the alleged harm cannot be thought of as a direct one. It might, then, be thought that the diligent citizens of Prudentistan are being penalized in the following way. These parents love their children, as seen among other things from the fact that they saved food and other resources (e.g., energy) for them. Their children's fates are of great concern to them, and therefore their children's flourishing affects their own. If the children fare ill, their own lives will have gone less well than they would otherwise. Moreover, these parents have admirably denied benefits from themselves for the sake of benefiting their children, only to see those benefits halved (in the best of cases) and taken away in order to subsidize the imprudent conduct of their neighbors. Global egalitarianism does not seem to be honoring their life project of providing adequate social determinants of health for the next generation.[46]

Recall, however, that we are discussing the issue of fairness here and are therefore setting aside the important question of disincentives for reckless conduct. That is crucial, since from the perspective of fairness, it hardly seems fair to punish the unlucky second generation of Imprudentia just so as to teach other people a general lesson about prudence. In doing so we would be punishing not the culprit but her very victim. Setting the forward-looking issue of incentives aside, is it really true, on an egalitarian reading, that the diligent elderly citizens of Prudentistan are being made worse off in spite of their prudence? I believe it is not. Assessments of an egalitarian distribution usually do not factor into one person's welfare balance whether or not the allocation of benefit to a third party is to that first person's liking. In other words, we set aside other-regarding factors like racism, envy, altruism, friendship, and parental love as determinants of people's bundles of goods. If that is correct, then splitting the resources left by the elderly citizens of Prudentistan (assuming this does not harm them directly) between their offspring and the offspring of Imprudentia should not count as harming the elderly. The cosmopolitan, then, need not deny that Prudentistanians love their children. She rather asserts that other people's children matter as well. Nor, I want to add, is splitting resources between the children of both nations disrespectful of the life project of the elderly Prudentistanians. Indeed, global redistribution of the social determinants of health may well give credit to the Prudentistanians' way of life. The global redistribution of these resources vindicates their prudent conduct in contrast to the reckless conduct of their neighbors and underscores the importance of promoting the health of future generations. In a way, this is a true way of honoring their life project of thrift and selflessness.

I hope to have shown in this section that it is reasonable to apply measures of egalitarian justice between contemporaneous generations across national borders. As such, the judgment that we should not hold people responsible for their health insomuch as it was bestowed upon them by other people (in this case, a previous generation) seems to hold.

V. Equality or Sufficiency in Global Health?

We can think of other objections to equalizing the health prospects of children worldwide, but ones that are not necessarily responsibility-based. Consider the following one. Let us suppose, along the global egalitarian position, that the huge gulf in life expectancy between a Zambian child and a Norwegian child is unjust. However, if that inequality is unjust, then so is, on the cosmopolitan-egalitarian logic, the minute discrepancy in life expectancy between the Norwegian child and her Swedish counterpart, say.[47] The fact that we do not commonly think of discrepancies in life expectancy that persist between wealthy nations as being unjust implies that the problem is not

one of equality but rather of sufficiency.[48] It follows, so a critic of global egalitarianism might say, that what is ethically troubling about the poor health of
the Zambian child is that it falls below some decent level of health, not that it
is worse than the health of the Norwegian child. The problem, in short, is one
of insufficiency, not of inequality.[49] Thus, humanitarians are arguably right to
characterize the gulf in life expectancy between the Norwegian child and the
Zambian child as one generating a mere humanitarian duty of aid rather than
the much stronger requirements of egalitarian distributive justice.

Suppose though, for the sake of argument, that we insist along with the
luck egalitarian position that it is always unfair for one person to be worse off
than others through no fault of her own. And suppose, correspondingly, that
it is unjust for the Norwegian child to be (slightly) worse off than the Swedish
child. If that were the case, funds would have to be transferred from Sweden
to Norway (provided, of course, that Sweden is at least as well off as Norway
GDP-wise; health, as we said in chapter 6, is not the only currency of egalitarianism, nor of global egalitarianism). Now, given that the difference in life
expectancy is not large, then presumably, the transfer of resources in question
would also not be large.[50] Furthermore, given the hugely superior health state
of developed countries (such as Sweden and Norway) compared to that of
many nations in the developing world, and given the priority we ought to give
to the worse off, it is the case that the transfer of resources between Sweden
and Norway would feature very low, if at all, on the global agenda of redistributing the burden of disease.[51] Once we bear this in mind, casting the inequality in life expectancy between Sweden and Norway as unjust becomes much
less counterintuitive than might initially appear. Thus, despite the initial appeal of the objection in question, egalitarians ought to simply bite the bullet
and insist that the inequality in life expectancy between Sweden and Norway
is an unjust one, albeit one that is dwarfed by more urgent (not just practically
but morally speaking) redistribution elsewhere.

Children (and successive generations more generally) should therefore
not be made to bear the cost of the domestic health-related policies in their
respective countries, and for *egalitarian* reasons. But this conclusion, and our
rejection of the sufficientarian case in global health, may present the luck
egalitarian cosmopolitan with at least two potential objections. The first is
that transferring funds from Sweden to Norway may be unjust toward those
in Sweden whose life expectancy is actually lower than that of the average
Norwegian (say, the Saamis who live in the north of Sweden). Notice, however, that the cosmopolitan analysis of the global burden of disease only con-
tingently speaks of discrepancies in life expectancy between *nations*. As a
matter of principle, the cosmopolitan is happy to adopt any level of analysis,
and in fact the smaller the better. If it were possible to assess individual life

expectancies, the cosmopolitan would demand equalizing those. The cosmopolitan is all the more happy with a health policy that taxes the healthy and wealthy *individual* and distributes to her poor and unhealthy counterpart. Of course, this raises all sorts of practical difficulties, but these are beside the principled point regarding justice. Alternatively, the cosmopolitan position would be content with endorsing regions or counties (as opposed to nations) as the appropriate level of analysis.[52] It is worth pointing out that something of this sort is effectively taking place with regard to the regional policy in the European Union. Under its regional development policy, the EU transfers subsidies to what it calls Objective 1 counties (not countries), those whose GDP falls below 75% of the EU average. Crucially, these counties are eligible for the subsidies independently of their nationality.[53] There is therefore no principled, or even practical, impediment to pursuing an egalitarian policy in global health on a smaller unit of distribution than the nation, thereby largely avoiding the alleged unfairness of the Saami example. It may however still be the case that the only practical way of redistributing the global burden of disease is by transferring funds from one nation to another, nations being currently the kind of agent that is sovereign over resources. In that case, average national life expectancies and national GDPPC are restored as the only plausible indices for calculating who owes whom what. That again may entail some unfairness toward those Saamis in Sweden. But crucially, that potential unfairness is offset by the greater urgency of benefiting the even worse off (on average) Norwegians.[54]

I mentioned a second objection to the egalitarian, rather than sufficientarian, case for global health. It might be objected that my argument captures too much. For what is true for children in Zambia is also true, to a certain degree at least, for black children born in New Orleans. On my account, these children should also be entitled to compensation from some global redistribution mechanism, by virtue of their disadvantaged position. Some may find this counterintuitive.[55] But consider this. The low life expectancy of the children in New Orleans is probably the result of socioeconomic inequality, of the absence of universal health care, and of the legacy of racism in the very wealthy nation within which they live. But if that is the case, then, is it still counterintuitive to suppose that a global redistribution mechanism would bypass the U.S. administration and transfer some resources to this disadvantaged population? It would appear that in the case of these worse-off individuals, the fact of their citizenship in a rich and developed nation does not translate into an improved health status (quite the contrary, in fact). It is not obvious, then, why the fact of their citizenship should in any way reduce their entitlement to compensation (on grounds of global justice). In other words, it seems consistent to hold that nationality, whether in a poor nation or in a rich but nonegalitarian nation, ought not to determine one's health status. Rather than demonstrating the weakness of the global egalitarian approach to health, this objection in fact seems to me to point to its consistency and strength.

What I have just said does not detract, of course, from the claim that the primary responsibility for the health of children in New Orleans rests, at least currently, with the U.S. administration, especially given the fact that it does not lack the resources with which to achieve this modest aim.[56] That, however, is a different question from the one raised by the objection above, namely, what is to be done *given* that the American state does not meet its obligations toward its own citizens? To that the luck egalitarian cosmopolitan reiterates that children should not be made to suffer worse health prospects due to national membership, something over which they have no control.

VI. Intergalactic Egalitarianism

The conclusion of the previous section was that the cosmopolitan insists that it is egalitarianism (in the form of priority to the worse off) rather than sufficientarianism that should govern global health policy. That, however, may open global egalitarianism, in health and in general, to another peculiar objection. Suppose, humanitarians may say, that we discover the long-searched-for intelligent life on Mars (or some other planet). Such a discovery would represent, they might say, a decisive problem for cosmopolitans, for cosmopolitans believe that such arbitrary facts as national (or terrestrial, for that matter) boundaries ought not to exclude someone from being the subject of egalitarian distributive justice. Accordingly, these newly discovered intelligent beings from Mars would have, on the cosmopolitan view, a claim on us for full-blown egalitarian redistribution (supposing their health is worse off than ours). This, critics of global egalitarianism might say, shows the cosmopolitan position to be counterintuitive. It is counterintuitive to suppose, so I would take this objection to imply, that we might owe so much to someone the existence of whom we only just discovered and who happens to reside many millions of kilometers from us.[57]

It is unclear, though, that this intergalactic objection is an objection to cosmopolitanism, of all things. Let me explain. The decisive issue at the heart of dealing with such an objection is the question of whether or not these newly discovered intelligent beings have a moral standing roughly equal to humans. Crucially, that is not a question for cosmopolitans, of all people, to answer. Cosmopolitans would only argue that we have obligations of distributive justice toward these Martians if it is concluded (not necessarily by cosmopolitans) that these Martians have a moral standing that is equal to that of humans. In that case, the timing of their discovery, as well as their physical location, is of no moral relevance, the luck egalitarian cosmopolitan would insist. But furthermore, in that case, it is not obvious that the discovery of these human-like Martians presents a challenge (if there is one) that is peculiar to cosmopolitans alone. (The discovery of the Martians may not present a challenge at all if they happen to be healthier and wealthier than we humans,[58] surely not a more outrageous supposition than the supposition about their discovery to begin with.[59]) For consider what the humanitarian position would entail here. Humanitarians are committed to not exploiting foreigners (those of human moral standing), to meeting their basic needs, and to guaranteeing that they enjoy a decent level of living. If the newly discovered Martians' health falls below some perceived threshold of a decent minimum, then global humanitarians such as Miller would be committed to sending them aid. Notice that if the Martians' health is substantially low, then the obligation to bring them up to the required minimal level of health may be quite costly. Even if their health falls only slightly below the level of decent minimum, merely sending the required aid over to Mars may be an operation potentially costing many billions of dollars. In short, even being merely Samaritans toward Martians can be quite costly.

Unless one is a libertarian, then, the intergalactic objection poses, if anything, almost as much of a problem for humanitarians as it does for cosmopolitans.

Conclusion

We may summarize our findings in this chapter in the following way. It is not unjust for the citizens of Imprudentia to suffer lower health prospects than the citizens of Prudentistan if and only if the following conditions apply. First, each generation of Imprudentia has the same opportunity as its contemporaries in Prudentistan to have the latter's GDPPC (whether in terms of the distribution of natural resources or otherwise). (In today's world, that condition may be satisfied already if Imprudentia had the same opportunity as Prudentistan to reach the mark of $6,000 GDPPC, even if Prudentistan is still much wealthier than that.[60]) The second condition is that Prudentistan does not interfere in Imprudentia's attempt to meet its population's health needs (e.g., by aggressively recruiting their neighbors' physicians and nurses, or by offering Imprudentia loans on the condition that it cut public spending on education and public health). Third, all citizens of Imprudentia have effective political means for shaping the nation's health-affecting policies (notice that this does not require Imprudentia to be a fully fledged democracy). Fourth, dissenters in Imprudentia otherwise benefit from the imprudent health-related policies enacted by its government. And finally, the equality of opportunity for health for the next generation of Imprudentia is restored through a global corrective health dividend (this is meant to correct for the worse health prospects that were bestowed on these Imprudentians by their parents' generation). Only if all these conditions together are met is it not unjust to let citizens of Imprudentia suffer worse health and health prospects than their prudent neighbors. Needless to say, in the real world, we are quite a long way away from meeting these conditions.

Conclusion

■

I began this book by saying that one of the merits of the luck egalitarian account of justice in health care and health is that it is quite simple and straightforward. Let us, then, try and summarize its recommendations and see if it lives up to that earlier depiction.

First, according to the theory proposed here, the provision of health care is justified not through an attempt to equalize individuals' opportunity to pursue their life plans or to equalize their political and civic capabilities. Rather, health care is justified by way of society's obligation to reverse individuals' disadvantaging biological conditions for which they are not responsible. This requirement applies both to interventions aimed at deficits to full health, and to ones aimed at enhancing one's physical performance beyond the normal species functioning. As for individuals (residents, rather than merely citizens) who can be said to be responsible for their medical condition, a luck egalitarian guide to policy (rather than a narrow luck egalitarian account of justice) would recommend meeting their basic medical needs. Second, luck egalitarians hold that the just distribution of health care is important, but that the just distribution of health proper is even more important. As far as considerations of distributive justice are concerned, health ought to be redistributed in such a way as to prioritize the health of an individual the less responsible she is for her illness (and for individuals who are equally responsible, to prioritize care to ones whose health is worse). Third, luck egalitarian justice in health and health care requires, for the most part, ignoring differences in culturally driven medical "tastes" and thus resists calls for the devolution of health care services. Globally, luck egalitarian justice in health favors redistributing the global burden of disease, giving priority to nations or regions whose health is worse, allowing for considerations of national responsibility only subject to a set of specific provisos that the world today is yet far from meeting.

The theory I attempted to provide here is rather comprehensive: it applies to health as well as health care, to health deficits as well as enhancements to full health, and to domestic as well as global policy. In doing so I advocated a pluralist approach. As much as we political philosophers would like it to, a sole moral principle cannot account for all our intuitions with regard to ethics and health. Distributive justice, I have said throughout the book, ought to be supplemented and traded off with other moral requirements such as the concern for basic needs, for maximizing utility, and for preserving solidarity.

My approach could be characterized as a pluralist one also with respect to the specific issue of egalitarian distribution. That is, the account provided here has made use of the various patterns of egalitarian distribution (equality, priority, and sufficiency). I have advocated strict equality with regard to the distribution of human enhancements; priority to the worse off with regard to health itself; and a sufficientarian pattern of distribution with respect to meeting basic needs.

In the introductory chapter I said that applying the luck egalitarian theory of justice to health and health care might have the important added value of teaching us something about the nature of justice itself. To quote Amartya Sen again: "there are some special considerations related to health that need to come forcefully into the assessment of overall justice. In doing this exercise, the idea of health equity motivates certain questions and some specific perspectives, which enrich the more abstract notion of equity in general."[1] Indeed, the endeavor to learn something about justice itself from theorizing about health care is nothing new. Sen, Kenneth Arrow, and Michael Walzer, have all used insights from health care in order to highlight what they saw as certain deficiencies in Rawls's theory of justice.[2] I have already admitted to harboring a similar ambition in setting out to write this book: the ambition of saying something new about justice in health care and health, but also the ambition to use that applied theory in order to perhaps gain some new insight about justice itself. It is not for me of course to say whether the former objective was achieved successfully in this book, but allow me to speculate in the remaining paragraphs on what we may have gained regarding the latter. In other words, what can the application of luck egalitarianism to health care and health teach us about the nature of justice itself? I'll try and point out two potential lessons.

One lesson that we might take from the first part of the book concerns the plurality of moral considerations in contrast to the narrowness of distributive justice. If my account of luck egalitarian justice in health care is attractive, then it may lend some credence to the idea that we must not confuse distributive justice with what might be called "principles of regulation." Recall that my strategy in averting the abandonment objection was to show that luck egalitarian distributive justice seeks to interpret only a narrow slice of morality. As such, its recommendations regarding that narrow sphere of distributive justice ought to be traded off with other values we might hold. If luck egalitarianism yields attractive judgments about what distributive justice requires with regard to health care, and if trading off justice with other values in the sphere of health care yields attractive principles of regulations, then this should count in favor of luck egalitarianism. In other words, a successful application of luck egalitarian justice to health care might reinforce the claim that it is correct and attractive to hold a narrow view of what distributive justice requires and then to trade it off with other values. We might say that this lesson concerns the *structure* of justice.

The second lesson that this book might teach us about justice concerns, in turn, the *substance* of justice. It was evident, especially in the second part of the book, that luck egalitarianism gives us a conception of equality of opportunity that is quite radical. In the first chapter I have contrasted the natural or cosmic nature of luck egalitarianism with the political nature of Rawlsian justice. That contrast, it should be evident now, bears on the scope of the very concept of equality of opportunity. Luck egalitarianism instructs us to take equality of opportunity toward its logical conclusion, wherever that may lead us, and certainly far beyond the conventional "political" sphere. The most obvious instance in which that contrast was evidenced was with regard to the inequalities between the sexes as well as with the suggestion that equality of opportunity might be best served through distributing genetic enhancements (fairly). If radical equality of opportunity in health is attractive, then this may reflect back on the attractiveness of luck egalitarianism proper. In particular, the application to health may show the "natural" understanding of equality of opportunity to be more attractive than, or at least as attractive as, the Rawlsian one (which, given the current dominance of Rawlsianism, would be an achievement in itself).

Without belaboring the same point, I shall note only briefly that a very similar lesson might be drawn also from the third part of the book. There, it was my hope to show that the application of nonpolitical luck egalitarian justice in health care and health to levels below, and especially beyond, the nation-state is attractive. If I was successful in doing so, that might reflect favorably also on the pure (that is, non-applied) theory and demonstrate the inherent cosmopolitanism of luck egalitarianism to be superior and more attractive than the anti-cosmopolitanism arguably inherent in Rawlsian justice.

Luck egalitarianism is sometimes criticized by people on the left for having forsaken the traditional leftist emphasis on social responsibility, and for having switched to the more traditionally right-wing focus on personal responsibility. The left, it is said, has generally been concerned with the injustice of the background social conditions and thus tended not to rest the blame for destitution on the shoulders of the disadvantaged individual agent. It is therefore curious and unfortunate, the critic may say, that egalitarianism has resorted in recent years to the typically rightist focus on personal responsibility and to "blaming the victim." Equally, it may be said, it is unfortunate that what has traditionally been the leftist concern with societal injustices has given way to a de-contextualized inquiry after the appropriateness of individual conduct. It seems to me that that claim has been a subtheme in my exploration of the contrasting Rawlsian and luck egalitarian approaches to health and health care. If my luck egalitarian account of justice in health and health care is in any way attractive, then it may provide luck egalitarians with a response to the abovementioned criticism . Luck egalitarians, I have tried to emphasize throughout this book, are only indirectly concerned with what individuals are responsible for. Their true concern is with the factors that shape our lives and for which we are not responsible. The ambition to neutralize luck, we saw, has radical implications for the extent of society's duties of justice. It allows us to say that society ought to address *every* disadvantage for which the individual is not responsible. That, we saw in various places in the book, may lead to extensive, never before taken, action by society to address disadvantages in the sphere of health. These include, for example, society's duty to reverse all natural disadvantaging features, its duty to fund genetic enhancements, and its duty toward people who are not members of our society. Rather than limiting the scope of social responsibility with regard to justice, the alleged focus of luck egalitarianism on individual responsibility in fact spells out a much more comprehensive agenda than ever before for making society just.

Notes

■

Introduction

1 Ronald Dworkin, who is a leading luck egalitarian, has written on the just distribution of health care, but the account he offers there is not premised on neutralizing luck. See his *Sovereign Virtue: The Theory and Practice of Equality* (Cambridge, MA: Harvard University Press, 2000), ch. 8.

2 Most notably Elizabeth Anderson, "What Is the Point of Equality?" *Ethics* 109 (1999): 287–337; Norman Daniels, *Just Health: Meeting Health Needs Fairly* (Cambridge: Cambridge University Press, 2008), p. 72.

3 It has been established, for example, that the patient's own behavior is the greatest determinant of her health. See Daniel Wikler, "Personal Responsibility for Illness," in D. Van De Veer and T. Regan (eds.), *Health Care Ethics* (Philadelphia: Temple University Press, 1987), p. 330.

4 In contrast, it might be argued that individuals who die young due to imprudent health-related conduct save all of us the burden of paying their pension and taking care of them in old age. See Pieter H. M. Van Baal et al., "Lifetime Medical Costs of Obesity: Prevention No Cure for Increasing Health Expenditure," *PLoS Medicine* 5, no. 2 (2008): 242–49. I shall engage this claim in chapter 5.

5 Subject to some extreme exceptions: health is only divisible through organ donation. It is only transferable when genes are bequeathed (in the case of good and bad health), and when diseases are communicated (in the case of bad health).

6 More generally, see Mary Shaw et al., "Increasing Mortality Differentials by Residential Area Level of Poverty: Britain 1981–1997," *Social Science and Medicine* 51, no. 1 (2000): 151–53.

7 As has been established in the famous Whitehall study, which found a steady gradient in health between civil servants, all of whom had identical access to health care. See Michael Marmot, Martin J. Shipley, and Geoffrey Rose, "Inequalities in Death-Specific Explanations of a General Pattern," *Lancet* 1984: 1003–6.

8 Indeed, on a strict egalitarian reading, universal health care might be *too much*. That is, if we only cared about raising the health of the worst-off person then we might do well to provide selective health care, that is, only to the weakest socioeconomic classes. See J. P. Mackenbach, K. E. Stronks, and A. E. Kunst, "The Contribution of Medical Care to Inequalities in Health," *Social Science and Medicine* 29 (1989): p. 376. I revisit this issue in chapter 2.

9 See Gopal Sreenivasan, "Health Care and Equality of Opportunity," *Hastings Center Report* 37 (2007): 31–41.

10 *Independent Inquiry into Inequalities in Health: Report* (London: Stationery Office, 1998).

11 Daniels, *Just Health*, p. 83.

Chapter 1: Justice, Luck, and Equality

1 The most canonical luck egalitarian texts are Richard J. Arneson, "Equality and Equal Opportunity for Welfare," in L. P. Pojman and R. Westmoreland (eds.),

Equality: Selected Readings (New York, Oxford: Oxford University Press, 1997), pp. 229–41; G. A. Cohen, "On the Currency of Egalitarian Justice," *Ethics* 99, no. 4 (1989): 906–44; Ronald Dworkin, *Sovereign Virtue: The Theory and Practice of Equality* (Cambridge, MA: Harvard University Press, 2000), esp. chs. 1, 2; and John E. Roemer, *Egalitarian Perspectives* (Cambridge: Cambridge University Press, 1994).

2 Ronald Dworkin, "What is Equality? Part I: Equality of Welfare," *Philosophy and Public Affairs* 10, no. 3 (1981): 185–246, and "Part II: Equality of Resources," *Philosophy and Public Affairs* 10, no. 4 (1981): 283–345.

3 John Rawls, *A Theory of Justice* (Oxford: Oxford University Press, 1971), p. 102.

4 See Will Kymlicka, *Contemporary Political Philosophy: An Introduction* (Oxford: Clarendon Press, 1990), pp. 73–76.

5 Thomas Nagel, "Equality," in his *Mortal Questions* (Cambridge: Cambridge University Press, 1979).

6 Harry Frankfurt, "Equality as a Moral Ideal," *Ethics* 98, no. 1 (1987): 21–22.

7 Arneson, "Equality and Equal Opportunity for Welfare," p. 234.

8 Cohen, "On the Currency of Egalitarian Justice," p. 908 (emphasis added).

9 S. L. Hurley, *Justice, Luck, and Knowledge* (Cambridge, MA: Harvard University Press, 2003), p. 141 (emphasis added).

10 Larry Temkin, *Inequality* (Oxford: Oxford University Press, 1993), p. 13 (emphasis added).

11 G. A. Cohen, "Luck and Equality: A Reply to Hurley," *Philosophy and Phenomenological Research* 72 (2) (2006), p. 444 (original emphasis).

12 Ibid. (original emphasis).

13 Richard J. Arneson, "Desert and Equality," in N. Holtug and K. Lippert-Rasmussen (eds.), *Egalitarianism* (Oxford: Oxford University Press, 2007), p. 264.

14 Richard J. Arneson, "Luck and Equality," *Proceedings of the Aristotelian Society*, Supplement 75 (2001): 73–90; Peter Vallentyne, "Brute Luck Equality and Desert," in S. Olsaretti (ed.), *Desert and Justice* (New York: Oxford University Press, 2003), pp. 171–72; 182. As Vallentyne notes, a student who studies hard for an exam might be prudentially more deserving of a high mark than a student who studied less hard because he was busy helping other people (and, thus, was morally more deserving).

15 See Serena Olsaretti's Introduction to her *Desert and Justice* (New York: Oxford University Press, 2003), pp. 14–16.

16 Shelly Kagan, "Equality and Desert," in L. Pojman and O. McLeod (eds.), *What Do We Deserve? A Reader on Justice and Desert* (New York: Oxford University Press, 1999), 298–314.

17 Notice that since we are discussing noncomparative judgments we are setting aside any impact that making A better off than she was would have on the comparison between her and B, who may now become worse off than A and through no fault of her own.

18 Among leading luck egalitarians, it is only Dworkin who comes close to endorsing that desert view. For example: "Our initial principle, that equality of resources requires that people pay the true cost of the lives that they lead, warrants rather than condemns these differences [inequalities—SS]." Dworkin, *Sovereign Virtue*, p. 76.

19 See Arneson's rebuttal of noncomparative desert in his "Desert and Equality," esp. p. 280. If everyone already has what they deserve, shows Arneson, and a new

batch of goods is discovered, "Deserterians" would advocate throwing these goods away, for to add benefits to people who already have what they deserve is bad on the desert view. This seems highly counterintuitive. This problem, note, is peculiar only to *non*comparative desert.

20 Shelly Kagan, "Comparative Desert," in Serena Olsaretti (ed.), *Desert and Justice* (New York: Oxford University Press, 2003), pp. 93–122.

21 Arneson suggests avoiding that unpalatable outcome by substituting prioritarianism for egalitarianism. See his "Desert and Equality," p. 281.

22 Vallentyne, "Brute Luck Equality and Desert," p. 176.

23 Of course, the story may be structured a little differently to say that Lazy has in fact taken a gamble that a fish will wash ashore. But I assume, as in Vallentyne's example, that the fish washing ashore was pure good *brute* luck.

24 Some recent luck egalitarian accounts are drawing near that conclusion, although not explicitly so. See Martin E. Sandbu, "On Dworkin's Brute-Luck-Option-Luck Distinction and the Consistency of Brute-Luck Egalitarianism," *Politics, Philosophy, and Economics* 3, no. 3 (2004): 297; Zofia Stemplowska, "Making Justice Sensitive to Responsibility," *Political Studies*, forthcoming.

25 On the claim that what counts as a responsible action would depend on what risks it is conventionally reasonable to undertake, see Arthur Ripstein, "Equality, Luck, and Responsibility," *Philosophy and Public Affairs* 23, no. 1 (1994): 3–23.

26 Cf. John E. Roemer, "A Pragmatic Theory of Responsibility for the Egalitarian Planner," *Philosophy and Public Affairs* 22, no. 2 (1993): 146–66.

27 Eric Rakowski, *Equal Justice* (Oxford: Oxford University Press, 1991), pp. 73–90.

28 Ibid., p. 79. See also Elizabeth Anderson, "What Is the Point of Equality?" *Ethics* 109 (1999): 296.

29 "We share an interest in people choosing to mine or farm, to work in areas prone to storms and earthquakes, to deposit their money in banks and provide for retirement in pensions." Elizabeth S. Anderson, "How Should Egalitarians Cope with Market Risks?" *Theoretical Inquiries in Law* 9 (2008): 255. Viewing choice of residence in an earthquake-prone area as a legitimate choice the consequences of which the individual should bear is typically a libertarian, not egalitarian, position. See Hillel Steiner, "How Equality Matters," *Social Philosophy and Policy* 19 (2002): 350–51.

30 See Seana Shiffrin, "Egalitarianism, Choice-Sensitivity, and Accommodation," in R. J. Wallace et al. (eds.), *Reason and Values: Themes from the Moral Philosophy of Joseph Raz* (Oxford: Oxford University Press, 2004), p. 278.

31 Following the conventional medical wisdom according to which having only one child increases the risk of breast cancer compared to having several children, or to having no children at all.

32 Anderson, "What Is the Point of Equality?" pp. 295–302.

33 Ibid., p. 296. See also Jules Coleman and Arthur Ripstein, "Mischief and Misfortune," *McGill Law Journal* 41 (1995): 111.

34 Allen Buchanan, "The Right to a Decent Minimum of Health Care," *Philosophy and Public Affairs* 13 (1984): 67; Shlomi Segall, "In Solidarity with the Imprudent: A Defense of Luck Egalitarianism," *Social Theory and Practice* 33, no. 2 (2007), sec. III.

35 Anderson, "What Is the Point of Equality?" p. 297.

36 Nir Eyal, "Egalitarian Justice and Innocent Choice," *Journal of Ethics and Social Philosophy* 2, no. 1 (2007): 1–18.

37 That way, we also avoid some of the problems pointed out by Vallentyne with regard to reasonable avoidability. Vallentyne's target of criticism is an idea focused on what it is reasonable for the agent to do, that is, what is in her best interests, whereas my criterion speaks of what it is reasonable for society to expect. The example Vallentyne offers is one where the agent has either the choice of acquiring education and thus leading a wonderful life, or acquiring the habit of drug use and thus succumbing to a horrible life. It would be unreasonable for her to choose the latter path, which makes the former a matter of brute luck. But to depict the choice resulting in the wonderful life as a matter of brute luck, Vallentyne says, "seems intuitively strange" (Peter Vallentyne, "Brute Luck, Option Luck, and Equality of Initial Opportunities," *Ethics* 112, no. 3 [2002]: 533). I do not quite see why. Suppose these are genuinely the only two options open to the agent, and suppose education would cost an X amount of dollars. It seems to me that it would be unjust not to compensate her in the sum of X given that she could not have reasonably avoided that course of action (acquiring education). If so, there is nothing intuitively wrong about brute luck as reasonable unavoidability.

38 Richard J. Arneson, "Luck Egalitarianism Interpreted and Defended," http://philosophyfaculty.ucsd.edu/faculty/rarneson/luckegalitarianism2.pdf (2005); "Luck Egalitarianism: A Primer," paper presented at the Harvard Law School, April 2007.

Chapter 2: Responsibility-*In*sensitive Health Care

1 Elizabeth S. Anderson, "What Is the Point of Equality?" *Ethics* 109 (1999), p. 296. See also Norman Daniels, "Democratic Equality: Rawls's Complex Egalitarianism," in S. Freeman (ed.), *The Cambridge Companion to Rawls* (Cambridge: Cambridge University Press, 2003), pp. 241–76, esp. pp. 254–55.

2 Both accounts can be described as Rawlsian. Indeed, Rawls's theory of justice is so dominant in thinking about just health care that it is often seen as the sole such available theory. See, for example, the exploration of theories of justice in health policy in Madison Powers and Ruth Faden, *Social Justice: The Moral Foundations of Public Health and Health Policy* (Oxford: Oxford University Press, 2006).

3 Norman Daniels, "Justice and Health Care," in D. Van De Veer and T. Regan (eds.), *Health Care Ethics* (Philadelphia: Temple University Press, 1987), p. 312.

4 Norman Daniels, "Fair Equality of Opportunity and Decent Minimums: A Reply to Buchanan," *Philosophy and Public Affairs* 14, no. 1 (1985): 107, *Am I My Parents' Keeper? An Essay on Justice between the Old and the Young* (New York: Oxford University Press, 1988), pp. 70–71, and *Justice and Justification: Reflective Equilibrium in Theory and Practice* (Cambridge: Cambridge University Press, 1996), pp. 187–88; Allen Buchanan et al., *From Chance to Choice: Genetics and Justice* (Cambridge: Cambridge University Press, 2000), p. 122.

5 For more literature critical of Daniels, see Allen Buchanan, "The Right to a Decent Minimum of Health Care," *Philosophy and Public Affairs* 13 (1984), 55–78; Lawrence Stern, "Opportunity and Health Care: Criticisms and Suggestions," *Journal of Medicine and Philosophy* 8 (1983): 339–62; Dan Brock, "Justice, Health Care, and the Elderly," *Philosophy and Public Affairs* 18, no. 3 (1989): 297–311; Sarah Marchand, "Liberal Theories and Health," unpublished manuscript.

6 J. P. Mackenbach, K. E. Stronks, and A. E. Kunst, "The Contribution of Medical Care to Inequalities in Health," *Social Science and Medicine* 29 (1989): 376.

7 Thomas Pogge, *Realizing Rawls* (Ithaca, NY: Cornell University Press, 1989), pp. 181–96.

8 John Rawls, *A Theory of Justice* (Oxford: Oxford University Press, 1971), p. 440.

9 Norman Daniels, "Health-Care Needs and Distributive Justice," *Philosophy and Public Affairs* 10, no. 2 (1981): 166.

10 The following two sections are largely reworked from my "Is Health Care (Still) Special?" *Journal of Political Philosophy* 15, no. 3 (2007): 342–63.

11 Jonathan Gruber, *Public Finance and Public Policy* (New York: Worth, 2005), p. 443.

12 Dan Brock advances a criticism to the same effect ("Justice, Health Care, and the Elderly," p. 305).

13 Daniels himself cites the fact of patients over 65 consuming 3.5 times more medical services (in terms of cost) compared with patients below that age. Norman Daniels, *Just Health Care* (Cambridge: Cambridge University Press, 1985), p. 86.

14 See Brock, "Justice, Health Care, and the Elderly," p. 309.

15 Cf. Daniels, *Just Health Care*, pp. 86–87.

16 This is Daniels's Prudential Life Span Account (see *Am I My Parents' Keeper?* pp. 90–91).

17 See also Aki Tsuchiya, "QALYs and Ageism: Philosophical Theories and Age Weighting," *Health Economics* 9, no. 1 (2000): 64; Brock, "Justice, Health Care, and the Elderly," pp. 303–4.

18 See also Daniel Callahan, *Setting Limits: Medical Goals in an Aging Society* (New York: Simon and Schuster, 1987). See Brock's review of this issue in "Justice, Health Care, and the Elderly."

19 Or even to younger patients who, willy-nilly, have completed their life plan, such as people on death row.

20 Cf. Daniels, "Justice, Health, and Healthcare," p. 5. To stress, Daniels's Prudential Life Span Account *is* able to accommodate long-term care for the elderly (provided it is not terribly expensive; see *Am I My Parents' Keeper?* pp. 106–11). My point, rather, is that the more fundamental "fair opportunity" account cannot do so.

21 Norman Daniels, Bruce Kennedy, and Ichiro Kawachi, "Health and Inequality, or, Why Justice Is Good for Our Health," in S. Anand, F. Peter, and A. Sen (eds.), *Public Health, Ethics, and Equity* (Oxford: Oxford University Press, 2004), p. 79.

22 Better yet, it may be suggested that dying in dignity is part of many people's life plan. And doing what it takes to prolong life, even at a very advanced age, is part of what it is to die with dignity. Dying while knowing that "everything possible" has been done is the way many people would want to exit this world, so the argument goes. Of course, for many people the exact opposite may be true. That is, terminal patients may view intrusive medical procedures that carry negligible expected medical benefit as conflicting with their view of what is a dignified way of dying. Still, sparing no effort to prolong one's life is yet another potential interpretation of people's life plan concerning the very last stages of life, and so my argument below applies to such life plans as well.

23 Daniels, *Just Health Care*, pp. 42–48, 104; "Justice and Health Care," p. 304, 314; *Am I My Parents' Keeper?* p. 74; *Justice and Justification*, pp. 189–92; *Just Health*, pp. 46–63.

24 Daniels, *Just Health Care*, p. 39, p. 46.

25 Rawls, *A Theory of Justice*, p. 84.

26 Ibid. For a critique of the lexical priority of the FEOP over the DP see Richard J. Arneson, "Against Rawlsian Equality of Opportunity," *Philosophical Studies* 93, no. 1 (1999): 77–112; Harry Brighouse and Adam Swift, "Equality, Priority, and Positional Goods," *Ethics* 116, no. 3 (2006), sec. V.

27 As Arneson points out, the argument from self-realization is probably the most persuasive, if ultimately flawed, reason provided by Rawls for the priority of the FEOP over the DP ("Against Rawlsian Equality of Opportunity," p. 97).

28 Arneson reconstructs some of these rationales in his "Against Rawlsian Equality of Opportunity," p. 80. See also Marchand, "Liberal Theories and Health," p. 16; Daniels, Kennedy, and Kawachi, "Why Justice Is Good for Our Health," p. 77; Robert S. Taylor, "Self-Realization and the Priority of Fair Equality of Opportunity," *Journal of Moral Philosophy* 1 (2004): 333–47. In my view, Arneson provides persuasive objections to all of these rationales. For the sake of argument, though, I will assume with Daniels the priority of the FEOP over the DP and focus, rather, on whether or not his arguments for that relationship, when applied to health care, are consistent with those provided by Rawls.

29 See, on this point, Lesley A. Jacobs, *Pursuing Equal Opportunities: The Theory and Practice of Egalitarian Justice* (Cambridge: Cambridge University Press, 2004), part I.

30 See also John Rawls, *Political Liberalism* (New York: University of Columbia Press, 1993), p. 184.

31 See, again, Daniels, *Just Health Care*, p. 104.

32 Daniels, *Just Health Care*, p. 33; *Am I My Parents' Keeper?* p. 70; *Justice and Justification*, p. 214. Arguably, as pointed out by Marchand, this feature already harbors a potentially serious problem for Daniels. For, where Rawls's FEOP seeks to remove *social* barriers in the competition for X, Daniels's (presumably) wishes also to remove *natural* barriers in the competition for X. In other words, to be consistent with the Rawlsian scheme, the only variances from normal species functioning that Daniels's theory could possibly correct would have to be those that are caused by social factors. I shall discuss this aspect of Daniels's theory more fully in chapter 7.

33 A rationale that Daniels acknowledges. See *Just Health Care*, p. 39. He also writes in Buchanan et al., *From Chance to Choice*, p. 127: "In effect, health care, like compensatory education programs, aims to produce 'normal *competitors*'" (emphasis added).

34 I have cast my argument in this section (for Daniels's impermissibility in using "life plan" in its broad interpretation) in Rawlsian terms. I did so in order to remain as faithful as possible to the framework constructed by Daniels himself. This may open my argument to the objection that my critique is only valid inasmuch as Daniels's argument depends on the Rawlsian framework. In response let me stress that the Rawlsian framework is central to Daniels, and his choice of Rawls's FEOP is not accidental. Chiefly, it allows Daniels to justify distributing health care in an equal, rather than a Pareto optimal (thus allowing for inequalities), way. Moreover, my objection applies to the very concept of "fair equality of opportunity," independently of its use by Rawls. Regulating *competitive* positions is inherent to the very notion of fair equality of opportunity (see, again, Jacobs, *Pursuing Equal Opportunities*, part I). And, it is due to that feature of fair equality

of opportunity that Daniels cannot subject noncompetitive pursuits, such as "leading a pain-free life," to that principle.

35 Anderson, "What Is the Point of Equality?" p. 306. See also Harry Frankfurt, "Equality as a Moral Ideal," *Ethics* 98, no. 1 (1987): 24.

36 As mentioned, the ideal of democratic or social equality is not new. Michael Walzer says: "The aim of political egalitarianism is a society free from domination." *Spheres of Justice: A Defense of Pluralism and Equality* (Oxford: Blackwell, 1983), p. xii. Cf. Miller's "equality of status, or simply social equality": "a society in which people regard and treat one another as equals, in other words a society that is not marked by status divisions such that one can place different people in hierarchically ranked categories." David Miller, "Equality and Justice," in A. Mason (ed.), *Ideals of Equality* (Oxford: Blackwell, 1998), p. 23. See also his "What Kind of Equality Should the Left Pursue?" in J. Franklin (ed.), *Equality* (London: Institute for Public Policy Research, 1997), p. 83. Still, each of these three ideals has a slightly different emphasis. Anderson highlights "oppression," Walzer "domination," and Miller "exclusion" and "alienation." Compare also with Scheffler's ideal of "social and political equality": "As a social ideal, it holds that a human society must be conceived of as a co-operative arrangement among equals, each of whom enjoys the same social standing. As a political ideal, it highlights the claims that citizens are entitled to make on one another by virtue of their status *as* citizens." Samuel Scheffler, "What Is Egalitarianism?" *Philosophy and Public Affairs* 31, no. 1 (2003): 22. (See also his "Choice, Circumstance, and the Value of Equality," *Philosophy, Politics, and Economics* 4, no. 1 [2005]: 5–28.) Finally, Daniels, at some point, complements his fair opportunity account by making use of a very similar ideal to Anderson's democratic equality: "Healthcare is of special moral importance, because it helps to preserve our status as fully functioning citizens." Norman Daniels, "Justice, Health, and Healthcare," *American Journal of Bioethics* 1, no. 2 (2001): 4.

37 Anderson, "What Is the Point of Equality?" p. 316.

38 Richard J. Arneson, "Luck Egalitarianism Interpreted and Defended," http://philosophyfaculty.ucsd.edu/faculty/rarneson/luckegalitarianism2.pdf (2005), p. 28. See also his "Disability, Priority, and Equal Opportunity," paper presented at the Bergen Workshop on Disability, June 2006, Bergen, Norway, p. 17.

39 "By necessaries I understand, not only the commodities which are indispensably necessary for the support of life, but whatever the custom of the country renders it indecent for creditable people, even of the lowest order, to be without. A linen shirt, for example, is, strictly speaking, not a necessary of life. [...] But in the present times, through the greater part of Europe, a creditable day-laborer would be ashamed to appear in publick without a linen shirt, the want of which would be supposed to denote that disgraceful degree of poverty, which, it is presumed, no body can well fall into without extreme bad conduct. Custom, in the same manner, has rendered leather shoes a necessary of life in England." Adam Smith, *The Wealth of Nations* (Glasgow: Glasgow University, 1976), pp. 869–70.

40 Paula Casal, "Why Sufficiency Is Not Enough," *Ethics* 117, no. 2 (2007): 296–326.

41 See Richard G. Wilkinson, *Unhealthy Societies: The Afflictions of Inequality* (London: Routledge, 1996); Michael Marmot and Richard G. Wilkinson, *Social Determinants of Health* (Oxford: Oxford University Press, 1999); Ichiro Kawachi, Bruce P. Kennedy, and Richard G. Wilkinson, *The Society and Health Reader: Income*

Inequality and Health (New York: The New Press, 1999). Cf. Angus Deaton, "Policy Implications of the Gradient of Health and Wealth," *Health Affairs* 21 (2002): 13–30. Deaton argues that the correct way of tackling health inequality is not by flattening the income gradient but by targeting the poor (since he fears the adverse effects of leveling down income). Furthermore, Deaton challenges the correlation of income with health, showing that often the correlation can be explained in the other direction, since low health often leads to low income. However, granted all that, even Deaton, a leading opponent of the idea that we should redistribute the social determinants of health equally, does not challenge the view that inequality, and not just poverty, generates low health and health inequalities. And he also does not claim that the effect of disease on earnings and education explains all the correlation between income and health. Thus, the view that health is determined by one's relative and not just absolute standing with regard to income and other indices of socioeconomic status seems to be unchallenged (although admittedly slightly weakened if Deaton is correct).

42 Michael Marmot, Martin J. Shipley, and Geoffrey Rose, "Inequalities in Death-Specific Explanations of a General Pattern," *Lancet* (1984): 1003–6.

43 Robert M. Sapolsky, Susan C. Alberts, Jeanne Altman, "Hypercortisolism Associated with Social Subordinance or Social Isolation among Wild Baboons," *Archives of General Psychiatry* 54 (1997): 1137–43; Robert M. Sapolsky, *Why Zebras Don't Get Ulcers: A Guide to Stress, Stress-Related Disease, and Coping* (New York: W. H. Freeman, 1998); Carol A. Shively and Thomas B. Clarkson, "Social Status and Coronary Artery Atherosclerosis in Female Monkeys," *Arteriosclerosis, Thrombosis, and Vascular Biology* 14 (1994): 721–26.

44 Wilkinson, *Unhealthy Societies*; Ichiro Kawachi, et al., "Social Capital, Income Inequality, and Mortality," *American Journal of Public Health* 87 (1997): 1491–98.

45 Michael Marmot, "Social Causes of Social Inequalities in Health," in S. Anand, F. Peter, and A. Sen (eds.), *Public Health, Ethics, and Equity*, pp. 37–62.

46 See Richard J. Arneson, "Egalitarianism and Responsibility," *Journal of Ethics* 3 (1999), p. 236; Casal, "Why Sufficiency Is Not Enough," p. 298.

47 See G. A. Cohen, "On the Currency of Egalitarian Justice," *Ethics* 99, no. 4 (1989): 919. This is a general criticism against capabilities-based approaches to equality, and specifically Amartya Sen's, whose "equality of capabilities" has probably inspired Anderson's democratic equality (see Amartya Sen, "Equality of What?" *The Tanner Lectures on Human Values* [Cambridge: Cambridge University Press, 1980], 197–220). For a similar point see also Thomas Christiano, "Comment on Elizabeth Anderson's "What Is the Point of Equality?" http://www.brown.edu/Departments/Philosophy/bears/9904chri.html. The point has been made also with regard to Daniels's focus on opportunities in what makes health care important. See Buchanan, "The Right to a Decent Minimum of Health Care"; Amy Gutmann, "For and against Equal Access to Health Care," *Milbank Memorial Fund Quarterly* 59 (1981): 542–60.

48 It is debatable, however, whether or not it is a health deficit. Some instances of pain cannot be properly seen as health deficits, for example, pain accompanying menstruation. I return to that point in chapter 9.

49 Anderson can perhaps respond by widening the definition of "participation in the life of the community" to include also participation in society's renewal and

survival, thus justifying compensation for fertility (as pointed out to me by Nir Eyal). Yet it seems to me that by doing so she would overstretch the democratic element of her "democratic equality."

50 That is, assuming we allow that Daniels's account requires equal opportunity for the pursuit of life plans. Having one's own biological children is part of many people's life plan. But this is of course contingent on Daniels's ability to actually justify applying Rawls's FEOP to this broad interpretation of a "life plan," something which, as was argued in the previous two sections, it is not obvious he can do.

51 "Negatively, people are entitled to whatever capabilities are necessary to enable them to avoid or escape entanglement in oppressive social relationships. Positively, they are entitled to the capabilities necessary for *functioning as an equal citizen in a democratic state.*" Anderson, "What Is the Point of Equality?" p. 316, emphasis added.

52 More accurately, they would lose their entitlement to that part of health care that does not eliminate oppression. See the previous note.

53 They may avoid that consequence by paternalistically guaranteeing democratic capabilities even to those who express no interest in ever participating. However, it would be difficult for democratic egalitarians to consistently hold such a position, as they themselves often accuse luck egalitarians of resorting to paternalism. See Anderson, "What Is the Point of Equality?" p. 301.

54 Frances Kamm makes a similar point about general entitlement to medical treatment. See Frances M. Kamm, "Health and Equality of Opportunity," *American Journal of Bioethics* 1, no. 2 (2001): 17. Anderson, in fact, explicitly states that convicted criminals should retain their entitlement to medical care, but she does not explain how doing so follows from her theory. "What Is the Point of Equality?" p. 327.

55 Anderson, "What Is the Point of Equality?" p. 313. Note that I leave aside the question of what a distributive theory premised on political participation would say about the entitlement of mentally incapacitated citizens to health care. The point has already been discussed in the literature, but it is even more relevant for the attempt to base distributive justice on democratic participation. (Cf. Richard Norman, "The Social Basis of Equality," in A. Mason [ed.], *Ideals of Equality* [Oxford: Blackwell, 1998], pp. 46–48.)

56 The point equally applies to a society governed through democracy by lot: according to democratic equality, this society would be obliged to allocate health care only to those drawn by the lot (a point made to me by Karl Widerquist).

57 And also "fetishistic," according to some. See Richard J. Arneson, "Luck Egalitarianism and Prioritarianism," *Ethics* 110, no. 2 (2000): 342.

58 For a similar argument about welfare policy in general, see Robert E. Goodin, *Reasons for Welfare: The Political Theory of the Welfare State* (Princeton, NJ: Princeton University Press, 1988), ch. 4.

59 He describes the ideal of social equality as "free-standing and independent of justice." Miller, "Equality and Justice," pp. 23, 31. See also Miller, "What Kind of Equality Should the Left Pursue?" pp. 84, 94.

60 Scheffler, "What Is Egalitarianism?" p. 26; "Equality as the Virtue of Sovereigns: A Reply to Ronald Dworkin," *Philosophy and Public Affairs* 31, no. 2 (2003): 203; "Choice, Circumstance, and the Value of Equality," p. 21.

61 See Miller, "What Kind of Equality Should the Left Pursue?" p. 94. Again, this is another aspect in which Miller's "social equality" seems to me to be superior to Anderson's "democratic equality" and Scheffler's ideal of "political equality."

Chapter 3: Ultra-Responsibility-Sensitive Health Care

1 Elizabeth S. Anderson, "What Is the Point of Equality?" *Ethics* 109 (1999): 301; cf. Ronald Dworkin, "Sovereign Virtue Revisited," *Ethics* 113, no. 1 (2002): 114. See also Paul Bou-Habib, "Compulsory Insurance without Paternalism," *Utilitas* 18, no. 3 (2006): 243–63.

2 Michael Otsuka, "Luck, Insurance, and Equality," *Ethics* 113 (2002): 41; Kasper Lippert-Rasmussen, "Egalitarianism, Option Luck, and Responsibility," *Ethics* 111 (2001): 548–79, and "Hurley on Egalitarianism and the Luck-Neutralizing Aim," *Politics, Philosophy and Economics* 4, no. 2 (2005): 259; Thomas Christiano, "Comment on Elizabeth Anderson's 'What Is the Point of Equality?'" http://www .brown.edu/Departments/Philosophy/bears/9904chri.html; Marc Fleurbaey, "Egalitarian Opportunities," *Law and Philosophy* 20, no. 5 (2001): 499–530, esp. pp. 513–22, and "Equal Opportunity or Equal Social Outcome?" *Economics and Philosophy* 11 (1995), 25–55; Alexander W. Cappelen and Bertil Tungodden, "A Liberal Egalitarian Paradox," *Economics and Philosophy* 22 (2006): 394; Cappelen and Tungodden, "Relocating the Responsibility Cut: Should More Responsibility Imply Less Redistribution?" *Politics, Philosophy, and Economics* 5, no. 3 (2006): 353–62; Alexander W. Cappelen and Ole F. Norheim, "Responsibility in Health Care: A Liberal Egalitarian Approach," *Journal of Medical Ethics* 31 (2005): 476–80; Alexander W. Cappelen, "Responsibility and International Distributive Justice," in A. Føllesdal and T. Pogge (eds.), *Real World Justice: Grounds, Principles, Human Rights, and Social Institutions* (Dordrecht: Springer, 2005), 215–28; Nicholas Barry, "Reassessing Luck Egalitarianism," *Journal of Politics* 70 (2008): 136–50. For the contrasting view that matching individuals' fates to the quality of their conduct (prudence-wise) is not required by equality but, if anything, by desert, see S. L. Hurley, *Justice, Luck, and Knowledge* (Cambridge, MA and London: Harvard University Press, 2003), p. 190; Robert E. Goodin, "Negating Positive Desert Claims," *Political Theory* 13 (1985): 585.

3 See, for example, Peter Vallentyne, "Brute Luck, Option Luck, and Equality of Initial Opportunities," *Ethics* 112, no. 3 (2002): 68.

4 Interestingly enough, this policy is also endorsed by Elizabeth Anderson, who is of course no friend of luck egalitarianism. See her "What Is the Point of Equality?" pp. 328–29.

5 Cappelen and Norheim, "Responsibility in Health Care," p. 478; See also Cappelen and Tungodden, "Relocating the Responsibility Cut," p. 356; Cappelen, "Responsibility and International Distributive Justice," p. 216; Alexander W. Cappelen, Ole F. Norheim, and Bertil Tungodden, "Genomics and Equal Opportunity Ethics," *Journal of Medical Ethics* 34 (2008): 361–64.

6 Nir Eyal makes a similar point in "Egalitarian Justice and Innocent Choice," *Journal of Ethics and Social Philosophy* 2, no. 1 (2007): 8.

7 See Lippert-Rasmussen, "Egalitarianism, Option Luck, and Responsibility," p. 555.

8 I am grateful to Daniel Attas for helping me clarify this point.

9 See also Richard J. Arneson, "Equality and Equal Opportunity for Welfare," in L. P. Pojman and R. Westmoreland (eds.), *Equality: Selected Readings* (New York, Oxford: Oxford University Press, 1997), pp. 239–40.

10 Lippert-Rasmussen, "Egalitarianism, Option Luck, and Responsibility," pp. 572–73.

11 For the argument that prudent gambles gone wrong should be understood as cases of bad brute luck rather than bad option luck, see Fleurbaey, "Egalitarian Opportunities," esp. pp. 513–22. In the example of Ned and Oliver as I gave it, not gambling is irrational. But as I state below, the argument holds not only for gambles that it would be *irrational* not to take, but also for ones that it would be *unreasonable* not to take. For example, it would be unreasonable not to gamble in something like the following: (A) 100% chance of receiving 100; (B) 50% chance of receiving 0, and 50% of 1,000. Since the expected utility of B is so much higher than A, it would be very reasonable to opt for B (i.e., gamble). Provided that ending up with 0 is not something catastrophic, opting for B and ending up unlucky may count as bad *brute* luck.

12 For a persuasive critique of the position that says that egalitarian justice is grounded on neutralizing luck as such, see Hurley, *Justice, Luck, and Knowledge*, esp. ch. 6.

13 Bernard Williams, "Moral Luck," in his *Moral Luck: Philosophical Papers 1973–1980* (Cambridge: Cambridge University Press, 1981); Thomas Nagel, "Moral Luck," in his *Mortal Questions* (Cambridge: Cambridge University Press, 1979).

14 David Enoch and Andrei Marmor, "The Case against Moral Luck," *Law and Philosophy* 26, no. 4 (2006): 405.

15 Arneson, "Luck Egalitarianism Interpreted and Defended," http://philosophy faculty.ucsd.edu/faculty/rarneson/luckegalitarianism2.pdf, p. 7. See also Fleurbaey, "Equal Opportunity or Equal Social Outcome?" pp. 40–41; Goodin, "Negating Positive Desert Claims," p. 585.

16 Notice that even the desert view may be committed to abandoning certain patients. For surely sometimes it would be the case that the punishment of leaving someone to bleed by the side of the road does, or nearly does, fit one's crime (think of a murderer who, following a car chase with the police, crashes his car and is gravely wounded). Most people would think that we still ought to treat him even though the fate he suffers fits, or at least approximates, his crime.

17 As pointed out by Arneson, "Luck Egalitarianism Interpreted and Defended," p. 1. It seems that Arneson and Cohen implicitly endorse the label, while Dworkin explicitly rejects it. See G. A. Cohen, "Luck and Equality: A Reply to Hurley," *Philosophy and Phenomenological Research* 72, no. 2 (2006): 439–46; Ronald Dworkin, "Equality, Luck and Hierarchy," *Philosophy and Public Affairs* 31, no. 2 (2003): 190.

18 Richard J. Arneson, "Equality and Equal Opportunity for Welfare," p. 234.

19 Ibid., p. 235.

20 He admits that when a person is responsible for her blindness, say, "it becomes questionable whether compensation is owed for the handicap." Richard J. Arneson, "Liberalism, Distributive Subjectivism, and Equal Opportunity for Welfare," *Philosophy and Public Affairs* 19, no. 2 (1990): 187. We can also safely count John Roemer as a "brute luck egalitarian," since he adopts Arneson's egalitarian ideal. (His concern is not so much to offer a basis for egalitarianism as to operational-

ize the concept of equality that he favors, i.e., that of Arneson's "Equality of Opportunity for Welfare.") See John E. Roemer, "A Pragmatic Theory of Responsibility for the Egalitarian Planner," *Philosophy and Public Affairs* 22, no. 2 (1993): 147, 149.

21 G. A. Cohen, "On the Currency of Egalitarian Justice," *Ethics* 99, no. 4 (1989): 916. See also his "Luck and Equality," n. 2.

22 Dworkin, "Equality, Luck and Hierarchy," p. 191.

23 The same can be said of another luck egalitarian, Eric Rakowski, since he sides with Dworkin's method of converting brute luck into option luck through the latter's famous hypothetical insurance mechanism (more on which in the next chapter). Rakowski therefore identifies justice as concerning eventualities for which individuals cannot be held responsible. This, again, denies that he is an all-luck egalitarian (see his *Equal Justice* [Oxford: Oxford University Press, 1991], pp. 80–81). Moreover, he explicitly writes that in his view justice does not require compensating victims of option luck (*Equal Justice*, pp. 74–75).

Chapter 4: Tough Luck? Why Egalitarians Need Not Abandon Reckless Patients

1 This chapter makes extensive use of (but also revises) material from my "In Solidarity with the Imprudent: A Defense of Luck Egalitarianism," *Social Theory and Practice* 33, no. 2 (2007): 177–98.

2 Elizabeth S. Anderson, "What Is the Point of Equality?" *Ethics* 109 (1999): 287–337. For criticism of Anderson, see Richard J. Arneson, "Luck Egalitarianism and Prioritarianism," *Ethics* 110, no. 2 (2000): 339–49; Thomas Christiano, "Comment on Elizabeth Anderson's "What Is the Point of Equality,'" http://www.brown.edu/Departments/Philosophy/bears/9904chri.html; David Sobel, "Comment on Elizabeth Anderson's "What Is the Point of Equality,'" http://www.brown.edu/Departments/Philosophy/bears/9904sobe.html. For sympathetic reviews, see Samuel Scheffler, "What Is Egalitarianism?" *Philosophy and Public Affairs* 31, no. 1 (2003): 5–39; Daniel Wikler, "Personal and Social Responsibility for Health," in S. Anand, F. Peter, and A. Sen (eds.), *Public Health, Ethics, and Equity*(Oxford: Oxford University Press, 2004), pp. 123–26.

3 "[J]ustice does not permit the exploitation or abandonment of anyone, even the imprudent." Anderson, "What Is the Point of Equality?" p. 298 (see also pp. 295–96). See also Scheffler: "[T]he fact that a person's urgent medical needs can be traced to his own negligence or foolishness or high-risk behavior is not normally seen as making it legitimate to deny him the care he needs" ("What Is Egalitarianism?" pp. 18–19); and his "Choice, Circumstance, and the Value of Equality," *Philosophy, Politics, and Economics* 4, no. 1 (2005): 15.

4 The term "imprudent" is Anderson's ("What Is the Point of Equality?" p. 298), yet it may inaccurately describe the array of cases she has in mind. I shall nevertheless follow Anderson in using "imprudence" to describe also incidents of prudent gambles that go wrong, and the case of informed negligence.

5 Peter Vallentyne, "Brute Luck, Option Luck, and Equality of Initial Opportunities," *Ethics* 112 (2002): 529–57. See also Marc Fleurbaey, "Egalitarian Opportunities," *Law and Philosophy* 20, no. 5 (2001): 499–530, esp. pp. 513–22. As mentioned in the previous chapter, Kasper Lippert-Rasmussen offers a somewhat similar argument for compensating bad option luck, but one that combines the current

response with the one surveyed in the previous chapter. (See his "Egalitarianism, Option Luck, and Responsibility," *Ethics* 111 [2001]: 548–79). In a recent unpublished manuscript, Richard Arneson has identified this group of philosophers as "desert luck egalitarians," for they hold that prudent risks (as well as altruistic conduct) convert a case of bad option luck into one deserving compensation. See his "Luck Egalitarianism Interpreted and Defended," http://philosophyfaculty .ucsd.edu/faculty/rarneson/luckegalitarianism2.pdf (2005), pp. 3–5.

6 Vallentyne, "Brute Luck, Option Luck, and Equality of Initial Opportunities," p. 556.

7 On the claim that what counts as a responsible action would depend on what risks it is conventionally reasonable to undertake, see Arthur Ripstein, "Equality, Luck, and Responsibility," *Philosophy and Public Affairs* 23, no. 1 (1994): 3–23.

8 Ronald Dworkin, *Sovereign Virtue: The Theory and Practice of Equality* (Cambridge, MA: Harvard University Press, 2000), chs. 2, 9. See also his "Foundations of Liberal Equality," *The Tanner Lectures on Human Values*, vol. 11 (Salt Lake City: University of Utah Press, 1990), p. 85; "Sovereign Virtue Revisited," *Ethics* 113, no. 1 (2002): 114; "Equality, Luck and Hierarchy," *Philosophy and Public Affairs* 31, no. 2 (2003): 192.

9 Anderson, "What Is the Point of Equality?" p. 301.

10 See "Sovereign Virtue Revisited," p. 114.

11 Dworkin acknowledges, at one point, this potential objection, noting that society cannot have a complaint against the imprudent who has purchased insurance against her eventual imprudence (*Sovereign Virtue*, p. 332).

12 Arneson, "Equality and Equal Opportunity for Welfare," in L. P. Pojman and R. Westmoreland (eds.), *Equality: Selected Readings* (New York, Oxford: Oxford University Press, 1997), p. 239. See also Anderson, "What Is the Point of Equality?" p. 300; Susan L. Hurley, *Justice, Luck, and Knowledge* (Cambridge, MA and London: Harvard University Press, 2003), pp. 187–90.

13 John E. Roemer, "A Pragmatic Theory of Responsibility for the Egalitarian Planner," *Philosophy and Public Affairs* 22, no. 2 (1993): 146–66.

14 Dworkin, *Sovereign Virtue*, p. 73.

15 David Miller, "What Kind of Equality Should the Left Pursue?" in J. Franklin (ed.), *Equality* (London: Institute for Public Policy Research, 1997), p. 91.

16 This response's only means of sidestepping such cases would be to assert that all cases of self-inflicted harm result, at bottom, from lack of true agency, and thus still fall under brute luck. But it is difficult to respond to such an assertion short of immersing ourselves "up to our necks in the free will problem," as Cohen has noted. "On the Currency of Egalitarian Justice," *Ethics* 99, no. 4 (1989): 934.

17 Nicholas Barry, "Defending Luck Egalitarianism," *Journal of Applied Philosophy* 23, no. 1 (2006): 99.

18 It is important, of course, to distinguish nonegalitarian considerations from anti-egalitarian ones. By "nonegalitarian considerations" I simply mean those that are compatible with egalitarian justice but that are not required by it.

19 Bernard Williams, "The Ideal of Equality," in L. P. Pojman and R. Westmoreland (eds.), *Equality: Selected Readings* (New York and Oxford: Oxford University Press, 1997), pp. 91–102.

20 Vallentyne has a useful exploration of the different components of justice in "Brute Luck, Option Luck, and Equality of Initial Opportunities," p. 530.

21 For explicit remarks to that effect see, for example, Arneson, "Liberalism, Distributive Subjectivism, and Equal Opportunity for Welfare," *Philosophy and Public Affairs* 19, no. 2 (1990): 176; "Welfare Should Be the Currency of Justice," *Canadian Journal of Philosophy* 30, no. 4 (2000): 497.

22 Cohen refers to this sentiment as the "primary egalitarian impulse" ("On the Currency of Egalitarian Justice," p. 908).

23 "One can defend luck egalitarianism not as a master moral principle but specifically as a principle for the distributive justice component of social justice" (Arneson, "Luck Egalitarianism Interpreted and Defended," p. 29). See also Cohen, "On the Currency of Egalitarian Justice," p. 908; "Facts and Principles," *Philosophy and Public Affairs* 31, no. 3 (2003): 244.

24 Cohen writes: "justice should not be the only guide to policy with respect to holdings." *Self-Ownership, Freedom, and Equality* (Cambridge: Cambridge University Press, 1995), p. 25. See also "Expensive Taste Rides Again," in J. Burley (ed.), *Dworkin and His Critics*, (Oxford: Blackwell, 2004), p. 4. Temkin similarly notes that "equality is not all that matters" (Larry Temkin, *Inequality* [Oxford: Oxford University Press, 1993], p. 282), and that "we should be pluralists about morality" ("Egalitarianism Defended," *Ethics* 113 [2003]: 782). McKerlie also points out that "equality is a matter of justice, but the theory of justice is pluralist and contains other principles, and the theory does not give equality lexical priority over the other values." Denis McKerlie, "Equality," *Ethics* 106, no. 2 (1996): 277. Thomas Scanlon writes, "we temper the demands of equality with other considerations. Equality is not our only concern" ("Nozick on Rights, Liberty, and Property," *Philosophy and Public Affairs* 6, no. 1 [1976]: 10). See also Derek Parfit, "Equality and Priority," A. Mason (ed.), *Ideals of Equality*, (Oxford: Blackwell, 1998), p. 4; Michael Walzer, "Response," in D. Miller and M. Walzer (eds.), *Pluralism, Justice, and Equality*, (Oxford: Oxford University Press, 1995), p. 293.

25 Thomas Nagel, *Mortal Questions* (Cambridge: Cambridge University Press, 1979), p. 107; Parfit, "Equality and Priority," p. 4.

26 Jonathan Wolff, "Fairness, Respect, and the Egalitarian Ethos," *Philosophy and Public Affairs* 27, no. 2 (1998): 97–122.

27 Cohen, "Expensive Taste Rides Again," p. 13.

28 G. A. Cohen, *If You're an Egalitarian, How Come You're So Rich?* (Cambridge, MA: Harvard University Press, 2000), p. 213.

29 See my discussion in the previous section.

30 One notable value that need not be traded off against egalitarian distributive justice is that of liberty, since it may already be incorporated within egalitarian considerations. Liberty, as luck egalitarians such as Dworkin and Cohen argue, is, in one sense at least, simply the license to discharge as one wishes with the goods and resources that are allocated through distributive justice. See Dworkin, *Sovereign Virtue*, ch. 3; "Do Liberal Values Conflict?" in M. Lilla, R. Dworkin, and R. B. Silvers (eds.), *The Legacy of Isaiah Berlin* (New York: New York Review Books, 2001), pp. 73–90. See also Arneson: "The luck egalitarian is wondering what we owe to one another, in general, by way of provision of the opportunities, *liberties* and resources that fall under the domain of distributive justice" ("Luck Egalitarianism Interpreted and Defended," p. 14, emphasis added).

31 Wolff says that it may be right to award unemployment benefits unconditionally despite this resulting in occasionally granting them to the undeserving lazy, so as

to avoid forcing "shameful revelation," i.e., the need to declare one's failure to find a job. Wolff, "Fairness, Respect, and the Egalitarian Ethos," pp. 113–15.

32 Arneson, "Welfare Should Be the Currency of Justice," p. 508; Nir Eyal, "Egalitarian Justice and Innocent Choice," *Journal of Ethics and Social Philosophy* 2, no. 1 (2007): 1–18.

33 Michael Otsuka, "Liberty, Equality, Envy, and Abstraction," in J. Burley (ed.), *Dworkin and His Critics* (Oxford: Blackwell, 2000), pp. 70–78.

34 Jonathan Wolff says that we must "be open to the possibility that the task of the egalitarian political philosopher is not completed by finding the fairest principles of justice." "Fairness, Respect, and the Egalitarian Ethos," p. 102.

35 As I noted in chapter 1, among luck egalitarians it is only Dworkin who may potentially hold a conflicting view, for he can sometimes be interpreted as saying that not only is society permitted to allow inequalities that result from bad option luck, it actually must do so. See Dworkin, *Sovereign Virtue*, pp. 74, 324. See also Kasper Lippert-Rasmussen, "Arneson on Equality of Opportunity for Welfare," *Journal of Political Philosophy* 7, no. 4 (1999): 480.

36 Susan Hurley hints at that possibility in her "On the What and the How of Distributive Justice and Health," in N. Holtug and K. Lippert-Rasmussen (eds.), *Egalitarianism* (Oxford: Oxford University Press, 2007), pp. 308–34.

37 Anderson, "What Is the Point of Equality?" p. 295.

38 Miller, "What Kind of Equality Should the Left Pursue?" p. 88.

39 Avishai Margalit, *The Decent Society* (Cambridge, MA, and London: Harvard University Press, 1996), ch. 13.

40 See also Wolff, "Fairness, Respect, and the Egalitarian Ethos," p. 102. We may do so even with regard to the case mentioned by Miller as his prime (and seemingly unassailable) example: suppressing justice in the name of security. Dworkin notes that in dealing with suspected terrorists sometimes the just policy is not necessarily the reasonable policy to undertake. "Ronald Dworkin Replies," in J. Burley (ed.), *Dworkin and His Critics* (Oxford: Blackwell, 2000), p. 344.

41 Otsuka, "Luck, Insurance, and Equality," *Ethics* 113 (2002): 48.

42 Dworkin, *Sovereign Virtue*, p. 1; "Sovereign Virtue Revisited," pp. 122–24; "Equality, Luck, and Hierarchy," p. 190.

43 Dworkin in fact hints at the possibility of trading off justice with other values, and specifically when the allocation of health care goods is concerned. See his "Justice in the Distribution of Health Care," *McGill Law Journal* 38, no. 4 (1993): 897.

44 Barry, "Defending Luck Egalitarianism," p. 98.

45 Norman Daniels himself recognizes that "we have a widely recognized moral obligation to meet people's medical needs." *Just Health: Meeting Health Needs Fairly* (Cambridge: Cambridge University Press, 2008), p. 111.

46 Thomas Scanlon, "Preference and Urgency," *Journal of Philosophy* 72 (1975): 655–69.

47 David Wiggins, *Needs, Values, Truth: Essays in the Philosophy of Value* (Oxford: Blackwell, 1988), ch. 1.

48 Allen Buchanan, "The Right to a Decent Minimum of Health Care," *Philosophy and Public Affairs* 13 (1984): 67–68.

49 This has been recognized also by Rawls in his most recent writing. Rawls writes of the social minimum: "the expectation of an assured provision of health care at a certain level (calculated by estimated cost) is included as part of that mini-

mum." John Rawls, *Justice as Fairness: A Restatement* (Cambridge, MA: Harvard University Press, 2001), p. 173. On the concept of social minimum more generally, see Stuart White, "Social Minimum," *Stanford Encyclopedia of Philosophy*, http://plato.stanford.edu/entries/social-minimum/, 2004.

50 Arneson, "Luck Egalitarianism Interpreted and Defended," http://philosophy faculty.ucsd.edu/faculty/rarneson/luckegalitarianism2.pdf, p. 7. See also Marc Fleurbaey, "Equal Opportunity or Equal Social Outcome?" *Economics and Philosophy* 11 (1995): 40–41; Robert E. Goodin, "Negating Positive Desert Claims," *Political Theory* 13 (1985): 585.

51 See for example, Daniels, *Just Health*, p. 298.

52 If our obligation toward the AIDS patient who contracted the disease while receiving transfusion is strong, our obligation toward the patient who has contracted it while *donating* blood (say, from an infected needle) is even stronger. Of course, things get a little complicated if we determine that the blood donation was a matter of option luck (the person chose to give blood) whereas the blood transfusion was one of brute luck (the patient had to have a blood transfusion). Yet, if giving blood is something that it would be unreasonable to expect people not to do, then we may cast the case of AIDS following a donation as one constituting a brute luck disadvantage. I am grateful to Kristin Voigt for helping me clarify this point.

53 Daniels, *Just Health*, p. 305.

54 I should say that I have in fact already given Daniels (at least) the benefit of trading off his theory of justice with other values. Recall that in chapter 2, section I, I raised the objection that equality of opportunity might in fact justify selective, and not universal, health care. And I then allowed that Daniels may escape that objection by coupling his theory of egalitarian justice with the concern for not harming the self-respect of those who would be denied public health care under selective health care.

Chapter 5 : Responsibility-Sensitive Universal Health Care

1 See Norman Daniels, *Just Health: Meeting Health Needs Fairly* (Cambridge: Cambridge University Press, 2008), p. 147.

2 See in particular Norman Daniels, "Health-Care Needs and Distributive Justice," *Philosophy and Public Affairs* 10, no. 2 (1981): 146–79.

3 In that, my account follows that of Buchanan. See Allen Buchanan, "The Right to a Decent Minimum of Health Care," *Philosophy and Public Affairs* 13 (1984): 55–78.

4 Daniels, *Just Health*, pp. 31–36.

5 On this point see also Buchanan, "The Right to a Decent Minimum of Health Care," p. 66.

6 Bodily health, bodily integrity, and physical survival are all cited by Nussbaum as part of the capabilities constituting the basic decent minimum. Martha Nussbaum, *Women and Human Development* (Cambridge: Cambridge University Press, 2000). Notice that my allusion to the capabilities approach is different in one significant way from the way in which it is usually alluded to. Many appeal to Sen's capabilities approach as an interpretation of the requirements of egalitarian distributive justice. Here, in contrast, I appeal to this set of capabilities, as representing basic needs, as part of a sufficientarian layer of distribution, and not one

of egalitarian distributive justice. Since the moral requirement to supply these capabilities is independent of *egalitarian* distributive justice, meeting them is not subject to the abandonment objection.

7 There is empirical evidence suggesting that most people believe that compulsory insurance for such cases is justified. See Paul Anand and Allan Wailoo, "Utilities versus Rights to Publicly Provided Goods: Arguments and Evidence from Health Care Rationing," *Economica* 67, no. 268 (2000): 563.

8 That is why a concern for the intrinsic value of the autonomy of the patient can justify medical *coverage* but it cannot justify forcing medical care. This consideration is sometimes overlooked in justifications of a universal minimum. See, for example, Paul Bou-Habib, "Compulsory Insurance without Paternalism," *Utilitas* 18, no. 3 (2006): 243–63.

9 Harald Schmidt, "Bonuses as Incentives and Rewards for Health Responsibility: A Good Thing?" *Journal of Medicine and Philosophy* 33 (2008): 216.

10 See, for example, David B. Resnik, "The Patient's Duty to Adhere to Prescribed Treatment: An Ethical Analysis," *Journal of Medicine and Philosophy* 30 (2005): 167–88. Resnik, though, has a peculiar emphasis on the reciprocal duties between the doctor and the patient, whereas it seems to me that reciprocity between the patient and all other actual and potential patients in society is the more relevant dimension of reciprocity in this case.

11 See also Bou-Habib, "Compulsory Insurance without Paternalism."

12 Notice that I speak of coverage, and not about care itself, as something that cannot be waived. For as we just saw, a person may waive her right to medical care at present, in the sense that no one could have a medical procedure performed on them without their prior and explicit consent. One may refuse care at a specific point of time, but one may not waive one's entitlement for general coverage.

13 See Bou-Habib, "Compulsory Insurance without Paternalism."

14 Stuart White has invoked the concept of "a normatively nonexcludable good" in a different context. See his *The Civic Minimum: On the Rights and Obligations of Economic Citizenship* (Oxford: Oxford University Press, 2003), p. 61.

15 Bou-Habib offers a very similar reason. "Compulsory Insurance without Paternalism," esp. p. 252.

16 Notice that I do not claim that the provision of health care is justified merely by physical proximity. Rather I claim that *insofar as* health care is seen as a public good on account of its normative nonexcludability, it then makes more sense to view that normative nonexcludability as spatial rather than as personal. Insomuch as society is committed to the idea that it is wrong to allow anyone's basic needs to go unmet, my claim is that that "anyone" refers to anyone inhabiting the territory and not merely to citizens. To do otherwise, I suggested, would run against the grain of normative nonexcludability.

17 For such an account of health care that sees value in personal responsibility and seeks to hold imprudent patients responsible, see Rob Houtepen and Ruud Ter Muelen, "New Types of Solidarity in the European Welfare State," *Health Care Analysis* 8 (2000): 329–40.

18 See Schmidt, "Bonuses as Incentives and Rewards for Health Responsibility."

19 "The cost of sloth, gluttony, alcoholic intemperance, reckless driving, sexual frenzy, and smoking is now a national, not an individual responsibility. This is justified as individual freedom—but one man's freedom in health is another

man's shackle in taxes and insurance premiums." John H. Knowles, "The Responsibility of the Individual," in J. H. Knowles (ed.), *Doing Better and Feeling Worse: Health in the United States* (New York: Norton, 1997), p. 59. Such an attitude, according to Daniel Wikler, amounts to "legalized moralism." Daniel Wikler, "Persuasion and Coercion for Health: Ethical Issues in Government's Effort to Change Lifestyle," *Milbank Memorial Fund Quarterly/Health and Society* 56, no. 3 (1978): 316, 332.

20 Margaret Whitehead, "The Concepts and Principles of Equity and Health," *Health Promotion International* 6, no. 3 (1991): 220.

21 A potential objection to Roemer's proposal is that since skiing is an activity that is typical to the rich, it would follow that the poor skier is more responsible than the rich skier (see Daniels, *Just Health*, p. 77). But notice that on Roemer's account finding the typical level of risk-taking characterizing a class of people is meant only to allow us to recognize what would count as an imprudent behavior *even* for members of this group (namely, anything that is above the mean). Crucial to Roemer's suggestion is the supposition that the mean level of risk-taking should be allowed to be higher the lower the socioeconomic class. This is based on the thought that we ought to make more concessions to individuals, in terms of imprudence, the worse off they are. That supposition, central to Roemer's proposal, allows us to avoid the counterintuitive conclusion that the poor skier is more responsible than the rich skier.

22 Pieter H. M. Van Baal et al., "Lifetime Medical Costs of Obesity: Prevention No Cure for Increasing Health Expenditure," *PLoS Medicine* 5, no. 2 (2008): 242–49.

23 See the excellent discussion in Schmidt, "Bonuses as Incentives and Rewards for Health Responsibility."

24 See again Schmidt (ibid., p. 211) on this latter point.

25 Ronald Dworkin, *Sovereign Virtue: The Theory and Practice of Equality* (Cambridge, MA: Harvard University Press, 2000), p. 61.

26 See, for example, Leslie A. Jacobs, "Justice in Health Care: Can Dworkin Justify Equal Access?" in J. Burley (ed.), *Dworkin and His Critics* (Oxford: Blackwell, 2004), p. 142. Although Dworkin's otherwise "ambition-sensitive" theory denies that possibility by introducing compulsory insurance in the case of health care. See Ronald Dworkin, "Ronald Dworkin Replies," in that same volume, p. 361; *Sovereign Virtue*, ch. 8.

27 Despite his assertion to the contrary in later work: Norman Daniels, "Justice, Health, and Healthcare," *American Journal of Bioethics* 1, no. 2 (2001): 4; *Justice and Justification: Reflective Equilibrium in Theory and Practice* (Cambridge: Cambridge University Press, 1996), p. 197.

28 That is, the non-Dworkinian version of luck egalitarianism that I employ in this book. As for Dworkin, he in fact bites the bullet and argues that in some cases patients should be allowed to opt out and receive the cash equivalent of their treatment. See "Ronald Dworkin Replies," p. 360.

Chapter 6: Why Justice in Health?

1 The next several paragraphs contain material from my "Is Health Care (Still) Special?" *Journal of Political Philosophy* 15, no. 3 (2007): 342–63.

2 Dan Brock, "Broadening the Bioethics Agenda," *Kennedy Institute of Ethics Journal* 10, no. 1 (2000): 31. See also Anthony J. Culyer, "Health, Health Expenditures,

and Equity," in E. van Doorslaer, A. Wagstaff, and F. Rutten (eds.), *Equity in the Finance and Delivery of Health Care* (Oxford: Oxford University Press, 1993), p. 301; Gopal Sreenivasan, "Health Care and Equality of Opportunity," *Hastings Center Report* 37 (2007): 31–41.

3 This was illustrated in the famous Whitehall study, which found a steady and steep gradient in morbidity and mortality across rank and socioeconomic status between British civil servants who all had more or less the same access to health care. See Michael G. Marmot, Martin J. Shipley, and Geoffrey Rose, "Inequalities in Death-Specific Explanations of a General Pattern," *Lancet* 1984: 1003–6.

4 Some, for example, are even more skeptical about health care than the studies cited by Brock, and estimate that health care accounts for only about one-sixth of life years gained in the previous century. See Jonathan M. Mann, "Medicine and Public Health, Ethics and Human Rights," *Hastings Center Report* 27 (1997): 8. On the other hand, Angus Deaton, whose work was mentioned in chapter 2, has argued that we should be skeptical of some of this literature. Dismissing the impact of health care on health inequalities, Deaton says, is motivated by the apparent correlation between income and health that exists even in societies that have universal health care. But this view, says Deaton, tends to overlook the fact that wealthier and more educated patients get more out of a universal system (I mention some of the reasons for this below). Thus, health care is of greater impact than is commonly assumed. Still, even Deaton does not dispute that some inequalities in health cannot be explained by inequalities with regard to health care, such as the inequalities in cardiovascular diseases discovered in Whitehall civil servants *prior to hospitalization*. See Angus Deaton, "Policy Implications of the Gradient of Health and Wealth," *Health Affairs* 21 (2002): 18. If Deaton is correct, it might be that the impact of health care on our health is greater than 20%.

5 Although we may plausibly hypothesize that the impact of clinical care on population health in developing countries is negligible compared to preventive public health measures. The latter, however, is not part of what is normally referred to by the term "social determinants of health." (I elaborate on that point below).

6 Richard Wilkinson and Michael Marmot, *Social Determinants of Health: The Solid Facts,* 2nd ed. (Geneva: WHO, 2003), p. 7 (emphasis added).

7 Norman Daniels, Bruce Kennedy, and Ichiro Kawachi, "Health and Inequality, or, Why Justice Is Good for Our Health," in S. Anand, F. Peter, and A. Sen (eds.), *Public Health, Ethics, and Equity* (Oxford: Oxford University Press, 2004), p. 87; also pp. 63, 68. See also Norman Daniels, Bruce Kennedy, and Ichiro Kawachi, "Justice Is Good for our Health," in J. Cohen and J. Rogers (eds.), *Is Inequality Bad for Our Health?* (Boston: Beacon Press, 2000), pp. 3–33; Daniels, *Just Health: Meeting Health Needs Fairly* (Cambridge: Cambridge University Press, 2008), p. 4.

8 See Norman Daniels, *Just Health Care* (Cambridge: Cambridge University Press, 1985), ch. 8; Allen Buchanan et al., *From Chance to Choice: Genetics and Justice* (Cambridge: Cambridge University Press, 2000), p. 122; Daniels, Kennedy, and Kawachi, "Health and Inequality," p. 75.

9 See Michael Marmot, *The Status Syndrome: How Social Standing Affects Our Health and Longevity* (New York: Times Books, 2004).

10 See Wilkinson and Marmot, *Social Determinants of Health*; Michael Marmot and Richard G. Wilkinson, *Social Determinants of Health*, 2nd ed. (Oxford: Oxford University Press, 2006). The latter source is particularly good on the *psychologi-*

cal effects of social exclusion, poverty, and unemployment, and their effect on our health.

11 This is of course most conspicuously evidenced in the shift of titles from Daniels's 1985 *Just Health Care* to his most recent *Just Health*. As for policy makers, see *Independent Inquiry into Inequalities in Health: Report* (London: Stationery Office, 1998).

12 Sreenivasan, "Health Care and Equality of Opportunity."

13 See for example, Norman Daniels, "Fair Equality of Opportunity and Decent Minimums: A Reply to Buchanan," *Philosophy and Public Affairs* 14, no. 1 (1985): 107; "A Reply to Some Stern Criticisms and a Remark on Health Care Rights," *Journal of Medicine and Philosophy* 8 (1983): 363; "Justice and Health Care," in D. Van De Veer and T. Regan (eds.), *Health Care Ethics*, (Philadelphia: Temple University Press, 1987), p. 312.

14 For that view, see, for example, Madison Powers and Ruth Faden, *Social Justice: The Moral Foundations of Public Health and Health Policy* (Oxford: Oxford University Press, 2006). Another statement of a "global," as opposed to "local," view of justice in health is offered in Marc Fleurbaey and Erik Schokkaert, "Unfair Inequalities in Health and Health Care," unpublished manuscript.

15 Daniels, *Just Health*, ch. 2; Amartya Sen, "Why Health Equity?" *Health Economics* 11 (2002): 659–66.

16 Daniels, *Just Health*, p. 4.

17 Sen, "Why Health Equity?"

18 As in Descartes's famous saying that the "preservation of health" is "chief of all goods." See Michael Walzer, *Spheres of Justice: A Defense of Pluralism and Equality* (Oxford: Blackwell, 1983), p. 87.

19 See Sen, "Why Health Equity?" p. 660. Cf. Powers and Faden (*Social Justice*), whose theory of just health resists depicting health as a separate sphere of justice.

20 Sen, "Why Health Equity?" p. 663. This is why, perhaps, the "nonideal" theory of justice in health offered by Powers and Faden is, in my view, not particularly helpful either in offering a theory of justice in health, or in providing insights about justice in general.

21 See Emanuela E. Gakidou, Christopher J. L. Murray, and Julio Frenk, "Defining and Measuring Health Inequality: An Approach Based on the Distribution of Health Expectancy," *Bulletin of the World Health Organization* 78 (2000): 42–54.

22 See Christopher J. L. Murray and Alan D. Lopez (eds.), *The Global Burden of Disease* (Cambridge, MA: Harvard School of Public Health, World Health Organization, World Bank, 1996). Note that, since "an individual life expectancy" is meaningless (see also Daniel M. Hausman, Yukiko Asada, and Thomas Hedemann, "Health Inequalities and Why They Matter," *Health Care Analysis* 10, no. 2 [2002], p. 186), on the account discussed here "health inequalities" are inevitably inequalities between groups. What counts as an appropriate group for the purposes of health inequalities, however, is left open here, and I return to that question only in the third part of the book.

Chapter 7: Luck Egalitarian Justice in Health

1 Anthony J. Culyer and Adam Wagstaff, "Equity and Equality in Health and Health Care," *Journal of Health Economics* 12 (1993): 431–57. Cf. Margaret White-

head, "The Concepts and Principles of Equity and Health," *Health Promotion International* 6, no. 3 (1991): 219. She discusses "a situation where everyone in the population has the same level of health, suffers the same type and degree of illness and dies after exactly the same life span. This is not an achievable goal, nor even a desirable one." But she never explains why this is unjust, let alone why this is not desirable.

2 Now, of course, it is highly probable that there will exist an inequality of health between a 20-year-old and a 70-year-old. But proponents of outcome equality in health need not characterize this state of affairs as unjust. Rather, outcome equality in health takes a lifetime view of equality, comparing individuals' health throughout their lives, say in the form of healthy life expectancy.

3 See for example, Norman Daniels, Bruce Kennedy, and Ichiro Kawachi, "Health and Inequality, or, Why Justice Is Good for Our Health," in S. Anand, F. Peter, and A. Sen (eds.), *Public Health, Ethics, and Equity* (Oxford: Oxford University Press, 2004), p. 73.

4 See Sarah Marchand, Daniel Wikler, and Bruce Landesman, "Class, Health, and Justice," *Milbank Quarterly* 76, no. 3 (1998): 463–65.

5 Others who hold that health inequalities that are owed to freely chosen lifestyle are not unjust include Julian Le Grand ("Equity, Health, and Health Care," *Social Justice Research* 1, no .3 [1987]: 257–74) and Margaret Whitehead ("The Concepts and Principles of Equity and Health"). For a review of health inequalities and responsibility for health, see Daniel Wikler, "Personal and Social Responsibility for Health," in S. Anand, F. Peter, and A. Sen (eds.), *Public Health, Ethics, and Equity* (Oxford: Oxford University Press, 2004), pp. 109–34, esp. pp. 113–17. See also Fabienne Peter, "Health Equity and Social Justice," in that same volume, pp. 94–95.

6 Amartya Sen, *Inequality Re-examined* (Cambridge, MA: Harvard University Press, 1992), ch. 6; "Why Health Equity?" in *Public Health, Ethics, and Equity*, eds. S. Anand, F. Peter, and A. Sen, pp. 21–33.

7 Note that I speak of inequalities in health between the "sexes," whereas some recent literature on health equity refers to "*gender* inequalities," "*gender* differences," and "*gender* discrimination" (Sudhir Anand, "The Concern for Equity in Health," in *Public Health, Ethics, and Equity*, eds. S. Anand, F. Peter, and A. Sen, p. 19; Sen, "Why Health Equity?" p. 30; Sen, *Development as Freedom* [Oxford: Oxford University Press, 1999], p. 20; Christopher J. L. Murray, "Rethinking DALYs," in *The Global Burden of Disease*, eds. C.J.L. Murray and A. D. Lopez [Cambridge, MA: Harvard School of Public Health, World Health Organization, World Bank, 1996], pp. 16, 18; Madison Powers and Ruth Faden, *Social Justice: The Moral Foundations of Public Health and Health Policy* [Oxford: Oxford University Press, 2006], p. 62). Now, "gender" usually refers to the social construct of sex. The Oxford English Dictionary defines it as "a euphemism for the sex of a human being, often intended to emphasize the social and cultural, as opposed to the biological, distinctions between the sexes." "Gender discrimination" or "gender inequalities" on that understanding, then, appear to be a tautology, for "gender" *already* implies "sex-based differences." It is therefore more accurate, I think, to speak of "inequalities between the sexes."

8 Interestingly, the idea that health equity should move from equality of outcome toward equality of opportunity is gaining ground also among health economists.

See Pedro Rosa Dias and Andrew M. Jones, "Giving Equality of Opportunity a Fair Innings," *Health Economics* 16 (2007): 109–12.

9   As I mentioned in chapter 4, section I, it is often pointed out that the level of effort an individual is able to exercise may itself be subject to morally arbitrary constraints. I should stress, then, that "effort" is here meant as a placeholder for whatever it is the reader considers to be within the individual's control.

10 Notice also that according to the stated principle it is also *not* unfair for the smoker and the jogger to end up having the exact same health outcome; unfairness only obtains when there is *in*equality in health (recall our discussion in chapter 1, section II). It is *only* unfair, according to the stated principle, if the person investing as much or more effort ends up being less healthy.

11 See for example, Richard J. Arneson, "Equality and Equal Opportunity for Welfare," in L. P. Pojman and R. Westmoreland (eds.), *Equality: Selected Readings* (New York: Oxford University Press, 1997), p. 234.

12 That is, effectively, the position held by Le Grand ("Equity, Health, and Health Care"). See also Robert M. Veatch, "Justice and the Right to Health Care: An Egalitarian Account," in T. J. Bole and W. B. Bondeson (eds.), *Rights to Health Care* (Dordrecht: Kluwer, 1991), pp. 83–102, esp. p. 83; Margaret Whitehead, *The Concepts and Principles of Equity and Health* (Copenhagen: World Health Organization, 1990), p. 9. Incidentally, in that respect, the luck egalitarian approach appears decisively less paternalistic than Daniels's Rawlsian approach. Daniels's Rawlsian approach, recall, sees the importance of health as contributing to equality of opportunity. The commitment to equality of opportunity thus generates the commitment to equalize health. Crucially, on the Rawlsian account, individuals cannot trade opportunities for jobs and careers for other goods, mainly for reasons having to do with self-respect. In its application to health, the principle of FEO generates a strong commitment to equalizing health and to preventing individuals from trading health for other goods. Arguably, this entails a breach of Rawls's own commitment to neutrality between conceptions of the good life. But Daniels in fact bites the bullet on this point. See his *Just Health: Meeting Health Needs Fairly* (Cambridge: Cambridge University Press, 2008), pp. 98–99.

13 Sen cites the interesting finding that female fetuses have higher chances of survival than male ones. See his *Development as Freedom*, p. 105.

14 John Rawls, *A Theory of Justice* (Oxford: Oxford University Press, 1971), sec. 14.

15 Supposing, for example, it were possible to distinguish different smokers' genetic propensity to contract lung cancer, Rawls's FEOP would warrant equalizing health within, and not between, these groups of smokers.

16 An approach to measuring health inequalities that in fact adopts something like the FEO for health is presented in Antoine Bommier and Guy Stecklov, "Defining Health Inequality: Why Rawls Succeeds Where Social Welfare Theory Fails," *Journal of Health Economics* 21 (2002): 497–513.

17 Notice that the link I draw between FEOP and health is of the opposite direction compared to the one drawn by Daniels. I look here at FEO *for* health, whereas Daniels proposes health *for the sake of* FEO (for life plans). Having said that, Daniels would probably also endorse FEO for health. The closest he comes to endorsing that position is in saying that society ought not be committed to "the

futile task of leveling all natural differences between persons." *Just Health Care* (Cambridge: Cambridge University Press, 1985), p. 46.

18 Rawls, *A Theory of Justice*, p. 84; *Political Liberalism* (New York: University of Columbia Press, 1993), p. 184.

19 See, for example, John E. Roemer, "A Pragmatic Theory of Responsibility for the Egalitarian Planner," *Philosophy and Public Affairs* 22, no. 2 (1993): 146–66.

20 So according to FEO for health, it is *not unfair* for a person of better genetic disposition (say, a female smoker compared to a male smoker) to end up having better health. In accordance with our discussion in chapter 1, section II, it is also not *un*fair if the female smoker and the male smoker end up having *equal* health. It *is* unfair if the female smoker ends up being *less* healthy than the male smoker.

21 See Anand, "The Concern for Equity in Health," p. 19; Sen, "Why Health Equity?" p. 23; Daniel M. Hausman, Yukiko Asada, and Thomas Hedemann, "Health Inequalities and Why They Matter," *Health Care Analysis* 10, no. 2 (2002): 177–91.

22 See, on a similar point, Sarah Marchand, "Liberal Theories and Health," unpublished manuscript.

23 Rawls, *A Theory of Justice*, sec.11.

24 Rawls's three lexically ordered principles are the principle of equal basic liberties, the FEOP, and the DP. See *A Theory of Justice*, p. 60.

25 Notice that in the first part of the book I argued for applying two supplementary patterns of distribution to health *care*: first, a luck egalitarian distribution of health care to those who suffer brute luck disadvantages, and second, a sufficientarian distribution of care to meet basic needs. In other words, whatever needs are not met under the first principle will be met under the second. There is therefore no conflict between my two principles as there would be here with regard to a Rawlsian distribution of health.

26 "[I]f some places were not open on a basis fair to all, those kept out would be right in feeling unjustly treated even though they benefited from the greater efforts of those who were allowed to hold them. They would be justified in their complaint not only because they were excluded from certain external rewards of office but because they were debarred from the realization of self which comes from a skilful and devoted exercise of social duties. They would be deprived of one of the main forms of human good." Rawls, *A Theory of Justice*, p. 84.

27 David Mechanic, "Disadvantage, Inequality, and Social Policy," *Health Affairs* 21 (2002): 48–59. The following example is often mentioned in this context. In the United States, black infant mortality rates were 64% higher than infant mortality rates for whites in 1954, and were proportionally even higher (130% higher) in 1998, even though white rates dropped by 20.8 per thousand and black rates dropped by 30.1 per thousand in that period. So while everyone's health has improved considerably, health inequalities were at the same time aggravated. (See also Angus Deaton, "Policy Implications of the Gradient of Health and Wealth," *Health Affairs* 21 (2002): 25.) Another example, cited by Daniels, is that stop-smoking campaigns may be more effective for individuals from higher socioeconomic groups compared to their effectiveness on those from lower socioeconomic groups. (See Elizabeth M. Barbeau, Nancy Krieger, and Mah-Jabeen Soobader, "Working Class Matters: Socio-Economic Disadvantage, Race/Ethnic-

ity, Gender, and Smoking in NIHS," *American Journal of Public Health* 94 [2004]: 269–87. Their research confirmed the hypothesis that socioeconomic resources are a key to helping the individual quit smoking.) An exception to the rule that public health interventions benefit the rich and healthy more than they do the poor and ill is the fluoridation of water. Many well-off people in the United States drink only bottled water, and so the fluoridation of water seems to be one type of health intervention that has a distinctly egalitarian effect, benefiting the poor more than it does the rich. I owe that observation to Eric Cavallero.

28 See also Sen, "Why Health Equity?" p. 25. Some may object to the use of the term "leveling down" in this context, for what is at stake is not leveling down *actual* levels of health (say, by stopping treatment of healthier patients, or even deliberately infecting them with some disease). Rather, my illustration so far only describes a case where the FEOP prevents us from exacerbating inequalities even when doing so would benefit the worse off. In effect, then, the case before us only concerns leveling down *potential* gains (to health) rather than current gains. While I do not dispute that observation, I cannot see how it affects, in any meaningful way, the undesirability of FEOP for health; leveling down potential gains to health is perhaps not as repugnant as leveling down current levels of health (for one thing, the latter may involve violating the self-ownership that individuals have over their own bodies whereas the former perhaps does not), but it is undesirable nevertheless.

29 Rawls, it seems, was aware of the leveling down effect of his FEOP, and his "second priority rule" (*A Theory of Justice*, p. 303) tries to address this problem. It says that "an inequality of opportunity must enhance the opportunities of those with the lesser opportunity." But of course that priority rule now conflicts with Rawls's earlier rationale for strict equality required by the FEOP (see again p. 84 of *A Theory of Justice*). It is therefore the case that opportunities are either to be treated like any other social primary good (and hence be regulated under a maximin principle), or must maintain their lexical priority over social primary goods and thus be distributed equally.

30 Rawls, *A Theory of Justice*, p. 84.

31 Richard J. Arneson, "Against Rawlsian Equality of Opportunity," *Philosophical Studies* 93, no. 2 (1999): 104–5.

32 Notice that the luck egalitarian EOP does not necessarily condemn outcome inequality in life expectancy between women and men (for that inequality might be the result of individuals' voluntary action). But EOP does condemn an inequality *in opportunity* between men and women as such. That is, it rules as unjust the fact that one's sex determines one's health prospects.

33 The thought that inequalities in life expectancy between the sexes are *not unjust* is the reason why, for example, the Human Development Index, which drew inspiration from Sen's capabilities approach, sets a different life expectancy target for men and women (82.5 and 87.5 respectively), while setting all other targets as equal between the sexes (The United Nations Development Program, *Human Development Report: Concept and Measurement of Human Development* [Oxford: Oxford University Press, 1990]). There is also some quantitative evidence for the public's preference for reducing health inequalities between socioeconomic groups and for *resisting* giving preference in medical treatment on the basis of sex. See Paul Dolan et al., "QALY Maximization and People's Preferences: A

Methodological Review of the Literature," *Health Economics* 14 (2005): 197–208; Paul Anand and Allan Wailoo, "Utilities versus Rights to Publicly Provided Goods: Argument and Evidence from Health Care Rationing," *Economica* 67, no .268 (2000): 543–77.

34　John Kekes, "A Question for Egalitarians," *Ethics* 107, no. 4 (1997): 662.

35　Aki Tsuchiya and Alan Williams, "A 'Fair Innings' between the Sexes: Are Men Being Treated Inequitably?" *Social Science and Medicine* 60, no. 2 (2005): 277–86; Alan Williams, "If We Are Going to Get a Fair Innings, Someone Will Need to Keep the Score!" in M. L. Barer, T. E. Getzen, and G. L. Stoddart (eds.), *Health, Health Care and Health Economics* (New York: Wiley, 1998), p. 327.

36　Murray, "Rethinking DALYs," p. 18. One could argue, I suppose, that even these ostensibly social factors are also in fact natural, for such reckless behavior may be the direct result of high levels of testosterone. (This is a possibility entertained by Tsuchiya and Williams. See their "A 'Fair Innings' between the Sexes," p. 281.) But it would be difficult to attribute all the aforementioned differences in lifestyle to genetic factors, leaving men no room for free will whatsoever (see the next numbered point).

37　Although that figure varies: the less developed a society is, the greater is the difference in life expectancy between men and women (Murray, "Rethinking DALYs," p. 18). This indicates, not surprisingly, that social factors have a stronger effect on the disparity in life expectancy between the sexes in developing countries.

38　*The World Health Report 2004* (Geneva: World Health Organization, 2004), pp. 120–25.

39　Tsuchiya and Williams, "A 'Fair Innings' between the Sexes," p. 280.

40　Sen, *Development as Freedom*, see esp. the introduction; Jonathan Wolff and Avner de-Shalit, *Disadvantage* (Oxford: Oxford University Press, 2007), esp. ch. 3.

41　See note 7 in this chapter.

42　Differences between men and women in percentage of deaths that could be attributed to alcohol or smoking (namely, deaths owed to cardiovascular diseases) are not so high (in the WHO sample of 2004 cardiovascular diseases accounted for 27.2% of all male deaths, as compared to 31.7% of all female deaths), compared to the differences in rates of deaths resulting from occupational hazard or violence (11.6% of all male deaths compared to 6.3% of all female deaths). *The World Health Report 2004*, pp. 120–25.

43　Daniels, Kennedy, and Kawachi entertain this thought experiment in "Health and Inequality," p. 83. See also Frances Kamm, "Health and Equity," in C.J.L. Murray et al. (eds.), *Summary Measures of Population Health: Concepts, Ethics, Measurement and Applications*, (Geneva: World Health Organization, 2002), p. 694.

44　Cf. Hausman, Asada, and Hedemann, "Health Inequalities and Why They Matter," p. 182; Daniel M. Hausman, "What's Wrong with Health Inequalities?" *Journal of Political Philosophy* 15, no. 1 (2007): 46–66.

45　Cf. Allen Buchanan et al., *From Chance to Choice: Genetics and Justice* (Cambridge: Cambridge University Press, 2000), p. 221.

46　If nothing else, doing so would promote the prospect of more heterosexual couples ending their lives at closer points of time than is currently the case. Pursuing equality in life expectancy between men and women, then, reduces the extent of widowhood, which is surely a desirable end.

47 Another reason why people may generally not be so troubled by differences in life expectancy between men and women is the following. It might be thought that comparing life expectancy between men and women does not capture the entire story. Women, it may be suggested, may live longer, but their health, over-all, is poorer. Women, especially in developing countries, suffer the various health effects of sexual intercourse (AIDS, rape), pregnancy, and childbirth. Strictly comparing life expectancy, then, skews the picture in favor of men. How-ever, it turns out that even when we compare *healthy* life expectancy (as we actu-ally do here) rather than life expectancy as such, it is still men who end up being worse off than women. See, for example, Christopher J. L. Murray, *U.S. Patterns of Mortality by County and Race: 1965–1994* (Cambridge: Harvard School of Pub-lic Health, 1998); Tsuchiya and Williams, "A 'Fair Innings' between the Sexes."

48 Hausman, "What's Wrong with Health Inequalities?" p. 59.

49 Amartya Sen, "Mortality as an Indicator of Economic Success and Failure," *Eco-nomic Journal* 108, no. 446 (1998): 1–25 (cited in Peter, "Health Equity and Social Justice").

50 An account that comes close to this luck egalitarian position without explicitly saying so is offered in Christopher J. L. Murray, Emanuela Gakidou, and Julio Frenk, "Health Inequalities and Social Group Differences: What Should We Measure?" *Bulletin of the World Health Organization* 77 (1999): 537–43; and Gaki-dou, Murray, and Frenk, "Defining and Measuring Health Inequality." Cf. Adam Wagstaff, Pierella Pact, and Eddy Van Doorslaer, "On the Measurement of In-equalities in Health," *Social Science and Medicine* 33, no. 5 (1991): 545–57. They conceive of health inequalities as being of moral concern only when they "reflect a socio-economic dimension," p. 556.

51 Sen, "Why Health Equity?" p. 30.

52 As Kekes, in his critique of egalitarianism, rightly points out. John Kekes, "A Question for Egalitarians," p. 664. See also Emmanuela Gakidou, Julio Frenk, and Christopher J. L. Murray, "A Health Agenda," in J. Cohen and J. Rogers (eds.), *Is Inequality Bad for Our Health?* (Boston: Beacon Press, 2000), pp. 71–78; Angus Deaton, "Policy Implications of the Gradient of Health and Wealth," p. 26.

Chapter 8: Equality or Priority in Health?

1 Philip Roth, *Everyman* (London: Vintage, 2006), pp. 100–101.

2 Richard J. Arneson, "Luck Egalitarianism and Prioritarianism," *Ethics* 110, no. 2 (2000): 341.

3 Derek Parfit, "Equality or Priority?" in M. Clayton and A. Williams (eds.), *The Ideal of Equality* (Basingstoke: McMillan, 2000), pp. 81–125. See also Dennis McKerlie, "Equality," *Ethics* 106, no. 2 (1996): 274–96; Thomas Nagel, *Mortal Questions* (Cambridge: Cambridge University Press, 1979), pp. 110, 118.

4 Who is the worse off for the purposes of medical treatment is obviously a com-plex matter (see Dan W. Brock, "Priority to the Worse Off in Health-Care Re-source Prioritization," in R. Rhodes, M. Battin, and A. Silvers (eds.), *Medicine and Social Justice*, [Oxford: Oxford University Press, 2002], pp. 362–72). In par-ticular, we may distinguish "need" from "urgency" as the determinants of the

worse-off position (Frances M. Kamm, *Morality, Mortality: Death and Whom to Save from It* [Oxford: Oxford University Press, 1993], ch. 8; Kamm, "Deciding Whom to Help, Health-Adjusted Life Years and Disabilities," in S. Anand, F. Peter, and A. Sen [eds.], *Public Health, Ethics, and Equity* [Oxford: Oxford University Press, 2004], pp. 225–42). For our purposes here, it is not essential to take a stand on that debate, and so I will simply speak of priority to "the worse off," whoever these individuals turn out to be.

5 Brock, "Priority to the Worse Off in Health-Care Resource Prioritization," p. 364; Susan L. Hurley, "On the What and the How of Distributive Justice and Health," in N. Holtug and K. Lippert-Rasmussen (eds.), *Egalitarianism: New Essays on the Nature and Value of Equality* (Oxford: Oxford University Press, 2007), pp. 308–33; Thomas M. Scanlon, "When Does Equality Matter?" http://law.usc.edu/academics/assets/docs/scanlon.pdf, p. 3; Norman Daniels, *Just Health: Meeting Health Needs Fairly* (Cambridge: Cambridge University Press, 2008), p. 310.

6 Larry S. Temkin, "Equality or Priority in Health Care Distribution," in D. Wikler and C.J.L. Murray (eds.), *Health, Well Being, Justice: Ethical Issues in Health Resource Allocation*, (Geneva: World Health Organization, forthcoming), p. 18.

7 Daniel M. Hausman, "Equality versus Priority: A Badly Misleading Distinction," and Marc Fleurbaey, "Equality vs. Priority: How Relevant Is the Distinction," both in D. Wikler and C.J.L. Murray (eds.), *Health, Well Being, Justice.*

8 John Broome, "Equality versus Priority: A Useful Distinction," in D. Wikler and C.J.L. Murray (eds.), *Health, Well Being, Justice.* Broome shows that when uncertainty is added into the picture, egalitarians and prioritarians would differ in their recommendations.

9 On that latter point, see also Marc Fleurbaey and Erik Schokkaert, "Unfair Inequalities in Health and Health Care," unpublished manuscript, p. 26.

10 The distinction between "intrinsic" and "instrumental" value was famously scrutinized by Christine Korsgaard (see her "Two Distinctions in Goodness," *Philosophical Review* 92 [1983]: 169–95; see also Andrew Mason, "Egalitarianism and the Leveling Down Objection," *Analysis* 61 [2001], pp. 247–48). For the purposes of my discussion I need not take a stand on that debate. The instrumental value of equality that I investigate below can also be understood as "the non-final value" of equality (to use Korsgaard's terminology). However, Parfit himself uses the terms "intrinsic" and "instrumental" here, and I shall follow him in doing so.

11 See also Samuel Scheffler, "Choice, Circumstance, and the Value of Equality," *Philosophy, Politics, and Economics* 4, no. 1 (2005): 19.

12 Thomas Scanlon, in contrast, does discuss some instrumental accounts of equality, but without clearly distinguishing those from the intrinsic value of equality. Thomas M. Scanlon, "The Diversity of Objections to Inequality," in his *The Difficulty of Tolerance: Essays in Political Philosophy* (Cambridge: Cambridge University Press, 2003), pp. 202–18.

13 Scanlon, "The Diversity of Objections to Inequality"; Scanlon, "When Does Equality Matter?"; David Miller, "Arguments for Equality," *Midwest Studies in Philosophy* 7, no. 1 (1982): 73–87.

14 See Elizabeth S. Anderson, "What Is the Point of Equality?" *Ethics* 109 (1999): 287–337.

15 See, for example, Richard G. Wilkinson, *Unhealthy Societies: The Afflictions of Inequality* (London: Routledge, 1996).

16 Thomas Pogge, *Realizing Rawls* (Ithaca, NY: Cornell University Press, 1989), pp. 181–96.

17 I say "in any meaningful way" for the following reason. If I suffer from some ailment I may derive some perverse satisfaction from witnessing others contract the same ailment, and the experience may indeed boost my self-esteem. But as the quotation from Philip Roth at the beginning of this chapter indicates, this is not something prevalent among "civilized persons."

18 Susan Hurley offers a different argument but one that has a similar effect to the argument presented here (see her "On the What and the How of Distributive Justice and Health"). The reason why it is sometimes desirable to level down income but never desirable to level down health, she says, is that equality in health "wastes excellence." "It is not just good for people to be healthy rather than unhealthy; it is also good in itself for there to be healthy people rather than unhealthy people." But it is unclear to me why it is not also good in itself for there to be richer, and thus arguably happier, individuals.

19 Although very few people would see this as a meaningful value (of equality in health). (See also Scanlon ["The Diversity of Objections to Inequality," p. 213] on this point.) Even fewer people, Temkin included, would see this as a reason to level down health. It seems more plausible to aim at breaking the correlation between deafness and stigma than at reducing the stigma by making more people deaf. On that latter point see Harry Brighouse and Adam Swift, "Equality, Priority, and Positional Goods," *Ethics* 116, no. 3 (2006), sec. VII.

20 A famous study in the 1980s found that in Norway, only 44% of people of the lowest socioeconomic group had their own teeth, compared with 86% of the highest income group. P. Maeside, "Norway," in R. Illsley and P. G. Svensson (eds.), *The Health Burden of Social Inequities* (Copenhagen: WHO, 1986), cited in Margaret Whitehead, "The Concepts and Principles of Equity and Health," *Health Promotion International* 6, no. 3 (1991): 218.

21 Another potential objection is this. Suppose that a certain person is the least healthy in society and moreover suffers from a certain illness afflicting only a few people. In our nonideal world that may well imply that the pharmaceutical industry would have a rather limited incentive to develop the suitable drug for that person's condition. Surely that ought to count as an instrumental disvalue of inequalities in health, the critic might say. Such cases, however, do not bear on my argument, for I have assumed a *just* distribution of health, and moreover, one that prioritizes the position of those who are worse off health-wise. Thus, my discussion excludes such cases of "double-jeopardy," where the fact of being worse off health-wise contributes, in itself, to having lower priority in medical treatment, as in the example here.

22 Although to think in that way would be to overlook its effect on widowhood, which does seem like an instrumental disvalue.

23 Norman Daniels, *Just Health Care* (Cambridge: Cambridge University Press, 1985).

24 Anand advances an argument to that effect (Sudhir Anand, "The Concern for Equity in Health," in S. Anand, F. Peter, and A. Sen [eds.], *Public Health, Ethics, and Equity*, [Oxford: Oxford University Press, 2004]).

25 Frances Kamm, "Health and Equity," in C.J.L. Murray et al. (eds.), *Summary Measures of Population Health: Concepts, Ethics, Measurement and Applications* (Geneva: World Health Organization, 2002), p. 687.

26 Arneson speaks of "the prioritarian branch of the family of *egalitarian* principles" ("Luck Egalitarianism and Prioritarianism," p. 343, emphasis added). For a useful typology of egalitarian principles, see his "Luck Egalitarianism Interpreted and Defended," http://philosophyfaculty.ucsd.edu/faculty/rarneson/luckegalitarianism2.pdf.

27 For a sufficientarian view of health equity, see Madison Powers and Ruth Faden, *Social Justice: The Moral Foundations of Public Health and Health Policy* (Oxford: Oxford University Press, 2006), esp. ch. 3. See also Roger Crisp, "Equality, Priority, and Compassion," *Ethics* 113, no. 4 (2003): 745–63. Cf. Richard J. Arneson, "Disability, Priority, and Equal Opportunity" (paper presented at the Bergen Workshop on Disability, June 2006, Bergen, Norway), sec. 4.6.

28 See Kenneth J. Arrow, "Some Ordinalist-Utilitarian Notes on Rawls's Theory of Justice," *Journal of Philosophy* 70, no. 9 (1973): 245–62; Daniels, *Just Health Care*, p. 44; Brock, "Priority to the Worse Off in Health-Care Resource Prioritization," p. 371.

29 The difference between absolutist and non-absolutist prioritarianism is captured by the following example. A: (2, 3, 7), B: (3, 3, 7), C: (2.5, 4, 7). Absolutist prioritarianism recommends B, whereas non-absolutist prioritarianism may recommend C. See Sarah Marchand, Daniel Wikler, and Bruce Landesman, "Class, Health, and Justice," *Milbank Quarterly* 76, no. 3 (1998): 461.

30 See also Richard J. Arneson, "Perfectionism and Politics," *Ethics* 111, no. 1 (2000): 58.

31 Here (and perhaps *only* here [see Dan W. Brock, "Ethical Issues in the Use of Cost Effectiveness Analysis for the Prioritization of Health Care Resources," in S. Anand, F. Peter, and A. Sen (eds.), *Public Health, Ethics, and Equity* (Oxford: Oxford University Press, 2004), p. 203]) public deliberation may be called upon. See Norman Daniels and James Sabin, "Limits to Health Care: Fair Procedures, Democratic Deliberation, and the Legitimacy Problem for Insurers," *Philosophy and Public Affairs* 26, no. 4 (1997): 303–50; Daniels, *Just Health*, ch. 4.

32 Arneson, "Luck Egalitarianism and Prioritarianism," p. 343. See also his "Egalitarianism and Responsibility," *Journal of Ethics* 3 (1999): 225–47; "Equality of Opportunity for Welfare Defended and Recanted," *Journal of Political Philosophy* 7, no. 4 (1999): 497; "Welfare Should Be the Currency of Justice," *Canadian Journal of Philosophy* 30, no. 4 (2000): 502; "Perfectionism and Politics," p. 57.

33 Arneson, "Luck Egalitarianism and Prioritarianism," p. 340.

34 Ibid., p. 343. See also his "Desert and Equality," in N. Holtug and K. Lippert-Rasmussen (eds.), *Egalitarianism* (Oxford: Oxford University Press, 2007), p. 263.

35 Note that Arneson sometime does revert to that differently ordered formulation of the luck prioritarian ideal, saying that we ought to give priority to the worse off, and of those, to those who are less rather than more responsible for their condition (e.g., "Luck Egalitarianism and Prioritarianism," p. 340). Arneson perhaps does not notice that he has two different formulations of luck prioritarianism, and moreover ones that are likely to produce different results. In any case, the formulation adopted here seems to me to better represent the luck prioritar-

ian ideal, which is, first to neutralize luck, and then to give priority to the worse off. In other words, it is luck first, prioritarianism second.

36 Recall the abandonment objection discussed in part I.

Chapter 9: Distributing Human Enhancements

1 Michael J. Sandel, *The Case against Perfection: Ethics in the Age of Genetic Engineering* (Cambridge, MA: Harvard University Press, 2007); Francis Fukuyama, *Our Posthuman Future: Consequences of the Biotechnology Revolution* (New York: Farrar, Straus and Giroux, 2002); Walter Glannon, *Genes and Future People* (Boulder, CO: Westview Press, 2001); Justine Burley, *The Genetic Revolution and Human Rights* (Oxford: Oxford University Press, 1999); John Harris, *Enhancing Evolution: The Ethical Case for Making Better People* (Princeton, NJ: Princeton University Press, 2007); Allen Buchanan et al., *From Chance to Choice: Genetics and Justice* (Cambridge: Cambridge University Press, 2000).

2 Buchanan et al., *From Chance to Choice* is a notable exception, more on which below.

3 See, for example, Harris, *Enhancing Evolution*. It seems to me, though, that Harris is too quick in dismissing the treatment/enhancement distinction. The fact that it may lack moral relevance, as he argues (a position to which I am on the whole sympathetic, see below), does not imply that the distinction itself is incoherent. What I attempt to do in this section, in fact, is to establish the validity of this distinction (in support of Daniels and *contra* Harris).

4 Norman Daniels, *Just Health: Meeting Health Needs Fairly* (Cambridge: Cambridge University Press, 2008), pp. 34–36; Daniels in Buchanan et al., *From Chance to Choice*, p. 109.

5 See Harris, *Enhancing Evolution*, p. 44. Of course, the fact that for one person Ritalin constitutes treatment whereas for the other it constitutes enhancement does not invalidate the coherence of the treatment/enhancement distinction, as Harris seems, erroneously, to imply.

6 An example might be drugs for treatment of Alzheimer's that may well be so effective as to boost normal memory capacity. See http://www.memorypharma.com/about.html. I am grateful to Ori Lev for pointing this out to me.

7 See also Harris, *Enhancing Evolution*, pp. 21, 56; Ori Lev and Ezekiel Emmanuel, "The Ethics of Biomedical Enhancement Research," unpublished manuscript. That is why I think Daniels is wrong to claim that "anything to do with maintaining normal function falls under the scope of 'treatment' as opposed to enhancement" (Norman Daniels, "Can Anyone Really Be Talking about Ethically Modifying Human Nature?" in J. Savulescu and N. Bostrom [eds.], *Human Enhancement* [Oxford: Oxford University Press, forthcoming]). But on that understanding, the futuristic genetic treatment I described that would allow us to roast our hands in the fire without ever getting a burn falls under the category of treatment rather than enhancement, which seems wrong.

8 Buchanan et al., *From Chance to Choice*, ch. 4. Although that book has four authors, its preface explicitly indicates that Daniels is the primary author of this particular chapter, which is why I reference it as Daniels's position rather than that of Buchanan et al. Moreover, at one point in that chapter the text indicates that some of the positions presented in it were not shared by some of the other

authors, and specifically the one regarding the moral relevance of the treatment/ enhancement distinction (p. 149), which happens to be my main focus of attention here. Daniels rehearses some of the main ideas in his recent *Just Health*, pp. 149–55.

9 I say "by and large" because Daniels makes the following exception for his resistance to funding enhancements: "It is possible, however, that some natural inequalities are not departures from normal species functioning but nonetheless so seriously limit an individual's opportunities that he or she is precluded from reaching the threshold of normal competition. In such cases, genetic intervention might be required if it were necessary to remove this barrier to opportunity." Buchanan et al., *From Chance to Choice*, p. 74. While I sympathize with this sentiment, it is difficult to see how one can espouse it and remain committed to the "normal function" view (see below).

10 Buchanan et al., *From Chance to Choice*, p. 122.

11 Ibid.

12 Leon R. Kass, *Life, Liberty, and the Defense of Dignity: The Challenge for Bioethics* (San Francisco: Encounter Books, 2002).

13 Sandel, *The Case against Perfection*.

14 Jurgen Habermas, *The Future of Human Nature* (Cambridge: Polity, 2003). Cf. Elizabeth Fenton, "Liberal Eugenics and Human Nature: Against Habermas," *Hastings Center Report* 36 (2006): 35–42.

15 This is John Harris's view in *Enhancing Evolution*.

16 Buchanan et al., *From Chance to Choice*, p. 115.

17 For example, Daniels, *Just Health*, p. 153.

18 Let us set aside the question of whether the parents themselves suffered from a deficient growth hormone, or simply had, in turn, short parents themselves, and so on.

19 I am grateful to Dani Attas for pointing out to me this potential objection.

20 If we are to believe the *New York Times* piece that followed the news about the recommendation made by an advisory panel to the Food and Drug Administration for the inclusion of synthetic growth hormone treatment, "men who are considerably shorter than the average American guy's height of 5-foot-9 ½ [...] are at elevated risk of dropping out of school, drinking heavily, dating sparsely, getting sick or depressed. They have a lower chance of marrying or fathering children than do taller men, and their salaries tend to be as modest as their stature." Natalie Angier, "Short Men, Short Shrift: Are Drugs the Answer?" *New York Times*, June 22, 2003.

21 In fact, and as Daniels himself points out, in 2004 the Food and Drug Administration did follow the abovementioned recommendation and approved the use of synthetic growth hormone treatment for idiopathically short children (children *not* suffering from growth hormone deficiency) who were in the bottom 1.5% of projected height. On this occasion then, policy seems to be adhering to the luck egalitarian view about disadvantage rather than to the "normal function" view.

22 I thank Nir Eyal and Dani Attas for helping me clarify this point.

23 The pain accompanying delivery, which is perhaps the reason why the process is called "labor" to begin with, is, we should recall, part and parcel of *normal* functioning in this case (see also Harris, *Enhancing Evolution*, p. 52).

24 Another, obvious example here would be treating the symptoms of aging, which, as I said in section I cannot be characterized as a departure from full normal

health. As John Harris puts the point against Daniels's account: "In old age, the diseases of old age are part of normal functioning; what is not normal in old age is to be disease free, have perfect vision and hearing and no increased vulnerability to colds, flu, and other diseases" (*Enhancing Evolution*, pp. 45, 52). But while Harris is certainly correct in this observation, it constitutes a much weaker critique of Daniels than he may think. For, Daniels is happy to bite this bullet and say that there may be reasons of fairness for denying (expensive) life-saving treatment to individuals who have exceeded the normal human life span. See Norman Daniels, *Am I My Parents' Keeper? An Essay on Justice between the Old and the Young* (New York: Oxford University Press, 1988); see also Alan Williams, "Intergenerational Equity: An Exploration of the 'Fair Innings' Argument," *Health Economics* 6 (1997): 117–32. That defense by Daniels, however, is clearly unavailable in the cases of pregnancy, labor, and menstruation. I therefore believe the critique of Daniels presented here is stronger than the one put forward by Harris.

25 It is worth recalling that the position I defended in part I says that luck egalitarian health care would provide treatment that meets basic needs whether or not the individual was responsible for her condition. Similarly, any enhancement that addresses a need rather than a mere disadvantage would be provided to the prudent and imprudent alike. A case in point would be vaccinations. Vaccinations prevent diseases that could be seen as harms. They therefore help prevent individuals from becoming needy. Thus, arguably, they would be justified for the prudent and imprudent alike. Only enhancements that do not address a basic need but rather rectify a disadvantage would be restricted for those who come to be disadvantaged in that way out of no fault of their own.

26 Notice again that Daniels could, of course, still justify vaccinations on other, non-justice-based, grounds, such as that it is cheaper to prevent these diseases than to treat them.

27 Daniels, "Can Anyone Really Be Talking about Ethically Modifying Human Nature?"

28 Buchanan et al., *From Chance to Choice*, p. 110; Daniels, *Just Health*, pp. 72–73, 150.

29 I say "generally" because there are obviously precautions that women can take in order to decrease the risk of breast cancer and thus reduce the risk of mastectomy (e.g., extending the duration of breast-feeding), but I shall leave these complications aside for the sake of argument.

30 With regard to the impact on self-esteem, see F. S. Faria et al., "Psychological Outcome and Patient Satisfaction following Breast Reduction Surgery," *British Journal of Plastic Surgery* 52, no. 6 (1999): 448–52.

31 Buchanan et al., *From Chance to Choice*, p. 144, Daniels, *Just Health*, pp. 150–54. Of course, the prevalence of moral hazard does not suffice to imply that there is no justice-based reason to provide to disadvantaged individuals the benefits of enhancement.

32 An interesting hypothetical case is that of mastectomy that results in symmetrical and normally shaped, albeit smaller than before, breasts. On the luck egalitarian reading the patient should be offered free reconstructive surgery, for she is worse off (supposing she is not pleased with the reduction in the size of her breasts), and due to no fault of her own. On Daniels's reading, in contrast, the

patient is not entitled to reconstructive surgery, for she suffers no departure from normal species functioning (she only suffers a departure from *her own* previous standard of functioning).

33 As in Louis Armstrong's memorable song: "My only sin is my skin. What did I do, to be so black and blue?" Words by Andy Razaf (1929).

34 See again Buchanan et al., *From Chance to Choice*, p. 221.

35 Harris, *Enhancing Evolution*, p. 92.

36 "Cuba Approves Free Sex-Change Operations," *Guardian*, June 7, 2008.

37 Larry S. Temkin, "Equality or Priority in Health Care Distribution," in D. Wikler and C.J.L. Murray (eds.), *Health, Well Being, Justice: Ethical Issues in Health Resource Allocation* (Geneva: World Health Organization, forthcoming), p. 18.

38 This question has been addressed by Colin Farrelly. However, Farrelly discusses leveling down genetic *interventions*, and thus lumps together gene therapy for health deficits with genetic enhancements to full normal health. That is why I think the conclusion he reaches—that we ought to be prioritarians with regard to genetic intervention as such—is mistaken. (See Colin Farrelly, "Genes and Equality," *Journal of Medical Ethics* 30, no. 4 [2004]: 587–92; see also Harris, *Enhancing Evolution*, pp. 28–29.) I believe that a more nuanced approach calls for a separate discussion of the value of equality in the distribution of health deficits and one in the distribution of enhancements to full health. That is what I will undertake here.

39 Glannon, *Genes and Future People*, p. 100. Francis Fukuyama also puts forward an argument to that effect in *Our Posthuman Future*. See also Michael J. Sandel, "The Case against Perfection: What's Wrong with Designer Children, Bionic Athletes, and Genetic Engineering," *Atlantic Monthly* 293, no. 3 (2004): 52.

40 I say "normally" because one could think of a hypothetical case whereby only one segment of the population is ever ill. In that case, that class of people might be cast as subhuman. But under a normal state of affairs, illness as such does not bestow on the unhealthy a status of being subhuman.

41 Harris, *Enhancing Evolution*, p. 63.

42 See Farrelly, "Genes and Equality," p. 591.

43 See also Harris, *Enhancing Evolution*, p. 30.

44 I say "current" because the normal human life span has obviously been extending throughout human existence (and has been extending even more so throughout history).

45 Adam Smith, *The Wealth of Nations* (Glasgow: Glasgow University, 1976), pp. 869–70.

46 See also G. A. Cohen, "Facts and Principles," *Philosophy and Public Affairs* 31, no. 3 (2003): 211–54.

Chapter 10 : Devolution of Health Care Services

1 This chapter is based on my "Why Devolution Upsets Distributive Justice," *Journal of Moral Philosophy* 4, no. 2 (2007): 259–74.

2 A greater demand for screening for Down syndrome may be the product of the choice to leave child bearing to a later age. On my account this should fall under choice rather than bad luck, but I leave such cases aside for the sake of argument. I am grateful to Jodi Beder for pointing this out to me.

3 More accurately, two conditions qualify this as an unfair state of affairs. First, it must be the case that the greater demand for expensive fetal screenings by the Jewish population disadvantages the Arab population in some way. Since resources, including medical resources, are usually scarce, the aforementioned unequal consumption results in rationing somewhere else within the system, and thus does disadvantage the Arab population. Second, it must be the case that the increased consumption of fetal screenings is the result of a voluntary choice, which I am assuming it is. That is, I assume there is no genetic or environmental cause that explains the discrepancy between Jews and Arabs in request for screenings, and that the sole reason for the discrepancy is a difference in cultural preference. (More on the latter below.)

4 Philippe Van Parijs, "Health Care in a Pluri-National Country," in S. Anand, F. Peter, and A. Sen (eds.), *Public Health, Ethics, and Equity* (Oxford: Oxford University Press, 2004), p. 164. I should hasten to say that in supporting this reform Van Parijs is in effect resisting, and attempting to preempt, the call for a more radical and separatist reform. More on which below.

5 See also Ronald Dworkin, *Sovereign Virtue: The Theory and Practice of Equality* (Cambridge, MA: Harvard University Press, 2000), p. 324.

6 I am content to use here David Miller's characterization of the group in question as "a set of people with a distinct set of cultural values and a shared language, who recognize their cultural kinship with one another, and engage in practices that set them apart from outsiders." David Miller, *Citizenship and National Identity* (Oxford: Polity, 2000), p. 127.

7 Van Parijs's argument may appear to amount to that of *subsidiarity*. "The 'principle of subsidiarity' regulates authority within a political order, directing that powers or tasks should rest with the lower-level sub-units of that order unless allocating them to a higher-level central unit would ensure higher comparative efficiency or effectiveness in achieving them." Andreas Føllesdal, "Subsidiarity," *Journal of Political Philosophy* 6, no. 2 (1998): 190. See also Hans M. Sass, "The New Triad: Responsibility, Solidarity and Subsidiarity," *Journal of Medicine and Philosophy* 20, no. 6 (1995): 591. In the EU, the principle of subsidiarity is responsible for, among other things, keeping the provision of health care with the member states (a policy that has recently come under challenge). See Panos Kanavos and Martin McKee, "Cross-Border Issues in the Provision of Health Services: Are We Moving towards a European Health Care Policy?" *Journal of Health Services Research and Policy* 5, no. 4 (2000): 231–36. I leave the issue of subsidiarity aside here, as it seems to be concerned not so much with distributive justice as with the values of self-determination, republican liberty, autonomy, and efficiency. See John Finnis, *Natural Law and Natural Rights* (Oxford: Clarendon Press, 1980), p. 146.

8 Devolving "welfare administration" often means that only transfers in kind are devolved while cash transfers are retained, as in the British case.

9 "Generous" is the term used by Van Parijs. I assume that by "generosity" Van Parijs refers to (and therefore I shall understand it to mean) the *number* of benefits and services the system distributes, independently of the net extent of *redistribution*.

10 Van Parijs, "Health Care in a Pluri-National Country," p. 176.

11 Ibid.

12 Ibid., p. 177.

13 Van Parijs's proposal is made with the particular case of Belgium in mind, but is universal in its appeal. A similar initiative was adopted in Quebec. In September 2004 the Canadian Health Accord included a special communiqué that exempted Quebec from some of the federal provisions. The exemption allowed for the government of Quebec to apply its own wait-time reduction plan and introduce its independent strategies for family and community care reform, home care, drug access strategies, health promotion, and chronic illness prevention. See http://www.hc-sc.gc.ca/english/hca2003/fmm/quebec_bk.html.

14 Donald L. Horowitz, "Constitutional Design: An Oxymoron?" *Nomos* 42 (2000): 253–84.

15 Harry Beran makes a similar comparison with regard to secession. "More Theory of Secession: A Response to Birch," *Political Studies* 36, no. 2 (1988): 318–19.

16 Unless one community is systematically discriminated against (rather than simply suffering from the other community's expensive medical tastes) in a way that cannot be repaired. So unless secession is likely to correct a severe case of ethnic discrimination, or unless the different communities are irreconcilably divided, secession should be resisted. This is a higher threshold than the one proposed by liberal nationalists like Miller, for whom it seems to be sufficient simply to have "two communities whose collective *identities* are radically at odds with one another." Miller, *Citizenship and National Identity*, p. 123.

17 See my "Unconditional Welfare Benefits and the Principle of Reciprocity," *Politics, Philosophy, and Economics* 4, no. 3 (2005), sec. 5.

18 Distribution according to need may take various forms, and primarily the following two. The "need principle" can refer to distribution *in proportion* to need, where the system equalizes the proportion of needs met. Alternatively, the system may *prioritize* those whose needs are greatest. In the latter case the equalisandum is the needs themselves, whereas in the former it is the proportion of needs met. For a discussion of this distinction, see David Miller, *Principles of Social Justice* (Cambridge, MA: Harvard University Press, 1999), pp. 213–21. What I have to say below applies to both interpretations of the need principle.

19 For a somewhat similar point, see Margaret Whitehead, "The Concepts and Principles of Equity and Health," *Health Promotion International* 6, no. 3 (1991): 221.

20 Alternatively, if distribution equalizes the needs themselves (rather than the proportion of needs met), then every citizen would end up at -3.

21 Or, in the case of equalizing needs, each member of B is fully cured, while each member of A is elevated to -6 at best (that is, if the residue from B is handed over to A).

22 It may be objected that the reform is still an egalitarian one, and for the following reason. Given the homogeneous nature of the medical needs in the regional communities, it would make economic sense to provide medical treatment locally. Each regional hospital is then allowed to specialize in the type of ailments that afflict that region. It therefore, so the objection runs, makes sense to devolve health care treatment to the different regions, as patients would see a greater share of their particular needs met (due to the local specialization in the types of illnesses that afflict them). Notice, however, that this form of service is not unique to a devolved system, and a unitary system may also operate in that manner. In fact, a unitary system that does not operate in that way, i.e., does not prioritize

medical treatment according to the needs of the particular communities it serves, would be failing its purpose.

23 See also Van Parijs, "Health Care in a Pluri-National Country," p. 166.

24 See Norman Daniels, *Just Health Care* (Cambridge: Cambridge University Press, 1985), p. 11. See also Thomas Scanlon, "Preference and Urgency," *Journal of Philosophy* 72 (1975): 655–69.

25 For my purposes in this chapter I am happy to allude again to Daniels's understanding of medical needs as "impairment to normal species functioning." Daniels, *Just Health Care*, p. 32; Daniels, "Justice and Health Care," in D. Van De Veer and T. Regan (eds.), *Health Care Ethics* (Philadelphia: Temple University Press, 1987), pp. 302–6.

26 (Ireland might be an exception here.) Or to take the case of Belgium more specifically, the stereotype is that the prudent Flemings's idea of "living well" is household decoration, whereas the more lighthearted Walloons' idea of living well is manifested through parades and feasting. See Kenneth D. McRae, *Conflict and Compromise in Multilingual Societies: Belgium* (Waterloo, ON: Wilfred Laurier University Press, 1986), p. 91.

27 Notice that when discussing medical needs (as opposed to preferences) I set aside the issue, discussed in part I, of whether, *individually*, these medical needs are the result of bad brute luck or, in contrast, of negligence. What matters for my discussion here is whether or not the patient's condition counts as a medical need, independently of how she ended up acquiring that need.

28 For the Jewish Israeli case see R. Landau, "Sex Selection for Social Purposes in Israel: Quest for the 'Perfect Child' of a Particular Gender or Centuries Old Prejudice against Women?" *Journal of Medical Ethics* 34 (2008): e10; L. Remennick, "The Quest after the Perfect Baby: Why Do Israeli Women Seek Prenatal Genetic Testing?" *Sociology of Health and Illness* 28 (2006): 21–53.

29 I acknowledge here the ambiguity regarding whether or not fertility treatments meet a medical need. But as I pointed out in chapter 2, we may say that although it does not, strictly speaking, answer a medical need, fertility treatment is a medical procedure that is needed for pursuing what for most people is a normal life plan. See Daniels, *Just Health Care*, pp. 42–48.

30 See again John E. Roemer, "A Pragmatic Theory of Responsibility for the Egalitarian Planner," *Philosophy and Public Affairs* 22, no. 2 (1993): 146–66.

31 A theme touched upon in Chinua Achebe's classic novel, *Things Fall Apart* (Oxford: Heinemann, 1986): "Among the Ibo the art of conversation is regarded very highly, and proverbs are the palm-oil with which words are eaten" (p. 5).

32 Daniels, "Justice and Health Care," p. 305; *Just Health*, p. 45.

33 I am grateful to Kristin Voigt for the example.

34 As noted above, I leave aside here the important question of the extent to which membership in a community with special medical *needs* can itself be considered an expensive taste. I have noted that Nigerian society should treat the Ibo speech impediment as constituting a greater need (than occurrences of that impediment in other cultural groups). But one may plausibly say then that in this case membership in Ibo culture itself becomes an expensive taste. It would follow that society need not treat that condition when it can simply require Ibo members who have a speech impediment to switch to another cultural group. Of course, a familiar reply to this type of suggestion is that it would be wrong to treat cultural

membership as a choice that could easily be revised. See Will Kymlicka, *Multicultural Citizenship: A Liberal Theory of Minority Rights* (Oxford: Clarendon Press, 1995). Cf. Brian Barry, *Culture and Equality: An Egalitarian Critique of Multiculturalism* (Cambridge, MA: Harvard University Press, 2001). Since I cannot resolve this important and complex debate within the confines of this chapter, let me simply say that culturally determined medical needs ought to be respected in cases where it would be unfair to ask individuals to give up their cultural membership.

35 Setting aside the possibility that male circumcision helps in curbing infection rates of HIV/AIDS.

36 Cf. Miller, *Principles of Social Justice*, pp. 212–13. To put this differently, to say that needs are to a large extent *socially determined* (in a way that is discernible to an outside observer) is not to say that needs are subjectively determined *by society* (as Michael Walzer erroneously, I think, suggests: *Spheres of Justice: A Defense of Pluralism and Equality* [Oxford: Blackwell, 1983], p. 65).

37 In the fourth type the particular community recognizes a certain "need" that society as a whole recognizes as only a taste or a preference. But suppose we turn the tables here. How does my argument so far reflect on a case where society as a whole recognizes a need that the subgroup in question recognizes only as a preference? A case in point would be deafness, where society at large may identify this as a handicap and as such, a medical need, to which the group in question may object (and rather advocate treating deafness as an alternative way of life, say). I have two, admittedly ad hoc, responses here. First, the deaf community does not normally constitute a geographical community, although it is possible to think of some local communities that are predominantly deaf (such as the Israeli Bedouin village of Al-Sayed, which purportedly has the highest percentage of deafness in a local community worldwide). However, such communities are unlikely to be large enough to justify mounting a claim for devolution, and so the case for devolution is unlikely to arise in the first place. Second, in turning the tables we would have lost the demand for *increased* spending. If the particular community objects to the depiction of X as a medical need, it follows that the group must demand a smaller, not larger, health care budget, and thus no problem of unfairness ought to arise.

38 Notice that my discussion would have, perhaps, yielded different results if health care remained unitary while other areas of policy, and particularly those bearing on public health, were devolved. The current ban on smoking in bars and restaurants in Scotland may imply that the English (so long as they fail to impose a full ban) have an "expensive taste" for medical treatment for cardiovascular diseases and lung cancer (for more on this dilemma, see the next chapter). For the sake of simplicity, then, I will assume that if health care remains unitary, then so do other areas of policy that bear on public health.

39 See my "Bringing the Middle Classes Back In: An Egalitarian Case for (Truly) Universal Public Services," *Ethics and Economics* 2, no. 1 (2004): 1–7.

40 William R. Morgan and Jack Sawyer, "Equality, Equity, and Procedural Justice in Social Exchange," *Social Psychology Quarterly* 42, no. 1 (1979): 71–75; Gerold Mikula and Thomas Schwinger, "Intermember Relations and Reward Allocation: Theoretical Considerations of Affects," in H. Brandstatter, J. H. Davis, and H. Schuler (eds.), *Dynamics of Group Decisions* (London: Sage, 1978), pp. 229–50;

Ivan D. Steiner, *Group Process and Productivity* (New York: Academic Press, 1972); Morton Deutsch, "The Effects of Co-operation and Competition upon Group Process," in D. Cartwright and A. Zander (eds.), *Group Dynamics* (New York: Harper & Row, 1968); *Distributive Justice: A Social-Psychological Perspective* (New Haven, CT: Yale University Press, 1985), p. 158. Further references to this conclusion are made in the review article by Karen S. Cook and Karen A. Hegtvedt, "Distributive Justice, Equity, and Equality," *Annual Review of Sociology* 9 (1983): 223.

41 David Miller, *On Nationality* (Oxford: Clarendon Press, 1995); *Principles of Social Justice*, ch. 2; *Citizenship and National Identity*, p. 32.

42 One typical objection I do not confront here says that we need not be concerned with the weakening of solidarity on a national level as it can easily be replaced by solidarity sustained by communities of a subnational level. See Michael Keating, "Social Inclusion, Devolution and Policy Divergence," *Political Quarterly* 74, no. 4 (2003): 430. It seems to me, though, that the benefits of solidarity are only readily available to the community of the level in which it is produced and sustained. Thus, it is only solidarity at the level of the political community that can strengthen those bonds crucial for the type of compromises and sacrifices needed when pursuing distributive justice. (See Andrew Mason, *Community, Solidarity and Belonging: Levels of Community and Their Normative Significance* [Cambridge: Cambridge University Press, 2000], p. 61.) It is the case, therefore, that the strengthening of Scottish solidarity, say, does not necessarily benefit the pursuit of distributive justice across Britain, and may actually hinder it.

43 The greater needs of the Walloons are owed to demographics (they are on average older), and economics (unemployment being higher in Wallonia). Van Parijs, "Health Care in a Pluri-National Country," p. 164.

44 As is the case, in principle, between England and Scotland.

45 The Barnett formula adopted in Britain is not based on the *changing* needs of the respective regions, and thus cannot respond to shifting demands for health care expenditure. See Scott L. Greer, "The Fragile Divergence Machine: Citizenship, Policy Divergence, and Devolution," in A. Trench (ed.), *Devolution and Power in the UK* (Manchester: Manchester University Press, forthcoming)].

46 See Theda Skocpol, *Social Policy in the United States: Future Possibilities in Historical Perspective* (Princeton, NJ: Princeton University Press, 1995), ch. 8.

47 It may be objected here that a unitary system also suffers from power bargaining over communal differences in needs, the reason being that within a unitary system, members of one community may refuse to recognize certain needs, or refuse to recognize certain conditions as constituting a more urgent need for members of the other community. That, admittedly, may still be the case, but the crucial advantage of the unitary system is that, to a large extent, this type of decision is taken out of the hands of politicians and constitutional lawyers and put into the hands of doctors and health care administrators. More generally, many pre-devolution unifying features of health care in the different regions are likely to disappear post-devolution as devolution leads, willy-nilly, to great divergence in health policy. See Greer, "The Fragile Divergence Machine."

48 A supposition that is different from the more plausible one made by Van Parijs, who claims that such an understanding is possible, but that it nevertheless results in a more limited list of agreed-upon needs.

49 I make here what I take to be a plausible assumption that citizens do not suspect that public officials *intentionally* falsify what counts as needs, although that obviously may sometimes take place.

50 Recall that by "generosity" I mean the number of benefits and services the system distributes, independently of the net extent of redistribution.

51 Van Parijs, "Health Care in a Pluri-National Country," p. 176.

52 The confusion results from my conforming to the way in which "thin" and "thick" are conventionally used in this context. See Michael Walzer, *Thick and Thin: Moral Argument at Home and Abroad* (Notre Dame, IN, and London: Notre Dame University Press, 1994).

53 Or as a critic of the special ("asymmetrical") provisions to the Quebec health care system succinctly put it: "it's hard to argue that Quebeckers have distinct diabetes and asymmetrical aortas." http://members.shaw.ca/nspector3/globe13.htm.

54 For more on "packing" and "un-packing," see my "Bringing the Middle Classes Back In."

55 On the justness of societies as depending also on the conduct of the individual actors, see G. A. Cohen, "Where the Action Is: On the site of Distributive Justice," *Philosophy and Public Affairs* 26, no. 1 (1997): 3–30.

56 I concede that to ask individuals to forego extra screenings for intelligence or Down syndrome (that they are otherwise about to take) for the sake of "distributive justice" is unlikely to alter the conduct of many prospective parents. That is why education, and a policy that takes these screenings off the menu to begin with, would be a more practical, and potentially a more successful, approach.

Chapter 11: Global Justice and National Responsibility for Health

1 *The Human Development Report 2005*, http://hdrstats.undp.org/countries/country_fact_sheets/cty_fs_ISL.html.

2 See Nir Eyal and Samia A. Hirst, "Physician Brain Drain—Can Nothing Be Done?" *Public Health Ethics*, 1, no. 2 (2008): 1–13.

3 Solomon R. Benatar, Abdallah S. Daar, and Peter A. Singer, "Global Health Ethics: The Rationale for Mutual Caring," *International Affairs* 79 (1) (2003): 110. See also James H. Flory and Philip Kitcher, "Global Health and the Scientific Research Agenda," *Philosophy and Public Affairs* 32, no. 1 (2004): 36–65.

4 John Rawls, *The Law of Peoples* (Cambridge, MA: Harvard University Press, 1999), pp. 117–18; David Miller, *National Responsibility and Global Justice* (Oxford: Oxford University Press, 2007).

5 Peter Singer, "Famine, Affluence, and Morality," *Philosophy and Public Affairs* 1, no. 3 (1972): 229–43; Thomas Pogge, "Moral Universalism and Global Economic Justice," *Politics, Philosophy, and Economics* 1 (2002): 29–58; Joshua Cohen and Charles Sabel, "Extra Rempublicam Nulla Justitia?" *Philosophy and Public Affairs* 34, no. 2 (2006): 147–75; Richard J. Arneson, "Do Patriotic Ties Limit Global Justice Duties?" *Journal of Ethics* 9 (2005): 127–50.

6 Rawls, *The Law of Peoples*; Thomas Nagel, "The Problem of Global Justice," *Philosophy and Public Affairs* 33, no. 2 (2005): 113–47; David Miller, "Justice and Global Inequality," in A. Hurrell and N. Woods (eds.), *Inequality, Globalization, and World Politics* (Oxford: Oxford University Press, 1999), pp. 187–210; Miller, *National Responsibility and Global Justice*; Michael Blake, "Distributive Justice,

State Coercion, and Autonomy," *Philosophy and Public Affairs* 30, no. 3 (2002): 257–96.

7 See Miller, "Justice and Global Inequality"; Miller, *Citizenship and National Identity* (Oxford: Polity, 2000), ch. 10, esp. pp. 174–78.

8 Thomas Pogge, "Relational Conceptions of Justice: Responsibilities for Health Outcomes," in S. Anand, F. Peter, and A. Sen (eds.), *Public Health, Ethics, and Equity* (Oxford: Oxford University Press, 2004), pp. 135–61.

9. Kok-Chor Tan, for example, uses that latter term. See his *Justice without Borders: Cosmopolitanism, Nationalism, and Patriotism* (Cambridge: Cambridge University Press, 2004), p. 61.

10 Charles Beitz, *Political Theory and International Relations* (Princeton, NJ: Princeton University Press, 1999). Cf. Brian Barry, "Humanity and Justice in Global Perspective," in J. R. Pennock and J. W. Chapman (eds.), *Ethics, Economics, and the Law*, Nomos 24 (New York: New York University Press, 1982), pp. 232–33; David Heyd, "Justice and Solidarity: The Contractarian Case against Global Justice," *Journal of Social Philosophy* 38, no. 1 (2007): 112–30. Barry and Heyd both argue that the global economic structure is not a mutually advantageous one and thus cannot fit the Rawlsian concept of "basic structure."

11 Thomas Pogge, "Eradicating Systematic Poverty: Brief for a Global Resource Dividend," in his *World Poverty and Human Rights: Cosmopolitans Responsibilities and Reforms* (Cambridge: Polity, 2002), pp. 196–215; Pogge, *Realizing Rawls* (Ithaca, NY: Cornell University Press, 1989), pp. 276–78; Iris Marion Young, "Responsibility and Global Justice: A Social Connection Model," *Social Philosophy and Policy* 23 (2006): 102–30.

12 See, for example, David A. J. Richards, "International Distributive Justice," in J. R. Pennock and J. W. Chapman (eds.), *Ethics, Economics, and the Law*, Nomos 24 (New York: New York University Press, 1982), 275–95.

13 Obviously, it is possible to be both a resource egalitarian and a luck egalitarian, Ronald Dworkin being the prime example. But I believe that in the context of global justice the distinction as I draw it stands.

14 Hillel Steiner, *An Essay on Rights* (Oxford: Blackwell, 1994), ch. 8; Steiner, "Territorial Justice," in S. Caney, D. George, and P. Jones (eds.), *National Rights, International Obligations* (Boulder, CO: Westview Press, 1996); Steiner, "Just Taxation and International Redistribution," in I. Shapiro and L. Brilmayer (eds.), *Global Justice*, Nomos 41 (New York: New York University Press, 1999); Brian Barry, "Humanity and Justice in Global Perspective."

15 Darrel Moellendorf, *Cosmopolitan Justice* (Boulder, CO: Westview Press, 2002), p. 55 (see also p. 64). See also Richards, "International Distributive Justice," p. 290; Simon Caney, "Cosmopolitan Justice and Equalizing Opportunities," in T. Pogge (ed.), *Global Justice* (Oxford: Blackwell, 2001), p. 125; Caney, "Global Equality of Opportunity and the Sovereignty of States," in A. Coates (ed.), *International Justice* (Aldershot: Ashgate, 2000); Joseph Carens, "Aliens and Citizens: The Case for Open Borders," *Review of Politics* 49 (1987): 83–99; Tan, *Justice without Borders*. Peter Singer's position (see his, "Famine, Affluence, and Morality") is also closely related to cosmopolitan luck egalitarianism in that he also emphasizes the moral arbitrariness and irrelevance of nationality for the duty to aid. I say "closely related" because Singer does not explicitly speak about distributive justice, but rather about the duty to aid. Thomas Pogge also subscribes to the

view that nationality is as morally arbitrary as race and sex (see his *Realizing Rawls*, p. 247). But I do not include him here because the conclusion he draws is not that opportunities should be equalized but rather that we ought to make sure that the global economic order does not harm the world's worst off.

16 I have said nothing about whether luck egalitarianism is necessarily cosmopolitan, nor can I fully defend that view here. Dworkin, for example, probably cannot be considered a cosmopolitan. At the same time, I believe that luck egalitarianism properly understood is necessarily cosmopolitan. This view is put forward by Arneson: "Luck egalitarianism in its core, unless encumbered with added moral commitments that do not arise from the internal development of its rationale but are instead just slapped on from outside, is a global cosmopolitan account of social justice." "Luck Egalitarianism: A Primer," unpublished manuscript, p. 14.

17 David Miller, "Holding Nations Responsible," *Ethics* 114, no. 2 (2004): 241.

18 See also Alexander Cappelen, "Responsibility and International Distributive Justice," in A. Føllesdal and T. Pogge (eds.), *Real World Justice: Grounds, Principles, Human Rights, and Social Institutions* (Dordrecht: Springer, 2005), pp. 218–19.

19 Miller, "Holding Nations Responsible," p. 242.

20 I distinguish here reparations from collective apologies. Reparations will generally be accompanied by an apology, but the converse is not necessarily the case. Sometimes an apology expresses a sense of shame in the actions of a previous generation, even when there is no institutional responsibility or consequent benefit (see below). Rather, apology in those cases would be justified by the fact that the current generation identifies for the most part with the previous generation and thus feels ashamed of some deeds committed by them. Current Germans may feel sufficiently alienated from their Nazi forbearers, in which case apology will express only some institutional responsibility. But current Americans may sufficiently identify with their ancestors to feel shamed by slavery or the treatment of Native Americans. See Miller, *National Responsibility and Global Justice*, pp. 158–59.

21 See Jeremy Waldron, "Superseding Historic Injustice," *Ethics* 103, no. 1 (1992): 4–28; Waldron, "Redressing Historic Injustice," *University of Toronto Law Journal* 52 (2002): 135–60; George Sher, "Ancient Wrongs and Modern Rights," in his *Approximate Justice: Studies in Non-Ideal Theory* (Lanham, MD: Rowman and Littlefield, 1997); A. J. Simmons, "Historical Rights and Fair Shares," in his *Justification and Legitimacy: Essays on Rights and Obligations* (Cambridge: Cambridge University Press, 2001); Jana Thompson, *Taking Responsibility for the Past: Reparation and Historical Injustice* (Cambridge: Cambridge University Press, 2002); Stephen Kershnar, *Justice for the Past* (Albany: State University of New York Press, 2004). For more references on the subject, see Miller, *National Responsibility and Global Justice*, pp. 137–38.

22 See Miller, "Justice and Global Inequality"; Miller, *National Responsibility and Global Justice*, p. 71; Rawls, *The Law of Peoples*, sec. 16.

23 Another general objection to global egalitarianism that we may mention here is that, as Miller suggests, it may undermine national self-determination. No national self-determination is sustainable, he argues, unless nations are given sufficient control over their natural and social assets (see *National Responsibility and Global Justice*, ch. 3). This is certainly true to some degree. Some sufficient level of resources is surely essential for national self-determination, no less than

it is essential for personal self-determination. Now, we must remember that, as Miller himself points out, global egalitarianism does not necessarily imply a world government, but can rather be attained through an equal distribution of resources among nation-states. (See for example, Tan, *Justice without Borders*, esp. chs. 4, 5.) This distinction is sometimes referred to as the one between *institutional* cosmopolitanism and *moral* cosmopolitanism. (See Charles Beitz, "International Liberalism and Distributive Justice: A Survey of Recent Thought," *World Politics* 51, no. 2 [1999]: 287.) Moral cosmopolitanism, then, implies an egalitarian distribution of resources among nations, and that, crucially, would surely lead to a more equal opportunity for nations to pursue national self-determination than is currently the case. Thus, to equalize the level of resources *across* nations would surely be in the interest of overall national self-determination, not against it. It is the case therefore that global egalitarianism and the concern for national self-determination actually go hand in hand (cf. Cecile Fabre, "Global Egalitarianism: An Indefensible Theory of Justice?" in D. Bell and A. de-Shalit [eds.], *Forms of Justice* [Lanham, MD: Rowman and Littlefield, 2003], pp. 327–28).

24 Miller, "Holding Nations Responsible," p. 242.

25 Beitz, "Rawls' Law of Peoples," p. 690.

26 Thomas Pogge, "Moral Universalism and Global Economic Justice."

27 Norman Daniels, *Just Health: Meeting Health Needs Fairly* (Cambridge: Cambridge University Press, 2008), p. 342. Notice though that a GDPPC of $8,000 is quite a high one. Above it lie only 70 out of the world's 177 nations, leaving out such populous nations as China and India and the whole of Africa save for Libya, South Africa, and Botswana. See the *Human Development Report 2007/2008*, http://hdrstats.undp.org/indicators/5.html. In other words, the correlation between income and health does seem to hold for the vast majority of humanity.

28 Daniels, *Just Health*, p. 334, pp. 342–43; Gopal Sreenivasan, "Health and Justice in Our Non-Ideal World," *Politics, Philosophy, and Economics* 6, no. 2 (2007): 218–36.

29 Pogge, *World Poverty and Human Rights*, p. 105; Pogge, "Relational Conceptions of Justice," p. 140; Pogge, "An Egalitarian Law of People's," *Philosophy and Public Affairs* 23, no. 3 (1994): 213–14; Beitz, "International Liberalism and Distributive Justice," p. 279; Beitz, "Social and Cosmopolitan Liberalism," *International Affairs* 73, no. 3 (1999): 525.

30 As Daniels mistakenly, I think, suggests. See his *Just Health*, pp. 338, 342.

31 Sudhir Anand and Martin Ravallion, "Human Development in Poor Countries: On the Role of Private Incomes and Public Services," *Journal of Economic Perspectives* 7 (1993): 133–50. Cf. Deon Filmer and Lant Pritchett, "The Impact of Public Spending on Health: Does Money Matter?" *Social Science and Medicine* 49, no. 10 (1999): 1309–23.

32 John Hobcraft, "Women's Education, Child Welfare, and Child Survival: A Review of the Evidence," *Health Transition Review* 3 (1993): 159–75; Kalanidhi Subbarao and Laura Raney, "Social Gains from Female Education: A Cross-National Study," *Economic Development and Cultural Change* 44, no. 1 (1995): 105–28; John C. Caldwell, "Routes to Low Mortality in Poor Countries," *Population and Development Review* 12, no. 2 (1986): 171–220. For additional relevant references, see Sreenivasan, "Health and Justice in our Non-Ideal World."

33 Pogge, *World Poverty and Human Rights*, p. 14. Daniels recounts how pressure from the IMF and World Bank has forced Cameroon to adopt budget-slashing

measures such as suspending the recruitment of health sector workers (including physicians), and mandatory retirement of such workers at the age of 50–55
(*Just Health*, p. 338).

34 Eyal and Hirst, "Physician Brain Drain—Can Nothing Be Done?"; Daniels, *Just Health*, p. 339.

35 See also Simon Caney, *Justice beyond Borders: A Global Political Theory* (Oxford: Oxford University Press, 2005), p. 130.

36 See Andrew Mason, *Leveling the Playing Field: The Idea of Equal Opportunity and Its Place in Egalitarian Thought* (Oxford: Oxford University Press, 2006), p. 202; Moellendorf, *Cosmopolitan Justice*, pp. 48–49; Fabre, "Global Egalitarianism," pp. 325–26; Beitz, "Social and Cosmopolitan Liberalism," pp. 526–28; Pogge, *Realizing Rawls*, pp. 252–53; Simon Caney, "Cosmopolitanism and the Law of Peoples," *Journal of Political Philosophy* 10, no. 1 (2002): 116–17; Tan, *Justice without Borders*, pp. 72–73.

37 Miller, "Justice and Global Inequality"; *National Responsibility and Global Justice*; "Holding Nations Responsible"; *On Nationality*, p. 108.

38 Miller, "Justice and Global Inequality," p. 195. For a similar view with regard to holding democratic nations in the third world responsible for their debts, see Alexander W. Cappelen, Rune Jansen Hagen, and Bertil Tungodden, "National Responsibility and the Just Distribution of Debt Relief," *Ethics and International Affairs* 21, no. 1 (2007): 69–83.

39 Miller draws a distinction between what he calls *outcome responsibility* and *remedial responsibility* (*National Responsibility and Global Justice*, ch. 4), but I think the conventional terms of "responsibility" and "liability" are more appropriate here.

40 I concede, however, that were immigration to be truly costless, the luck egalitarian *would* be compelled to hold a dissenter responsible for her decision not to immigrate to another country in search of better health. I thank Jonathan Quong for pointing this out to me.

41 It is an open question whether we should introduce some mechanism by which those who voted against a policy but still get to benefit from it are held *somewhat less* liable than those who voted for it. I shall leave that complication aside. I also set aside the question of the moral responsibility of abstainers.

42 Miller, "Justice and Global Inequality," p. 195.

43 Another argument we could mention in this context is the one put forward by Alexander Cappelen. He argues that new children are born every day, and that on the logic presented here it would never be possible to hold nations responsible, an outcome he finds impossible to accept. ("Responsibility and International Distributive Justice," pp. 221–22.) I do not share the intuition. If the only way to hold a nation responsible for its actions is in a way that would affect the life prospects of its children, then it may very well be the case that it is always wrong to hold nations responsible. In the absence of a reason to think otherwise, it is difficult to accept that that outcome in itself shows the cosmopolitan position to be incorrect.

44 This makes, I think, for an overall more coherent approach to global justice and national responsibility. Consider this. Since generation Y does not have a positive claim on resources left to it by the preceding generation X, then by the same token, Y also does not inherit an obligation of restitution for some injustice per-

petrated by X toward Z (provided, of course, that Y does not benefit from that past injustice). Cf. Miller, *National Responsibility and Global Justice*, p. 155.

45 Miller, *National Responsibility and Global Justice*, pp. 71–72.

46 See ibid., pp. 144–45.

47 Life expectancy in Norway is 79.7 and in Sweden, 80.6 (Source: U.S. Census Bureau, International database, 2007).

48 Miller, "Justice and Global Inequality." This argument is similar in structure to Harry Frankfurt's "abundance objection" to egalitarianism. See his "Equality as a Moral Ideal," *Ethics* 98, no. 1 (1987): 35.

49 Miller, *National Responsibility and Global Justice*, esp. ch. 3. For a sufficientarian account of global justice, see Henry Shue, *Basic Rights: Subsistence, Affluence, and U.S. Foreign Policy* (Princeton, NJ: Princeton University Press, 1996). One internal problem with the sufficientarian objection to global egalitarianism is that it may still lead to conclusions that are too cosmopolitan for the global humanitarian's taste. Consider this. Sufficientarians believe that raising people above some threshold matters over and above the ideal of equality. But that would imply that citizens of affluent nations must give priority to raising individuals in the developing world above that threshold before they can start thinking about meeting their co-nationals' claim for equal treatment. So a consistent sufficientarian position might yield results that are unpalatable for the anti-cosmopolitan. See Paula Casal, " Why Sufficiency Is Not Enough," *Ethics* 117, no. 2 (2007): 303–4.

50 I should qualify this: in relative terms the transfer *would be* quite large, for it is much more expensive to raise someone's life expectancy from 79 to 80 than from 45 to 46. Still, in absolute terms the amount of transfer between Sweden and Norway would be overshadowed by the redistribution from the developed world to the developing world. I thank Richard Child for drawing my attention to this.

51 For a similar argument, see Larry Temkin, "Egalitarianism Defended," *Ethics* 113 (2003): 770; Casal, " Why Sufficiency Is Not Enough," p. 311.

52 This is already practiced by Christopher Murray and his colleagues with regards to the United States. See Christopher J. L. Murray et al., "Eight Americas: Investigating Mortality Disparities across Races, Counties, and Race-Counties in the United States," *PLOS Medicine* 3, no. 9 (2006): e260.

53 http://ec.europa.eu/regional_policy/policy/object/index_en.htm.

54 Arneson makes an argument to a similar effect in his "Do Patriotic Ties Limit Global Justice Duties?"

55 Daniels, *Just Health*, p. 344.

56 On that point I agree with Daniels. *Just Health*, p. 344.

57 Some take this intergalactic objection to show the falseness of telic egalitarianism (that is, roughly, the idea of equality as an end-state rather than as a constraint on procedural distribution) in general, and not just of global egalitarianism. See Daniel M. Hausman, "Equality versus Priority: A Badly Misleading Distinction," in D. Wikler and C. J. L. Murray (eds.), *Health, Well Being, Justice: Ethical Issues in Health Resource Allocation* (Geneva: World Health Organization, forthcoming), p. 3.

58 A possibility entertained by Roger Crisp, "Equality, Priority, and Compassion," *Ethics* 113, no. 4 (2003): 762.

59 As pointed out to me by Hillel Steiner.

60 Since, as we said, national wealth above that mark seems not to correlate with life expectancy.

Conclusion

1 Amartya Sen, "Why Health Equity?" *Health Economics* 11 (2002): 663.

2 Arrow did so with regard to the bottomless pit objection to Rawls's difference principle; Sen with regard to the currency of egalitarian justice; and Walzer used health care in order to illustrate his communitarian criticism of Rawls's de-contextualized social primary goods. See Kenneth J. Arrow, "Some Ordinalist-Utilitarian Notes on Rawls's Theory of Justice," *Journal of Philosophy* 70, no. 9 (1973): 245–62; Amartya Sen, "Equality of What?" *The Tanner Lectures on Human Values* (Cambridge: Cambridge University Press, 1980): 195–220; Michael Walzer, *Spheres of Justice: A Defense of Pluralism and Equality* (Oxford: Blackwell, 1983), pp. 86–90.

Bibliography

Achebe, Chinua. 1986. *Things Fall Apart*. Oxford: Heinemann.

Anand, Paul, and Allan Wailoo. 2000. Utilities versus Rights to Publicly Provided Goods: Argument and Evidence from Health Care Rationing. *Economica* 67, no. 268: 543–77.

Anand, Sudhir. 2004. The Concern for Equity in Health. In *Public Health, Ethics, and Equity*, eds. Sudhir Anand, Fabienne Peter, and Amartya Sen, 15–20. Oxford: Oxford University Press.

Anand, Sudhir, and Martin Ravallion. 1993. Human Development in Poor Countries: On the Role of Private Incomes and Public Services. *Journal of Economic Perspectives* 7: 133–50.

Anderson, Elizabeth S. 1999. What Is the Point of Equality? *Ethics* 109: 287–337.

———. 2008. How Should Egalitarians Cope with Market Risks? *Theoretical Inquiries in Law* 9: 239–70.

Angier, Natalie. 2003. Short Men, Short Shrift: Are Drugs the Answer? *New York Times*, June 22.

Arneson, Richard J. 1990. Liberalism, Distributive Subjectivism, and Equal Opportunity for Welfare. *Philosophy and Public Affairs* 19, no. 2: 158–94.

———. 1997. Equality and Equal Opportunity for Welfare. In *Equality: Selected Readings*, eds. Louis P. Pojman and Robert B. Westmoreland, 229–41. Oxford: Oxford University Press.

———. 1999. Against Rawlsian Equality of Opportunity. *Philosophical Studies* 93, no. 1: 77–112.

———. 1999. Egalitarianism and Responsibility. *Journal of Ethics* 3: 225–47.

———. 1999. Equality of Opportunity for Welfare Defended and Recanted. *Journal of Political Philosophy* 7, no. 4: 488–97.

———. 2000. Luck-Egalitarianism and Prioritarianism. *Ethics* 110, no. 2: 339–49.

———. 2000. Perfectionism and Politics. *Ethics* 111, no. 1: 37–63.

———. 2000. Welfare Should Be the Currency of Justice. *Canadian Journal of Philosophy* 30, no. 4: 497–524.

———. 2001. Luck and Equality. *Proceedings of the Aristotelian Society*, Supplement 75, no. 1: 73–90.

———. 2002. Review of "Sovereign Virtue: The Theory and Practice of Equality" by Ronald Dworkin. *Ethics* 112: 367–71.

———. 2005. Do Patriotic Ties Limit Global Justice Duties? *Journal of Ethics* 9: 127–50.

———. 2005. Luck Egalitarianism Interpreted and Defended. http://philosophyfaculty.ucsd.edu/faculty/rarneson/luckegalitarianism2.pdf.

———. 2006. Disability, Priority, and Equal Opportunity. Paper presented at the Bergen Workshop on Disability, June, 2006, Bergen, Norway.

———. 2007. Desert and Equality. In *Egalitarianism*, eds. Nils Holtug and Kasper Lippert-Rasmussen, 262–94. Oxford: Oxford University Press.

———. 2007. Luck Egalitarianism—A Primer. Paper presented at the Harvard Law School, April.

Arrow, Kenneth J. 1973. Some Ordinalist-Utilitarian Notes on Rawls's Theory of Justice. *Journal of Philosophy* 70, no. 9: 245–63.

Barbeau, Elizabeth M., Nancy Krieger, and Mah-Jabeen Soobader. 2004. Working Class Matters: Socio-Economic Disadvantage, Race/Ethnicity, Gender, and Smoking in NIHS. *American Journal of Public Health* 94: 269–87.

Barry, Brian. 1982. Humanity and Justice in Global Perspective. In *Ethics, Economics, and the Law,* Nomos 24, eds. James R. Pennock and John W. Chapman, 219–25. New York: New York University Press.

———. 2001. *Culture and Equality: An Egalitarian Critique of Multiculturalism.* Cambridge, MA: Harvard University Press.

Barry, Nicholas. 2006. Defending Luck-Egalitarianism *Journal of Applied Philosophy* 23, no. 1: 89–107.

———. 2008. Reassessing Luck Egalitarianism. *Journal of Politics* 70: 136–50.

Beitz, Charles. 1999. International Liberalism and Distributive Justice: A Survey of Recent Thought. *World Politics* 51, no. 2: 269–96.

———. 1999. *Political Theory and International Relations.* Princeton, NJ: Princeton University Press.

———. 1999. Social and Cosmopolitan Liberalism. *International Affairs* 73, no. 3: 515–29.

———. 2000. Rawls's "Law of Peoples." *Ethics* 110, no. 4: 669–96.

Benatar, Solomon R., Abdallah S. Daar, and Peter A. Singer. 2003. Global Health Ethics: The Rationale for Mutual Caring. *International Affairs* 79, no. 1: 107–38.

Beran, Harry. 1988. More Theory of Secession: A Response to Birch. *Political Studies* 36, no. 2: 316–23.

Blake, Michael. 2002. Distributive Justice, State Coercion, and Autonomy. *Philosophy and Public Affairs* 30, no. 3: 257–96.

Bommier, Antoine, and Guy Stecklov. 2002. Defining Health Inequality: Why Rawls Succeeds Where Social Welfare Theory Fails. *Journal of Health Economics* 21: 497–513

Bou-Habib, Paul. 2006. Compulsory Insurance without Paternalism. *Utilitas* 18, no. 3: 243–63.

Brighouse, Harry, and Adam Swift. 2006. Equality, Priority, and Positional Goods. *Ethics* 116, no. 3: 471–97.

Brock, Dan W. 1989. Justice, Health Care, and the Elderly. *Philosophy and Public Affairs* 18, no. 3: 297–312.

———. 2000. Broadening the Bioethics Agenda. *Kennedy Institute of Ethics Journal* 10, no. 1: 21–38.

———. 2002. Priority to the Worse Off in Health-Care Resource Prioritization. In *Medicine and Social Justice,* eds. Rosamond Rhodes, Margaret Battin and Anita Silvers, 362–72. Oxford: Oxford University Press.

———. 2004. Ethical Issues in the Use of Cost Effectiveness Analysis for the Prioritization of Health Care Resources. In *Public Health, Ethics, and Equity,* eds. Sudhir Anand, Fabienne Peter, and Amartya Sen, 201–24. Oxford: Oxford University Press.

Broome, John. Forthcoming. Equality versus Priority: A Useful Distinction. In *Health, Well Being, Justice: Ethical Issues in Health Resource Allocation,* eds. Daniel Wikler and Christopher J. L. Murray. Geneva: World Health Organization.

Buchanan, Allen. 1984. The Right to a Decent Minimum of Health Care. *Philosophy and Public Affairs* 13: 55–78.

Buchanan, Allen, Dan W. Brock, Norman Daniels, and Daniel Wikler. 2000. *From Chance to Choice: Genetics and Justice*. Cambridge: Cambridge University Press.

Burley, Justine. 1999. *The Genetic Revolution and Human Rights*. Oxford: Oxford University Press.

Caldwell, John C. 1986. Routes to Low Mortality in Poor Countries. *Population and Development Review* 12, no. 2: 171–220.

Callahan, Daniel. 1987. *Setting Limits: Medical Goals in an Aging Society*. New York: Simon and Schuster.

Caney, Simon. 2000. Global Equality of Opportunity and the Sovereignty of States. In *International Justice*, ed. Anthony J. Coates, 130–49. Aldershot: Ashgate.

———. 2001. Cosmopolitan Justice and Equalizing Opportunities. In *Global Justice*, ed. Thomas Pogge, 123–44. Oxford: Blackwell.

———. 2002. Cosmopolitanism and the Law of Peoples. *Journal of Political Philosophy* 10, no. 1: 95–123.

———. 2005. *Justice beyond Borders: A Global Political Theory*. Oxford: Oxford University Press.

Cappelen, Alexander W. 2005. Responsibility and International Distributive Justice. In *Real World Justice: Grounds, Principles, Human Rights, and Social Institutions*, eds. Andreas Føllesdal and Thomas Pogge, 215–28. Dordrecht: Springer.

Cappelen, Alexander W., Rune J. Hagen, and Bertil Tungodden. 2007. National Responsibility and the Just Distribution of Debt Relief. *Ethics and International Affairs* 21, no. 1: 69–83.

Cappelen, Alexander W., and Ole F. Norheim. 2005. Responsibility in Health Care: A Liberal Egalitarian Approach. *Journal of Medical Ethics* 31: 476–80.

Cappelen, Alexander W., Ole F. Norheim, and Bertil Tungodden. 2008. Genomics and Equal Opportunity Ethics. *Journal of Medical Ethics* 34: 361–64.

Cappelen, Alexander W., and Bertil Tungodden. 2006. A Liberal Egalitarian Paradox. *Economics and Philosophy* 22: 393–408.

———. 2006. Relocating the Responsibility Cut: Should More Responsibility Imply Less Redistribution? *Politics, Philosophy, and Economics* 5, no. 3: 353–62.

Carens, Joseph. 1987. Aliens and Citizens: The Case for Open Borders. *Review of Politics* 49: 83–99.

Casal, Paula. 2007. Why Sufficiency Is Not Enough. *Ethics* 117, no. 2: 296–326.

Christiano, Thomas. 1999. Comment on Elizabeth Anderson's "What Is the Point of Equality?" http://www.brown.edu/Departments/Philosophy/bears/9904chri.html.

Cohen, G. A. 1989. On the Currency of Egalitarian Justice. *Ethics* 99, no. 4: 906–44.

———. 1995. *Self-Ownership, Freedom and Equality*. Cambridge: Cambridge University Press.

———. 1997. Where the Action Is: On the Site of Distributive Justice. *Philosophy and Public Affairs* 26, no. 1: 3–30.

———. 2000. *If You're an Egalitarian, How Come You're So Rich?* Cambridge, MA: Harvard University Press.

———. 2003. Facts and Principles. *Philosophy and Public Affairs* 31, no. 3: 211–54.

———. 2004. Expensive Taste Rides Again. In *Dworkin and His Critics*, ed. Justine Burley, 3–29. Oxford: Blackwell.

———. 2006. Luck and Equality: A Reply to Hurley. *Philosophy and Phenomenological Research* 72, no. 2: 439–46.

Cohen, Joshua, and Charles Sabel. 2006. Extra Rempublicam Nulla Justitia? *Philosophy and Public Affairs* 34, no. 2: 147–75.

Coleman, Jules, and Arthur Ripstein. 1995. Mischief and Misfortune. *McGill Law Journal* 41: 91–130.

Cook, Karen S., and Karen A. Hegtvedt. 1983. Distributive Justice, Equity, and Equality. *Annual Review of Sociology* 9: 217–41.

Crisp, Roger. 2003. Equality, Priority, and Compassion. *Ethics* 113, no. 4: 745–63.

Culyer, Anthony J. 1993. Health, Health Expenditures, and Equity. In *Equity in the Finance and Delivery of Health Care*, eds. Eddy Van Doorslaer, Adam Wagstaff, and Frans Rutten, 299–319. Oxford: Oxford University Press.

Culyer, Anthony J., and Adam Wagstaff. 1993. Equity and Equality in Health and Health Care. *Journal of Health Economics* 12: 431–57.

Dahlgren, Goran, and Margaret Whitehead. 1991. *Politics and Strategies to Promote Social Equality in Health.* Stockholm: Institute of Future Studies.

Daniels, Norman. 1981. Health-Care Needs and Distributive Justice. *Philosophy and Public Affairs* 10, no. 2: 146–79.

———. 1985. Fair Equality of Opportunity and Decent Minimums: A Reply to Buchanan. *Philosophy and Public Affairs,* 14, no. 1: 106–10.

———. 1985. *Just Health Care.* Cambridge: Cambridge University Press.

———. 1987. Justice and Health Care. In *Health Care Ethics*, eds. Donald Van De Veer and Tom Regan, 302–6. Philadelphia: Temple University Press.

———. 1988. *Am I My Parents' Keeper? An Essay on Justice between the Old and the Young.* New York: Oxford University Press.

———. 1996. *Justice and Justification: Reflective Equilibrium in Theory and Practice.* Cambridge: Cambridge University Press.

———. 2001. Justice, Health, and Healthcare. *American Journal of Bioethics* 1, no. 2: 2–16.

———. 2003. Democratic Equality: Rawls's Complex Egalitarianism. In *The Cambridge Companion to Rawls*, ed. Samuel Freeman, 241–76. Cambridge: Cambridge University Press.

———. 2008. *Just Health: Meeting Health Needs Fairly.* Cambridge: Cambridge University Press.

———. Forthcoming. Can Anyone Really Be Talking about Ethically Modifying Human Nature? In *Human Enhancement*, eds. Julian Savulescu and Nick Bostrom. Oxford: Oxford University Press.

Daniels, Norman, Bruce Kennedy, and Ichiro Kawachi. 2000. Justice Is Good for Our Health. In *Is Inequality Bad for Our Health?* eds. Joshua Cohen and Joel Rogers, 3–33. Boston: Beacon Press.

———. 2004. Health and Inequality, or, Why Justice Is Good for Our Health. In *Public Health, Ethics, and Equity*, eds. Sudhir Anand, Fabienne Peter, and Amartya Sen, 63–92. Oxford: Oxford University Press.

Daniels, Norman, and James Sabin. 1997. Limits to Health Care: Fair Procedures, Democratic Deliberation, and the Legitimacy Problem for Insurers. *Philosophy and Public Affairs* 26, no. 4: 303–50.

Deaton, Angus. 2002. Policy Implications of the Gradient of Health and Wealth. *Health Affairs* 21: 13–30.

Deutsch, Morton. 1968. The Effects of Co-operation and Competition upon Group Process. In *Group Dynamics*, eds. Dorwin Cartwright and Alvin Zander, 461–82. New York: Harper & Row.

———. 1985. *Distributive Justice: A Social-Psychological Perspective*. New Haven, CT: Yale University Press.

Dolan, Paul, Rebecca Shaw, Aki Tsuchiya, and Alan Williams. 2005. QALY Maximization and People's Preferences: A Methodological Review of the Literature. *Health Economics* 14: 197–208.

Dworkin, Ronald. 1981. What Is Equality? Part I: Equality of Welfare. *Philosophy and Public Affairs* 10, no. 3: 185–246.

———. 1981. What Is Equality? Part II: Equality of Resources. *Philosophy and Public Affairs* 10, no. 4: 283–345.

———. 1990. Foundations of Liberal Equality. *The Tanner Lectures on Human Values*, vol. 11 (Salt Lake City: University of Utah Press), 3–119.

———. 1993. Justice in the Distribution of Health Care. *McGill Law Journal* 38, no. 4: 883–97.

———. 2000. Ronald Dworkin Replies. In *Dworkin and His Critics*, ed. Justine Burley, 339–95. Oxford: Blackwell.

———. 2000. *Sovereign Virtue: The Theory and Practice of Equality*. Cambridge, MA: Harvard University Press.

———. 2001. Do Liberal Values Conflict? In *The Legacy of Isaiah Berlin*, eds. Mark Lilla, Ronald Dworkin, and Robert B. Silvers, 73–90. New York: New York Review of Books.

———. 2002. Sovereign Virtue Revisited. *Ethics* 113, no. 1: 106–43.

———. 2003. Equality, Luck and Hierarchy. *Philosophy and Public Affairs* 31, no. 2: 190–98.

Enoch, David, and Andrei Marmor. 2006. The Case against Moral Luck. *Law and Philosophy* 26, no. 4: 405–36.

European Commission. N.d. Regional Policy, Key Objectives, http://ec.europa.eu/regional_policy/policy/object/index_en.htm.

Eyal, Nir. 2007. Egalitarian Justice and Innocent Choice. *Journal of Ethics and Social Philosophy* 2, no. 1: 1–18.

Eyal, Nir, and Hirst, Samia A. 2008. Physician Brain Drain—Can Nothing Be Done? *Public Health Ethics* 1, no. 2: 1–13.

Fabre, Cecile. 2003. Global Egalitarianism: An Indefensible Theory of Justice? In *Forms of Justice*, eds. Daniel Bell and Avner de-Shalit, 315–30. Lanham, MD: Rowman and Littlefield.

Faria, F. S., E. Guthrie, E. Brandbury, and A. N. Brain. 1999. Psychological Outcome and Patient Satisfaction following Breast Reduction Surgery. *British Journal of Plastic Surgery* 52, no. 6: 448–52.

Farrelly, Colin. 2004. Genes and Equality. *Journal of Medical Ethics* 30, no. 4: 587–92.

Fenton, Elizabeth. 2006. Liberal Eugenics and Human Nature: Against Habermas. *Hastings Center Report* 36: 35–42.

Filmer, Deon, and Lant Pritchett. 1999. The Impact of Public Spending on Health: Does Money Matter? *Social Science and Medicine* 49, no. 10: 1309–23.

Finnis, John. 1980. *Natural Law and Natural Rights*. Oxford: Clarendon Press.

Fleurbaey, Marc. 1995. Equal Opportunity or Equal Social Outcome? *Economics and Philosophy* 11: 25–55.

———. 2001. Egalitarian Opportunities. *Law and Philosophy* 20, no. 5: 499–530.

———. Forthcoming. Equality vs. Priority: How Relevant Is the Distinction. In *Health, Well Being, Justice: Ethical Issues in Health Resource Allocation*, eds. Daniel Wikler and Christopher J. L. Murray. Geneva: World Health Organization.

Fleurbaey, Marc, and Schokkaert, Erik. N.d. Unfair Inequalities in Health and Health Care. Unpublished manuscript.

Flory, James H., and Philip Kitcher. 2004. Global Health and the Scientific Research Agenda. *Philosophy and Public Affairs* 32, no. 1: 36–65.

Føllesdal, Andreas. 1998. Subsidiarity. *Journal of Political Philosophy* 6, no. 2: 190–218.

Frankfurt, Harry. 1987. Equality as a Moral Ideal. *Ethics* 98, no. 1: 21–43.

Fukuyama, Francis. 2002. *Our Posthuman Future: Consequences of the Biotechnology Revolution*. New York: Farrar, Straus and Giroux.

Gakidou, Emmanuela, Julio Frenk, and Christopher J. L. Murray. 2000. A Health Agenda. In *Is Inequality Bad for Our Health?* eds. Joshua Cohen and Joel Rogers, 71–78. Boston: Beacon Press.

Gakidou, Emmanuela, Christopher J. L. Murray, and Julio Frenk. 2000. Defining and Measuring Health Inequality: An Approach Based on the Distribution of Health Expectancy. *Bulletin of the World Health Organization* 78: 42–54.

Glannon, Walter. 2001. *Genes and Future People*. Boulder, CO: Westview Press.

Goodin, Robert E. 1985. Negating Positive Desert Claims. *Political Theory* 13: 575–98.

———. 1988. *Reasons for Welfare: The Political Theory of the Welfare State*. Princeton, NJ: Princeton University Press.

Greer, Scott L. Forthcoming. The Fragile Divergence Machine: Citizenship, Policy Divergence, and Devolution. In *Devolution and Power in the UK*, ed. A. Trench. Manchester: Manchester University Press.

Gruber, Jonathan. 2005. *Public Finance and Public Policy*. New York: Worth.

Gutmann, Amy. 1981. For and against Equal Access to Health Care. *Milbank Memorial Fund Quarterly* 59: 542–60.

Habermas, Jurgen. 2003. *The Future of Human Nature*. Cambridge: Polity.

Harris, John. 2007. *Enhancing Evolution: The Ethical Case for Making Better People*. Princeton, NJ: Princeton University Press.

Hausman, Daniel M. 2007. What's Wrong with Health Inequalities? *Journal of Political Philosophy* 15, no. 1: 46–66.

———. Forthcoming. Equality versus Priority: A Badly Misleading Distinction. In *Health, Well Being, Justice: Ethical Issues in Health Resource Allocation*, eds. Daniel Wikler and Christopher J. L. Murray. Geneva: World Health Organization.

Hausman, Daniel M., Yukiko Asada, and Thomas Hedemann. 2002. Health Inequalities and Why They Matter. *Health Care Analysis* 10, no. 2: 177–91.

Heyd, David. 2007. Justice and Solidarity: The Contractarian Case against Global Justice. *Journal of Social Philosophy* 38, no. 1: 112–30.

Hobcraft, John. 1993. Women's Education, Child Welfare, and Child Survival: A Review of the Evidence. *Health Transition Review* 3: 159–75.

Horowitz, Donald L. 2000. Constitutional Design: An Oxymoron? *Nomos* 42: 253–84.

Houtepen, Rob, and Ruud Ter Muelen. 2000. New Types of Solidarity in the European Welfare State. *Health Care Analysis* 8: 329–40.

The Human Development Report 2005, http://hdrstats.undp.org/countries/country_fact_sheets/cty_fs_ISL.html.

The Human Development Report 2007/2008, http://hdrstats.undp.org/indicators/5.html.

Hurley, Susan L. 2003. *Justice, Luck, and Knowledge*. Cambridge, MA: Harvard University Press.

———. 2007. On the What and the How of Distributive Justice and Health. In *Egalitarianism: New Essays on the Nature and Value of Equality*, eds. Nils Holtug and Kasper Lippert-Rasmussen, 308–34. Oxford: Oxford University Press.

Independent Inquiry into Inequalities in Health: Report. London: Stationery Office, 1998.

Jacobs, Lesley A. 2004. Justice in Health Care: Can Dworkin Justify Equal Access? In *Dworkin and His Critics*, ed. Justine Burley, 134–49. Oxford: Blackwell.

———. 2004. *Pursuing Equal Opportunities: The Theory and Practice of Egalitarian Justice*. Cambridge: Cambridge University Press.

Kagan, Shelly. 1999. Equality and Desert. In *What Do We Deserve? A Reader on Justice and Desert*, eds. Louis P. Pojman and Owen McLeod, 298–314. New York: Oxford University Press.

———. 2003. Comparative Desert. In *Desert and Justice*, ed. Serena Olsaretti, 93–122. New York: Oxford University Press.

Kamm, Frances M. 1993. *Morality, Mortality: Death and Whom to Save from It*. Oxford: Oxford University Press.

———. 2001. Health and Equality of Opportunity. *American Journal of Bioethics* 1, no. 2: 17–19.

———. 2002. Health and Equity. In *Summary Measures of Population Health: Concepts, Ethics, Measurement and Applications*, eds. Christopher J. L. Murray, Joshua A. Solomon, Colin D. Mathers, and Alan D. Lopez, 685–706. Geneva: World Health Organization.

———. 2004. Deciding Whom to Help, Health-Adjusted Life Years and Disabilities. In *Public Health, Ethics, and Equity*, eds. Sudhir Anand, Fabienne Peter, and Amartya Sen, 225–42. Oxford: Oxford University Press.

Kanavos, Panos, and Martin McKee. 2000. Cross-Border Issues in the Provision of Health Services: Are We Moving towards a European Health Care Policy? *Journal of Health Services Research and Policy* 5, no. 4: 231–36.

Kass, Leon R. 2002. *Life, Liberty, and the Defense of Dignity: The Challenge for Bioethics*. San Francisco: Encounter Books.

Kawachi, Ichiro K., Bruce P. Kennedy, K. Lochner, and D. Prothrow-Stith. 1997. Social Capital, Income Inequality, and Mortality. *American Journal of Public Health* 87: 1491–98.

Kawachi, Ichiro K., Bruce P. Kennedy, and Richard G. Wilkinson. 1999. *The Society and Health Reader: Income Inequality and Health*. New York: The New Press.

Keating, Michael. 2003. Social Inclusion, Devolution and Policy Divergence. *Political Quarterly* 74, no. 4: 429–38.

Kekes, John. 1997. A Question for Egalitarians. *Ethics* 107, no. 4: 658–69.

Kershnar, Stephen. 2004. *Justice for the Past*. Albany: State University of New York Press.

Knight, Carl. 2005. In Defense of Luck Egalitarianism. *Res Publica* 11, no. 1: 55–73.

Knowles, John H. 1997. The Responsibility of the Individual. In *Doing Better and Feeling Worse: Health in the United States*, ed. John H. Knowles, 57–80. New York: Norton.

Korsgaard, Christine. 1983. Two Distinctions in Goodness. *Philosophical Review* 92: 169–95.

Kymlicka, Will. 1990. *Contemporary Political Philosophy: An Introduction.* Oxford: Clarendon Press.

———. 1995. *Multicultural Citizenship: A Liberal Theory of Minority Rights.* Oxford: Clarendon Press.

Landau, R. 2008. Sex Selection for Social Purposes in Israel: Quest for the "Perfect Child" of a Particular Gender or Centuries Old Prejudice against Women? *Journal of Medical Ethics* 34: e10.

Le Grand, Julian. 1987. Equity, Health, and Health Care. *Social Justice Research* 1, no. 3: 257–74.

Lev, Ori, and Ezekiel Emmanuel. N.d. The Ethics of Biomedical Enhancement Research. Unpublished manuscript.

Lippert-Rasmussen, Kasper. 1999. Arneson on Equality of Opportunity for Welfare. *Journal of Political Philosophy* 7, no. 4: 478–87.

———. 2001. Egalitarianism, Option Luck, and Responsibility. *Ethics* 111: 548–79.

———. 2005. Hurley on Egalitarianism and the Luck-Neutralizing Aim. *Politics, Philosophy and Economics* 4, no. 2: 249–65.

Mackenbach, J. P., K. E. Stronks, and A. E. Kunst. 1989.The Contribution of Medical Care to Inequalities in Health. *Social Science and Medicine* 29: 369–76.

Mann, Jonathan M. 1997. Medicine and Public Health, Ethics and Human Rights. *Hastings Center Report* 27: 6–13.

Marchand, Sarah. N.d. Liberal Theories and Health. Unpublished manuscript.

Marchand, Sarah, Daniel Wikler, and Bruce Landesman. 1998. Class, Health, and Justice. *Milbank Quarterly* 76, no. 3: 449–67.

Margalit, Avishai. 1996. *The Decent Society.* Cambridge, MA, and London: Harvard University Press.

Marmot, Michael. 2004. Social Causes of Social Inequalities in Health. In *Public Health, Ethics, and Equity*, eds. Sudhir Anand, Fabienne Peter and Amartya Sen, 37–62. Oxford: Oxford University Press.

———. 2004. *The Status Syndrome: How Social Standing Affects Our Health and Longevity.* New York: Times Books.

Marmot, Michael, Martin J. Shipley, and Geoffrey Rose. 1984. Inequalities in Death-Specific Explanations of a General Pattern. *Lancet* 1: 1003–6.

Marmot, Michael, and Richard G. Wilkinson. 2006. *Social Determinants of Health.* Oxford: Oxford University Press; 2nd ed.

Mason, Andrew. 2000. *Community, Solidarity and Belonging: Levels of Community and Their Normative Significance.* Cambridge: Cambridge University Press.

———. 2001. Egalitarianism and the Leveling Down Objection. *Analysis* 61: 246–54.

———. 2006. *Leveling the Playing Field: The Idea of Equal Opportunity and Its Place in Egalitarian Thought.* Oxford: Oxford University Press.

McKerlie, Dennis. 1996. Equality. *Ethics* 106, no. 2: 274–96.

McRae, Kenneth D. 1986. *Conflict and Compromise in Multilingual Societies: Belgium.* Waterloo, Ontario: Wilfred Laurier University Press.

Mechanic, David. 2002. Disadvantage, Inequality, and Social Policy. *Health Affairs* 21: 48–59.

Mikula, Gerold, and Thomas Schwinger. 1978. Intermember Relations and Reward Allocation: Theoretical Considerations of Affects. In *Dynamics of Group Decisions*, eds. Hermann Brandstatter, James H. Davis, and Heinz Schuler, 229–50. London: Sage.

Miller, David. 1982. Arguments for Equality. *Midwest Studies in Philosophy* 7, no. 1: 73–87.

———. 1995. *On Nationality*. Oxford: Clarendon Press.

———. 1997. What Kind of Equality Should the Left Pursue? In *Equality*, ed. Jane Franklin, 83–100. London: Institute for Public Policy Research.

———. 1998. Equality and Justice. In *Ideals of Equality*, ed. Andrew Mason, 21–36. Oxford: Blackwell.

———. 1999. Justice and Global Inequality. In *Inequality, Globalization and World Politics*, eds. Andrew Hurrell and Ngaire Woods, 187–210. Oxford: Oxford University Press.

———. 1999. *Principles of Social Justice*. Cambridge, MA: Harvard University Press.

———. 2000. *Citizenship and National Identity*. Oxford: Polity.

———. 2004. Holding Nations Responsible. *Ethics* 114, no. 2: 240–68.

———. 2007. *National Responsibility and Global Justice*. Oxford: Oxford University Press.

Moellendorf, Darrel. 2002. *Cosmopolitan Justice*. Boulder, CO: Westview Press.

Morgan, William R., and Jack Sawyer. 1979. Equality, Equity, and Procedural Justice in Social Exchange. *Social Psychology Quarterly* 42, no. 1: 71–75.

Murray, Christopher J. L. 1996. Rethinking DALYs. In *The Global Burden of Disease*, eds. Christopher J. L. Murray and Alan D. Lopez, 1–98. Cambridge, MA: Harvard School of Public Health, World Health Organization, World Bank.

———. 1998. *U.S. Patterns of Mortality by County and Race: 1965–1994*. Cambridge, MA: Harvard School of Public Health.

Murray, Christopher J. L., Emanuela Gakidou, and Julio Frenk. 1999. Health Inequalities and Social Group Differences: What Should We Measure? *Bulletin of the World Health Organization* 77: 537–43.

Murray, Christopher J. L., Sandeep C. Kulkarni, Catherine Michaud, Niels Tomijima, Maria T. Bulazacchelli, Terrell J. Iandiorio, and Majid Ezzati. 2006. Eight Americas: Investigating Mortality Disparities across Races, Counties, and Race-Counties in the United States. *PLOS Medicine* 3, no. 9: e260.

Murray, Christopher J. L., and Alan D. Lopez (eds.). 1996. *The Global Burden of Disease*. Cambridge, MA: Harvard School of Public Health, World Health Organization, World Bank.

Nagel, Thomas. 1979. *Mortal Questions*. Cambridge: Cambridge University Press.

———. 2005. The Problem of Global Justice. *Philosophy and Public Affairs* 33, no. 2: 113–47.

Norman, Richard. 1998. The Social Basis of Equality. In *Ideals of Equality*, ed. Andrew Mason, 37–51. Oxford: Blackwell.

Nussbaum, Martha. 2000. *Women and Human Development*. Cambridge: Cambridge University Press.

Olsaretti, Serena. 2003. Introduction: Debating Desert and Justice. In *Desert and Justice*, ed. Serena Olsaretti, 1–24. New York: Oxford University Press.

Otsuka, Michael. 2000. Liberty, Equality, Envy, and Abstraction. In *Dworkin and His Critics*, ed. Justine Burley, 70–78. Oxford: Blackwell.

———. 2002. Luck, Insurance, and Equality. *Ethics* 113: 40–54.

Parfit, Derek. 1998. Equality and Priority. In *Ideals of Equality*, ed. Andrew Mason, 1–20. Oxford: Blackwell.

———. 2000. "Equality or Priority?" In *The Ideal of Equality*, eds. M. Clayton and A. Williams 81–125. Basingstoke: McMillan.

Peter, Fabienne. 2004. Health Equity and Social Justice. In *Public Health, Ethics, and Equity*, eds. Sudhir Anand, Fabienne Peter, and Amartya Sen, 93–106. Oxford: Oxford University Press.

Pogge, Thomas. 1989. *Realizing Rawls*. Ithaca, NY: Cornell University Press.

———. 1994. An Egalitarian Law of Peoples. *Philosophy and Public Affairs* 23, no. 3: 195–224.

———. 2002. Moral Universalism and Global Economic Justice. *Politics, Philosophy, and Economics* 1: 29–58.

———. 2002. *World Poverty and Human Rights: Cosmopolitans Responsibilities and Reforms*. Cambridge: Polity.

———. 2004. Relational Conceptions of Justice: Responsibilities for Health Outcomes. In *Public Health, Ethics, and Equity*, eds. Sudhir Anand, Fabienne Peter, and Amartya Sen, 135–61. Oxford: Oxford University Press.

Powers, Madison, and Ruth Faden. 2006. *Social Justice: The Moral Foundations of Public Health and Health Policy*. Oxford: Oxford University Press.

Rakowski, Eric. 1991. *Equal Justice*. Oxford: Oxford University Press.

Rawls, John. 1971. *A Theory of Justice*. Oxford: Oxford University Press.

———. 1993. *Political Liberalism*. New York: University of Columbia Press.

———. 1999. *The Law of Peoples*. Cambridge, MA: Harvard University Press.

———. 2001. *Justice as Fairness: A Restatement*. Cambridge, MA: Harvard University Press.

Remennick, L. 2006. The Quest after the Perfect Baby: Why Do Israeli Women Seek Prenatal Genetic Testing? *Sociology of Health and Illness* 28: 21–53.

Resnik, David B. 2005. The Patient's Duty to Adhere to Prescribed Treatment: An Ethical Analysis. *Journal of Medicine and Philosophy* 30: 167–88.

Richards, David A. J. 1982. International Distributive Justice. In *Ethics, Economics, and the Law*, Nomos 24, eds. James R. Pennock and John W. Chapman, 275–94. New York: New York University Press.

Ripstein, Arthur. 1994. Equality, Luck, and Responsibility. *Philosophy and Public Affairs* 23, no. 1: 3–23.

Roemer, John E. 1993. A Pragmatic Theory of Responsibility for the Egalitarian Planner. *Philosophy and Public Affairs* 22, no. 2: 146–66.

———. 1994. *Egalitarian Perspectives*. Cambridge: Cambridge University Press.

Rosa Dias, Pedro, and Andrew M. Jones. 2007. Giving Equality of Opportunity a Fair Innings. *Health Economics* 16: 109–12.

Sandbu, Martin E. 2004. On Dworkin's Brute-Luck-Option-Luck Distinction and the Consistency of Brute-Luck Egalitarianism. *Politics, Philosophy, and Economics* 3, no. 3: 283–312.

Sandel, Michael J. 2004. The Case against Perfection: What's Wrong with Designer Children, Bionic Athletes, and Genetic Engineering. *Atlantic Monthly* 293, no. 3: 50–62.

———. 2007. *The Case against Perfection: Ethics in the Age of Genetic Engineering*. Cambridge, MA: Harvard University Press.

Sapolsky, Robert M. 1998. *Why Zebras Don't Get Ulcers: A Guide to Stress, Stress-Related Disease, and Coping*. New York: W. H. Freeman.

Sapolsky, Robert M., Susan C. Alberts, and Jeanne Altman. 1997. Hypercortisolism Associated with Social Subordinance or Social Isolation among Wild Baboons. *Archives of General Psychiatry* 54: 1137–43.

Sass, Hans M. 1995. The New Triad: Responsibility, Solidarity and Subsidiarity. *Journal of Medicine and Philosophy* 20, no. 6: 587–94.

Scanlon, Thomas M. 1975. Preference and Urgency. *Journal of Philosophy* 72: 655–69.

———. 1976. Nozick on Rights, Liberty, and Property. *Philosophy and Public Affairs* 6, no. 1: 3–25.

———. 2003. *The Difficulty of Tolerance: Essays in Political Philosophy*. Cambridge: Cambridge University Press.

———. 2004. When Does Equality Matter? http://law.usc.edu/academics/assets/docs/scanlon.pdf, 1–38.

Scheffler, Samuel. 2003. Equality as the Virtue of Sovereigns: A Reply to Ronald Dworkin. *Philosophy and Public Affairs* 31, no. 2: 199–206.

———. 2003. What Is Egalitarianism? *Philosophy and Public Affairs* 31, no. 1: 5–39.

———. 2005. Choice, Circumstance, and the Value of Equality. *Philosophy, Politics, and Economics* 4, no. 1: 5–28.

Schmidt, Harald. 2008. Bonuses as Incentives and Rewards for Health Responsibility: A Good Thing? *Journal of Medicine and Philosophy* 33: 198–220.

Segall, Shlomi. 2004. Bringing the Middle Classes Back In: An Egalitarian Case for (Truly) Universal Public Services. *Ethics and Economics* 2 no. 1 (2004): 1–7.

———. 2005. Unconditional Welfare Benefits and the Principle of Reciprocity. *Politics, Philosophy, and Economics* 4, no. 3: 331–54.

———. 2007. In Solidarity with the Imprudent: A Defense of Luck Egalitarianism. *Social Theory and Practice* 33, no. 2: 177–98.

———. 2007. Is Health Care (Still) Special? *Journal of Political Philosophy* 15, no. 3: 342–63.

———. 2007. Why Devolution Upsets Distributive Justice. *Journal of Moral Philosophy* 4, no. 2: 259–74.

Sen, Amartya. 1980. Equality of What? In *The Tanner Lectures on Human Values*, 197–220. Cambridge: Cambridge University Press.

———. 1992. *Inequality Re-examined*. Cambridge, MA: Harvard University Press.

———. 1998. Mortality as an Indicator of Economic Success and Failure. *Economic Journal* 108, no. 446: 1–25.

———. 1999. *Development as Freedom*. Oxford: Oxford University Press.

———. 2002. Why Health Equity? *Health Economics* 11: 659–66.

———. 2004. Why Health Equity? In *Public Health, Ethics, and Equity*, eds. Sudhir Anand, Fabienne Peter, and Amartya Sen, 21–33. Oxford: Oxford University Press.

Shaw, Mary, David Gordon, Danny Dorling, Richard Mitchell, and George Davy Smith. 2000. Increasing Mortality Differentials by Residential Area Level of Poverty: Britain 1981–1997. *Social Science and Medicine* 51, no. 1: 151–53.

Sher, George. 1997. *Approximate Justice: Studies in Non-Ideal Theory*. Lanham, MD: Rowman and Littlefield.

Shiffrin, Seana V. 2004. Egalitarianism, Choice-Sensitivity, and Accommodation. In *Reason and Values: Themes from the Moral Philosophy of Joseph Raz*, eds. R. Jay Wallace, Philip Pettit, Samuel Scheffler, and Michael Smith, 270–302. Oxford: Oxford University Press.

Shively, Carol A., and Thomas B. Clarkson. 1994. Social Status and Coronary Artery Atherosclerosis in Female Monkeys. *Arteriosclerosis, Thrombosis, and Vascular Biology* 14: 721–26.

Shue, Henry. 1996. *Basic Rights: Subsistence, Affluence, and U.S. Foreign Policy*. Princeton, NJ: Princeton University Press.

Simmons, A. John. 2001. *Justification and Legitimacy: Essays on Rights and Obligations*. Cambridge: Cambridge University Press.

Singer, Peter. 1972. Famine, Affluence, and Morality. *Philosophy and Public Affairs* 1, no. 3: 229–43.

Skocpol, Theda. 1995. *Social Policy in the United States: Future Possibilities in Historical Perspective.* Princeton, NJ: Princeton University Press.

Smith, Adam. 1976. *The Wealth of Nations.* Glasgow: Glasgow University.

Sobel, David. 1999. Comment on Elizabeth Anderson's "What Is the Point of Equality." In http://www.brown.edu/Departments/Philosophy/bears/9904sobe.html.

Sreenivasan, Gopal. 2007. Health and Justice in Our Non-Ideal World. *Politics, Philosophy, and Economics* 6, no. 2: 218–36.

———. 2007. Health Care and Equality of Opportunity. *Hastings Center Report* 37: 31–41.

Steiner, Hillel. 1994. *An Essay on Rights.* Oxford: Blackwell.

———. 1996. Territorial Justice. In *National Rights, International Obligations,* eds. Simon Caney, David George, and Peter Jones, 139–48. Boulder, CO: Westview Press.

———. 1999. Just Taxation and International Redistribution. In *Global Justice,* Nomos 41, eds. Ian Shapiro and Lea Brilmayer, 171–91. New York: New York University Press.

———. 2002. How Equality Matters. *Social Philosophy and Policy* 19: 342–56.

Steiner, Ivan D. 1972. *Group Process and Productivity.* New York: Academic Press.

Stemplowska, Zofia. Forthcoming. Making Justice Sensitive to Responsibility. *Political Studies.*

Stern, Lawrence. 1983. Opportunity and Health Care: Criticisms and Suggestions. *Journal of Medicine and Philosophy* 8: 339–62.

Subbarao K., and Laura Raney. 1995. Social Gains from Female Education: A Cross-National Study. *Economic Development and Cultural Change* 44, no. 1: 105–28.

Tan, Kok-Chor. 2004. *Justice without Borders: Cosmopolitanism, Nationalism, and Patriotism.* Cambridge: Cambridge University Press.

Taylor, Robert S. 2004. Self-Realization and the Priority of Fair Equality of Opportunity, *Journal of Moral Philosophy* 1: 333–47.

Temkin, Larry S. 1993. *Inequality.* Oxford: Oxford University Press.

———. 2003. Egalitarianism Defended. *Ethics* 113: 764–82.

———. Forthcoming. Equality or Priority in Health Care Distribution. In *Health, Well Being, Justice: Ethical Issues in Health Resource Allocation,* eds. Daniel Wikler and Christopher J. L. Murray. Geneva: World Health Organization.

Thompson, Jana. 2002. *Taking Responsibility for the Past: Reparation and Historical Injustice.* Cambridge: Cambridge University Press.

Tsuchiya, Aki. 2000. QALYs and Ageism: Philosophical Theories and Age Weighting. *Health Economics* 9, no. 1: 57–68.

Tsuchiya, Aki, and Alan Williams. 2005. A "Fair Innings" between the Sexes: Are Men Being Treated Inequitably? *Social Science and Medicine* 60, no. 2: 277–86.

United Nations Development Program. 1990. *Human Development Report: Concept and Measurement of Human Development.* Oxford: Oxford University Press.

Vallentyne, Peter. 2002. Brute Luck, Option Luck, and Equality of Initial Opportunities. *Ethics* 112, no. 3: 529–57.

———. 2003. Brute Luck Equality and Desert. In *Desert and Justice,* ed. Serena Olsaretti, 169–86. New York: Oxford University Press.

Van Baal, Pieter H. M., John J. Polder, G. Ardine de Wit, Rudolf T. Hoogenveen, Talitha L. Feenstra, Hendrick C. Boshuizen, Peter M. Engelfriet, and Werner B. F.

Brouwer. 2008. Lifetime Medical Costs of Obesity: Prevention No Cure for Increasing Health Expenditure, *PLoS Medicine* 5, no. 2: 242–49.

Van Parijs, Philippe. 1995. *Real Freedom for All: What (If Anything) Can Justify Capitalism?* Oxford: Clarendon Press.

———. 2004. Health Care in a Pluri-National Country. In *Public Health, Ethics, and Equity*, eds. Sudhir Anand, Fabienne Peter and Amartya Sen, 163–80. Oxford: Oxford University Press.

Veatch, Robert M. 1991. Justice and the Right to Health Care: An Egalitarian Account. In *Rights to Health Care*, eds. Thomas J. Bole and William B. Bondeson, 83–102. Dordrecht: Kluwer.

Wagstaff, Adam, Pierella Pact, and Eddy Van Doorslaer. 1991. On the Measurement of Inequalities in Health. *Social Science and Medicine* 33, no. 5: 545–57.

Waldron, Jeremy. 1992. Superseding Historic Injustice. *Ethics* 103, no. 1: 4–28.

———. 2002. Redressing Historic Injustice. *University of Toronto Law Journal* 52: 135–60.

Walzer, Michael. 1983. *Spheres of Justice: A Defense of Pluralism and Equality*. Oxford: Blackwell.

———. 1994. *Thick and Thin: Moral Argument at Home and Abroad*. Notre Dame, IN, and London: Notre Dame University Press.

———. 1995. Response. In *Pluralism, Justice, and Equality*, eds. David L. Miller and Michael Walzer, 281–98. Oxford: Oxford University Press.

White, Stuart. 2003. *The Civic Minimum: On the Rights and Obligations of Economic Citizenship*. Oxford: Oxford University Press.

———. 2004. Social Minimum. *Stanford Encyclopedia of Philosophy*, http://plato .stanford.edu/entries/social-minimum/.

Whitehead, Margaret. 1990. *The Concepts and Principles of Equity and Health*. Copenhagen: World Health Organization.

———. 1991. The Concepts and Principles of Equity and Health. *Health Promotion International* 6, no. 3: 217–28.

Wiggins, David. 1988. *Needs, Values, Truth: Essays in the Philosophy of Value*. Oxford: Blackwell.

Wikler, Daniel. 1978. Persuasion and Coercion for Health: Ethical Issues in Government's Effort to Change Lifestyle. *Milbank Memorial Fund Quarterly/Health and Society* 56, no. 3: 303–38.

———. 1987. Personal Responsibility for Illness. In *Health Care Ethics: An Introduction*, eds. Donald Van De Veer and Tom Regan, 326–58. Philadelphia: Temple University Press.

———. 2004. Personal and Social Responsibility for Health. In *Public Health, Ethics, and Equity*, eds. Sudhir Anand, Fabienne Peter, and Amartya Sen, 109–34. Oxford: Oxford University Press.

Wilkinson, Richard G. 1996. *Unhealthy Societies: The Afflictions of Inequality*. London: Routledge.

Wilkinson, Richard G., and Michael Marmot. 2003. *Social Determinants of Health: The Solid Facts*, 2nd ed. Geneva: WHO.

Williams, Alan. 1997. Intergenerational Equity: An Exploration of the "Fair Innings" Argument. *Health Economics* 6: 117–132.

———. 1998. If We Are Going to Get a Fair Innings, Someone Will Need to Keep the Score! In *Health, Health Care and Health Economics*, eds. Morris L. Barer, Thomas E. Getzen, and Greg L. Stoddart, 319–30. New York: Wiley.

Williams, Bernard. 1981. *Moral Luck: Philosophical Papers 1973–1980*. Cambridge: Cambridge University Press.

———. 1997. The Ideal of Equality. In *Equality: Selected Readings*, eds. Louis P. Pojman and Robert B. Westmoreland, 91–101. Oxford: Oxford University Press.

Wolff, Jonathan. 1998. Fairness, Respect, and the Egalitarian Ethos. *Philosophy and Public Affairs* 27, no. 2: 97–122.

Wolff, Jonathan, and Avner de-Shalit. 2007. *Disadvantage*. Oxford: Oxford University Press.

The World Health Report 2004. Geneva: World Health Organization.

Young, Iris Marion. 2006. Responsibility and Global Justice: A Social Connection Model. *Social Philosophy and Policy* 23: 102–30.

Index